Capsule Endoscopy

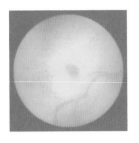

Capsule Endoscopy

Edited by

Douglas O Faigel MD
Professor of Medicine
Director of Endoscopy
Department of Gastroenterology
Oregon Health and Science University
Portland, Oregon
USA

David R Cave, MD, PhD
Professor of Medicine
Director of Clinical Gastroenterology Research
University of Massachusetts Memorial Medical Center
Worcester, Massachusetts
USA

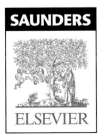

SAUNDERS

ELSEVIER

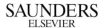

SAUNDERS
ELSEVIER

An imprint of Elsevier Inc.

On behalf of many of the authors in this book, we would like to acknowledge the support of Given Imaging, via research grants, which have enabled us to exploit this emerging imaging technology and explore its potential.

Douglas O Faigel MD
David R Cave MD, PhD

ISBN: 978-1-4160-3402-5

British Library Cataloguing in Publication Data
A catalogue record for this book is available from the British Library

Library of Congress Cataloguing in Publication Data
A catalog record of this book is available from the Library of Congress

---

Notice

Medical knowledge is constantly changing. Standard safety precautions must be followed, but as new research and clinical experience broaden our knowledge, changes in treatment and drug therapy may become necessary or appropriate. Readers are advised to check the most current product information provided by the manufacturer of each drug to be administered to verify the recommended doses and the best treatment for each individual patient. Neither the publisher nor the author assumes any liability for any injury and/or damage to persons or property arising from this publication.

The publisher

ELSEVIER your source for books, journals and multimedia in the health sciences
www.elsevierhealth.com

Working together to grow libraries in developing countries

www.elsevier.com | www.bookaid.org | www.sabre.org

ELSEVIER | **BOOK AID International** | **Sabre Foundation**

Commissioning Editor: Rolla Couchman
Development Editor: Joanne Scott
Project Manager: Cheryl Brant
Design: Stewart Larking
Illustration Manager: Bruce Hogarth
Illustrator: Antbits
Marketing Manager(s) (UK/USA): Clara Tombs; William Veltre

Printed in China

Last digit is the print number: 9 8 7 6 5 4 3 2 1

The publisher's policy is to use **paper manufactured from sustainable forests**

Contents

The modern history of gastroenterology has been marked by our ability to peer ever deeper, and less invasively, into the alimentary canal. Rigid instruments, really no more than stiff metal tubes with a light, gave us our initial looks into the most proximal and distal portals of the GI tract. These gave way to semi flexible instruments followed in turn by the development of fiberoptics and to the fully flexible video endoscopes that we have today.

Flexible video endoscopes have changed little in the last 20 years, showing incremental improvements in endoscope design and imaging. But the basic endoscopic procedure is the same. Flexible endoscopy is not non-invasive, but is "minimally invasive" in the sense that no tissue planes are traversed. It is limited by loop formation, and it is this constraint that makes these procedures uncomfortable, requiring conscious sedation in most cases. To be truly non-invasive, the insertion shaft and umbilical cord tying the endoscope to the outside world would have to be cut.

There can be no doubt that capsule endoscopy represents the single most profound change in the performance of endoscopy in our time. This self-contained swallowable imaging device is capable of the wireless transmission of thousands of high quality video images from deep within the gastrointestinal tract. All with no more discomfort than is involved with swallowing a large vitamin pill.

The initial clinical use of capsule endoscopy, and still the most common indication, is the examination of the small intestine. Prior to capsule endoscopy, this tortuous 15-20 foot-long organ had resisted complete examination by all but the most patient and persistent of endoscopists. Now, less than 6 years since FDA approval, capsule endoscopy forms the mainstay of our ability to diagnose diseases of the jejunum and ileum.

But capsule endoscopy is not limited to the small intestine. An esophageal capsule is FDA approved and has been shown to be comparable to conventional endoscopy in the detection of Barrett's esophagus, esophagitis and varices. A colonic capsule is currently in clinical trials and may be useful for colon cancer screening. Capsules optimized to image the stomach and duodenum cannot be far away. Steerable capsules, that can take biopsies or provide therapy, are under development.

This book will provide the clinician with the most up-to-date information on the state-of-the-art in capsule endoscopy. It provides technical information on the procedure with clinically relevant guidance on how capsule endoscopy may be used to facilitate the diagnosis and management of diseases of the small intestine. Still images are contextualized by the accompanying CD which provides videos of many of the images that are in each chapter. We believe that this is a key element of the book, since interpretation is based on image recognition. 'What you see is what you get' is what differentiates capsule endoscopy from conventional endoscopy which allows the practitioner to change position, poke, prod and biopsy. It is the ability to examine extraordinary images, usually enhanced by the presence of an aqueous environment, in previously inaccessible anatomy, that is so exciting. The ability to dynamically image disease processes in vivo, in a non invasive manner, has already proven to be of great value in improving management of our patients.

As early investigators in the application of capsule endoscopy and as physician educators, we are well aware of the interpretive pitfalls encumbent in this technology. There is a learning curve and interpretation will at least for the time being remain subjective. As consensus develops, the quality of interpretation will improve along with patient management. We regard this book as a contribution to that effort.

We hope you enjoy *Capsule Endoscopy*, and find it useful to your practice.

Douglas O Faigel MD
David R Cave MD, PhD

Contributors

Carla Abbiati, MD
Specialist in Gastroenterology and Gastrointestinal
    Endoscopy
Gastroenterology and Gastrointestinal Endoscopy Service
Ospedale Policlinico IRCCS
Milan, Italy

Douglas G Adler, MD
Assistant Professor of Medicine, Director of Therapeutic
    Endoscopy
Huntsman Cancer Center
University of Utah School of Medicine
Salt Lake City
Utah, USA

Gizela Beccari, MD
Specialist in Gastroenterology and Gastrointestinal
    Endoscopy
Gastroenterology and Gastrointestinal Endoscopy Service
Ospedale Policlinico IRCCS
Milan, Italy

David R Cave, MD PhD
Professor of Medicine
Director of Clinical Gastroenterology Research
University of Massachusetts Memorial Medical Center
Worcester
Massachusetts, USA

Guido Costamagna, MD FACG
Professor of Surgery and Director of Digestive
    Endoscopy Unit
Digestive Endoscopy Unit
"Agostino Gemelli" University Hospital
Catholic University of Rome
Rome, Italy

Glenn M Eisen MD MPH
Professor of Medicine
Oregon Health and Science University
Portland
Oregon, USA

Roberto de Franchis MD
Professor of Medical Sciences
Department of Internal Medicine
University of Milan
Director, 3rd Gastroenterology Unit
IRCCS Ospedale Maggiore Policlinico
Milan, Italy

Michel Delvaux MD
Staff Physician
Department of Internal Medicine and Digestive Pathology
CHU de Nancy
Hôpital de Brabois
Tour Drouet
Vandoeuvre les Nancy, France

Douglas O Faigel MD
Professor of Medicine
Director of Endoscopy
Department of Gastroenterology
Oregon Health and Science University
Portland
Oregon, USA

Victor L Fox MD
Assistant Professor of Pediatrics
Harvard Medical School
Director Gastroenterology Procedure Unit
Division of Gastroenterology and Nutrition
Children's Hospital Boston
Boston
Massachusetts, USA

Moti Frisch PhD
Director of Future Products and Product Management
Given Imaging Ltd
New Industrial Park
Yoqneam, Israel

Gerard Gay MD PhD
Department of Internal Medicine and Digestive Pathology
CHU de Nancy
Hôpital de Brabois
Tour Drouet
Vandoeuvre les Nancy, France

Peter H R Green MD, FRACP, FACG
Professor of Clinical Medicine
Columbia University College of Physicians and Surgeons
New York
New York, USA

Martin Keuchel MD
Consultant Gastroenterologist
1st Medical Department
Department of Medicine
Altona General Hospital
Hamburg, Germany

Tanja Kühbacher, MD PhD
Gastroenterologist
University Hospital Schleswig-Holstein
Campus Kiel
Clinic for General Internal Medicine
Kiel, Germany

Calvin W Lee, MD MPH
Gastroenterology Fellow
University of Massachusetts Medical School
Department of Gastroenterology
Worcester
Massachusetts, USA

Jonathan A Leighton, MD
Associate Professor of Medicine
Division of Gastroenterology and Hepatology
Mayo Clinic
Scottsdale
Arizona, USA

Blair S Lewis MD
Clinical Professor of Medicine
The Mount Sinai School of Medicine
New York
New York, USA

Klaus Mergener, MD PhD FACP FACG
Digestive Health Specialists
Tacoma
Washington, USA

Douglas Morgan, MD MPH
Assistant Professor of Medicine
Division of Gastroenterology and Hepatology
University of North Carolina
Chapel Hill
North Carolina, USA

Marco Pennazio, MD
Chief of Small Bowel Diseases Section
Gastroenterology 2
Department of Gastroenterology and Clinical Nutrition
San Giovanni A.S. Hospital
Turin, Italy

Maria Elena Riccioni MD
Clinical Assistant of Surgery
Digestive Endoscopy Unit
Catholic University
Rome, Italy

Emanuele Rondonotti MD
Department of Medical Sciences
University of Milan
3rd Gastroenterology Unit
IRCCS Ospedale Maggiore Policlinico
Elena Foundation
Milan, Italy

Moshe Rubin, MD
Associate Clinical Professor of Medicine
Columbia University College of Physicians and Surgeons
New York
New York, USA

Neal J Schamberg, MD
Fellow, Division of Gastroenterology and Hepatology
New York Presbyterian Hospital
Weill Cornell Medical Center
New York, USA

Felice Schnoll-Sussman, MD
Assistant Professor of Medicine
Division of Gastroenterology and Hepatology
Weill Medical College of Cornell University
Gastroenterologist, The Jay Monahan Center for
  Gastrointestinal Health
Presbyterian Hospital
New York, USA

Stefan Schreiber MD
Professor of Gastroenterology
Klinik für Innere Allgemeinemedizin
Kiel, Germany

Warwick Selby, MD MB BS FRACP
Clinical Associate Professor Department of Medicine,
  The University of Sydney
Senior Visiting Gastroenterologist, Royal Prince
  Alfred Hospital
Sydney
New South Wales, Australia

Syed Shah, MD MRCP
Consultant Physician/Gastroenterologist
Department of Gastroenterology
Pinderfields General Hospital
Wakefield, UK

Virender K Sharma, MD
Associate Professor of Medicine
Division of GI Hepatology
Mayo Clinic
Scottsdale
Arizona, USA

Clementina Signorelli MD
GI Fellow
Department of Medical Sciences
University of Milan
3rd Gastroenterology Unit
IRCCS Ospedale Maggiore Policlinico and
  Regina Elena Foundation
Milan, Italy

Christiano Spada MD
Clinical Assistant of Gastroenterology
Digestive Endoscopy Unit

Catholic University
Rome, Italy

Paul Swain MD
Professor of Oncology
Department of Surgical Oncology and Technology
Imperial College
London, UK

Stuart L Triester MD
Senior Fellow
Division of Gastroenterology and Hepatology
Mayo Clinic

Scottsdale
Arizona, USA

Federica Villa MD
GI Fellow
Department of Medical Sciences
University of Milan
3rd Gastroenterology Unit
IRCCS Ospedale Maggiore Policlinico and
    Regina Elena Foundation
Milan, Italy

Dedication:

I would like to dedicate this book to my wife, Kristin, and our daughters Madeleine, Olivia and Eliza who are always my greatest sources of inspiration.

Douglas O Faigel MD

I would like to dedicate this book to my wife Anne, who has been a continuous source of support and encouragement during its production.

David R Cave MD PhD

Acknowledgements

We would like to thank Joanne Scott for her tireless efforts in getting this book into production. It was no easy task cajoling a panel of busy physicians from all over the world into submitting state of the art information along with images and videos, many of whom have never previously been challenged with this format.

Section ONE

Performance of Capsule Endoscopy

CHAPTER **1**

History and Future

Paul Swain

A personal history of the development of wireless capsule

Two groups working independently on this project in Israel and London joined forces in 1997 to complete the technical development and clinical application of the wireless capsule endoscope.[1,2]

It became obvious in the early 1990s, when looking into shop windows, that video cameras were becoming smaller and that wireless transmitters were also available in small sizes (Table 1.1; Figures 1.1, 1.2). We had some fun finding out about these devices and set about exploring this technology and acquiring the smallest video cameras and transmitters then available to use them for experimental endoscopy. The problem was to find components and devices that were more or less small enough to swallow.

Most of the very small video cameras came from Japanese manufacturers. In 1993 we appointed Feng Gong to work with us. He was to do a PhD at University College on the development of endoscopic sewing machines and related technology. We had a grant for his project from Science and Engineering Research Council (SERC), a government body that funds scientific research in the UK.

The grant application mentioned sewing device development but did not mention our wireless capsule ambitions. Because he was Chinese, Feng could read Japanese script and we began to search Japanese trade journals for the

Table 1.1 Milestones in development of wireless capsule endoscopy

1949 Invention of transistor — Bardeen, Brattain and Shockley (Nobel Prize 1956)
1954 Hopkins — fiberoptic image transmission
1957 Zworkin, Mackay, Noller — radio-pills (temperature, pressure, pH)
1969 Smith and Boyle — charge coupled device (CCD)
1994 Fossum — CMOS improvements
First publication on feasibility
1996 First live pictures from pig GI tract with a wireless device
Co-development with Israeli Group (GivenImaging)
1999 Ethical committee approval for human use
2000 Publication in *Nature*, *NEJM* 2001
2001 CE mark and FDA approval
2005 200 000 patients examined

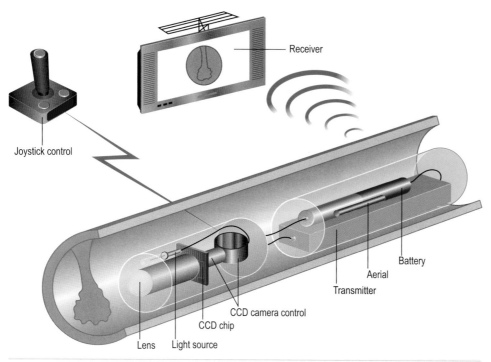

FIGURE 1.1 Early conceptual drawing of a wireless capsule endoscope. Early capsule image of a large villous rectal adenoma taken by an experimental colonic capsule endoscope.

smallest new video cameras and processors. We had almost no money, of course, but started to buy the cheapest smallest cameras and processors that were available for bench and animal testing.

We also contacted technical firms who worked with the BBC and became aware that low light level TV transmission had revolutionized battlefield television journalism. Cameras were now small enough to be concealed in tie-pins or handbags for covert journalism. We visited some of the so-called "spy shops" in London that supplied transmitters and small video cameras for installation in bedrooms

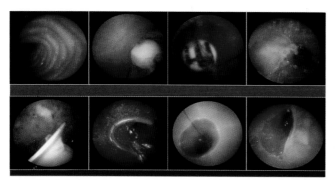

FIGURE 1.2 Early wireless capsule images acquired during a canine study prior to FDA approval. Right to left top row: (a) normal small intestine, (b) spherical bead sewn to small intestine, (c) flat button bead with burn markings sewn to small intestine, (d) nodule in small intestine. Bottom row left to right: (e) white plastic ingested material in cecum, (f) ascaris worm (the first unexpected pathological finding by a capsule), (g) black hair of a black dog, (h) superficial small intestinal ulceration.

by private detectives or other users. Most of these oddly transmit on illegal frequencies but are sold openly and we acquired a couple of these. Some could tune through a variety of frequencies. For the security and surveillance market some small video cameras were becoming available at surprisingly low cost. We also contacted a specialist firm that had developed sports video equipment. They had buried a video camera in a cricket stump using a prism so that the trajectory of the ball could be followed as it approached the batsman. A cricket stump is less than 3 centimeters wide so we knew it would be almost possible to pass a device like this through the esophagus. This firm hired us equipment. We acquired our first miniature microwave transmitter and receiver from them, and began to test them.

I was invited to talk on the uses of microwaves in gastroenterology at a world congress in Los Angeles in 1994. We had developed a microwave device for treating gastrointestinal bleeding and cancer but chose also to talk in public for the first time there on the possibility of using microwaves for transmission of images from a robotic capsular camera. We were using microwaves, which still may have some advantages — in particular the bandwidth allows transmission of larger amounts of data when compared with radio waves. The first abstract on this topic was also published in *Gut* in 1994 entitled "An endorobot for flexible endoscopy, a feasibility study".[3] It was presented as a poster at the British Society of Gastroenterology and did not attract much attention (Figure 1.1).

We started to make crude devices to see if we could transmit moving images with some of these fairly small cameras and transmitters. We began in 1996 to wrap our video camera and wireless transmitter devices in post-mortem tissue to test transmission through the stomach wall as well as surgical implantation of large devices.[4] We studied batteries and available light sources. Our first device used a miniature bulb as a light source. The principle of transmitting video images through the human body was tested by placing the device in a box through which microwaves could not penetrate and pressing a window, cut in the box, against the abdomen. Color video images were obtained by placing a receiver behind the body of the volunteer.

We inserted a large prototype device using a video camera, microwave transmitter and light source with batteries into a live pig stomach surgically. The device used a dome-shaped wire cage to keep the tissue away from the lens (Video 1.1); because of the airless nature of this endoscopy the whole device was sometimes placed in a transparent plastic bag. The stomach and abdomen was closed surgically. The device worked and we could see the pylorus open and close. At that stage we were acquiring images at 30 frames a second and could run this device for about 20 minutes.[4]

Although the cheapest available charge coupled device (CCD) chip cameras were now small enough to swallow and some had fairly low power requirements, the processor boards were larger — flat and square or rectangular — and the smallest we could purchase was 25 mm square, which was a bit too large to swallow. We knew that we could get all the components into a device that could be swallowed but that we would have to get it made and asked the electronics section of the Medical Physics department to do this for us. They agreed to do this for £7000, which was a lot of money for us at that time.

At about this time Gavriel Meron and Gavriel Iddan in Israel contacted us. It was obvious to me that progress would be much faster if our groups joined forces. They also knew about developments in complementary oxide silicone (CMOS) imaging, which meant that good quality images could be acquired using substantially less power than with CCD technology. We did not know about this development, which was crucial at that time to the manufacture of a realistic device. I visited their offices and workshop in Yoqneam in Israel and we experimented with wired devices in excised pig small intestine.

In London we did more work with conical, dome and cage shapes to test the idea that airless endoscopy was feasible.[5] We applied for ethical committee approval to test the device in human volunteers.

Together with the Israeli group we visited the Federal Drug Administration (FDA) in Bethesda. Prior to this we had advice on what we should say. "Don't mention screening" was the advice and we did not mention screening. The meeting went pretty well — I had to improvise the outline of an animal study, which was to be performed in pigs in the UK. We were going to inject colored inks into the small intestine to mark areas at endoscopy and then see how many of these could be recognized at wireless capsule and push enteroscopy. It turned out that all anesthetic agents which we used completely abolished peristalsis in pigs, that gastric emptying times were about 12 hours, and that push enteroscopy as a means of delivering capsules into the duodenum was much more difficult than I had imagined. Meantime we found that by using thread and sewing small beads at various sites in the small intestine we had developed the model we needed to test the capsule. We elected to do the study in dogs in Israel. We found that the anesthetic agents usually did not abolish peristalsis in these animals, and we developed a hydraulic device, like the cup of an acorn on a catheter, for delivering capsules through the pylorus into the duodenum in dogs.

The ethics committee at the Royal London Hospital approved my request to conduct the initial testing of the wireless capsule endoscope in myself in August 1999. They were amused and curious about some of the paradoxes of approving a protocol for volunteer self-experimentation. I had to designate a surgeon who could remove the device, if it got stuck.

I swallowed the first capsule in October 1999 (Video 1.2) and the second capsule the next day. The capsule at this stage was 11×33 mm in diameter with only two light emitting diodes (LEDs). The aerial reception was a single dipole arranged in a ring; it was hand held over the abdomen and we had to move this device to optimize reception. Two green rings on an oscilloscope had to be superimposed in order to get the best reception. Because we had had substantial difficulty with delayed gastric emptying in early animal studies we were worried that the device would not leave the stomach. I remember thinking that this was rather a large pill but was able to swallow it easily with the first gulp. We began to acquire our first images. I was able to compare the completely painless swallowing of the capsule with the experience of a conventional gastroscopy. We had a celebratory lunch in my hotel with views over the Mediterranean Sea.

Arkady Glukovsky, director of the R&D group of engineers at Given, who had made the first capsule for human use, took me to a medical clinic and asked if they could take a plain x-ray to show the position of the capsule. The x-ray showed that the capsule had reached my cecum. Oddly, the doctors in the clinic offered to do a barium enema on me to help get the capsule out. We declined this offer and returned to my hotel with the x-ray. The second capsule was swallowed the next morning in my hotel room. The hotel was swarming with armed security guards and military personnel because a Jordanian prince was staying there on a State visit. We brought a large amount of electronic equipment into my room through this security screen. On this occasion all the technical aspects worked really well. We were now practiced at optimizing the reception, and the capsule and I sat in the sunshine looking at the sea doing this experiment. The second capsule transmitted for more than six hours. When it ran out, we ordered sandwiches on room service. The engineers were able to process the images before I flew back to the UK the next day and they looked pretty good. We had a substantial length of small intestinal imaging with a lot of artifact on the first run. The second was much better and the capsule reached the cecum. I had to pass through the fairly rigorous Israeli airport security at Tel Aviv with the second capsule still possibly transmitting inside me. Their detectors did not find it. I retrieved this capsule in the toilet at my hospital in London the next morning.

I made several subsequent visits to Yoqneam and Haifa in order to help with the animal study that the FDA had wanted and to continue to help on the further development. The animal study turned out to be fairly demanding, using a push enteroscope and our hydraulic delivery system to deliver the capsules through the pylorus of the dogs. The trick was to identify the pylorus and press the capsule against it, then wait for the pylorus to open and push the catheter forwards when a wave of antral contraction opened the pylorus.

We became excited when we were able to see moving ascaris in these animals, which could not be seen on push enteroscopy. This was the first time I saw pathology using wireless capsule endoscopy that could not be seen by other means. The engineers had become so slick that we could retrieve capsules with the LEDs still flashing, replace the batteries, and reuse the capsules again within an hour.

By this time we had been granted ethics approval for a human volunteer study with larger numbers and also had ethics approval for the first patient studies at the Royal London Hospital. Meantime we wrote and submitted in December 1999 the abstract for presentation of our work at Digestive Disease Week (DDW) in San Diego in 2000. In April we carried out the first patient trials with the wireless capsule in four patients with obscure recurrent gastrointestinal bleeding. A small intestinal bleeding source was found in three of these. We also wrote the workup for publication and thought that we would try *Nature* since the first paper on flexible endoscopy by Hopkins had been published in that journal in 1954. The editors of *Nature* were quick to point out that there had been no subsequent papers in *Nature* on endoscopic topics but agreed to get referee's comments and after consideration agreed to publish it. *Nature* insists that there is no disclosure or publicity prior to publication. We had a period of anxiety when they lost our illustrations and the publication was delayed by a week, which by chance caused the publication in *Nature* and the DDW presentation to occur on the same day. The editors of *Nature* had added as a header to our article "The discomfort on internal endoscopy may soon be a thing of the past" and had released the article to the press with a moratorium on publication until the article in *Nature* was published.[6] There was substantial television and radio and press interest and the presentation in San Diego seemed to be well received by the endoscopists present. *Gastrointestinal Endoscopy* published the account of our efforts in London to develop this technology[7] a few days after the publication of the *Nature* article, *Gastroenterology* published our experimental animal study in December 1999,[8] and the *New England Journal of Medicine* report of our first four patients was published a month later.[9] The device received a CE mark and FDA approval in August 2000. The wireless capsule endoscope was launched.

Future innovations

Wireless capsule technology is an incompletely developed technology that might change endoscopy forever and has the capacity to replace a good deal of conventional endoscopy.

Will capsule endoscopy replace much of conventional upper gastrointestinal endoscopy and colonoscopy? The answer is probably "yes" but the timeframe is unclear. Will capsule endoscopy be able to deliver therapy? This is also probable.

There are two major challenges to the expansion of capsule technology into a position where it can challenge conventional diagnostic gastroscopy and colonoscopy. The first challenge is power management. At present the M2A capsule contains two small 3 volt hearing aid batteries which allow about 8 hours of continuous imaging at 2 frames per second. The use of CMOS technology for the video has the advantage of requiring extremely low power levels when compared with a CCD. Slowing the video frame rate to 2 frames per second also increased the lifespan of the capsule. The recently introduced esophageal capsule takes 14 frames a second and has a lifespan of about 20 minutes. More batteries or more efficient batteries would help but these might increase the size and weight of the capsule. The two small silver oxide batteries are not the most efficient in terms of power weight ratios but were chosen because of their safety record. Lithium batteries could run the capsule for longer periods. There has been a "breakthrough" in battery design with the advent of carbon nanotubes and Buckytubes which have the intrinsic characteristics desired in material used as electrodes in batteries and capacitors, two technologies of rapidly increasing importance. Buckytubes have a tremendously high surface area ($\sim$ 1000 m^2/g), good electrical conductivity, and their linear geometry makes their surfaces highly accessible to the electrolyte. It may be that better battery design and clever power management will give the capsule the power required for additional performance and functions.

The development of external power transmission methods using electrical field induction, radiofrequency, microwaves or ultrasound technology could free the capsule from the requirement for batteries. This would substantially lighten the capsule and allow space and power for other functions such as biopsy or drug delivery but above all would allow the capsule to be powered for indefinite periods which would allow increases in the current rather low frame rate and in particular make the problem of capsule colonoscopy much easier to solve (Table 1.2).

The development of the capsule endoscopy was made possible by miniaturization of digital chip camera technology, especially CMOS chip technology. The continued reduction in size, increases in pixel numbers, and improvements in imaging with the two rival technologies — CCD and CMOS — are likely to change the nature of endoscopy. The current differences outlined in Table 1.3 are becoming blurred and hybrids are emerging.

The main pressure to reduce the component size will be to release space that could be used for other capsule functions, for example biopsy, coagulation, or therapy. New engineering methods for constructing tiny moving parts and miniature actuators or even motors into capsules have been described.

Although semiconductor lasers exist which are small enough to swallow, the nature of lasers which have typical inefficiencies of 100–1000% makes the idea of a remote

Table 1.2 Capsule endoscope technology

1.	Technology of capsule endoscope	Compact, low power-consumption imaging technology, wireless transmission technology
2.	Capsule guidance system	Navigates freely within the gastrointestinal tract
3.	Wireless power supply system	Eliminates constraints on operating time and energy levels
4.	Drug delivery system	Administers drugs directly to the affected area
5.	Body fluid sampling technology	Extracts body fluid for diagnosis and analysis
6.	Self-propelled capsule	Propels freely within the gastrointestinal tract
7.	Ultrasound capsule	Ultrasound scanning from inside the body

laser in a capsule stopping bleeding or cutting out a tumour seem something of a pipe dream at present, because of power requirements. The construction of an electrosurgical generator small enough to swallow and powered by small batteries is conceivable but currently difficult because of the limitations imposed by the internal resistance of batteries. Small motors are currently available to move components such as biopsy devices but need radio-controlled activators. One limitation is the low mass of the capsule endoscope. A force exerted on tissue, for example by biopsy forceps, may push the capsule away from the tissue.

Future diagnostic developments are likely to include capsule colonoscopy, attachment to the gut wall, ultrasound imaging, biopsy and cytology, propulsion methods, and therapy including tissue coagulation.

Table 1.3 Comparison of CMOS and CCD technology

- CCD sensors create high-quality, low-noise images. CMOS sensors, traditionally, are more susceptible to noise

- Because each pixel on a CMOS sensor has several transistors located next to it, the light sensitivity of a CMOS chip tends to be lower. Many of the photons hitting the chip hit the transistors instead of the photodiode

- CCDs use a process that consumes lots of power. CCDs consume as much as 100 times more power than an equivalent CMOS sensor

- CMOS chips can be fabricated on just about any standard silicon production line, so they tend to be extremely inexpensive compared to CCD sensors

- CCD sensors have been mass produced for a longer period of time, so they are more mature. They tend to have higher quality and more pixels

- CCD requires application of several clock signals, clock levels, and bias voltages, complicating system integration and increasing power consumption, overall system size, and cost

- CMOS architecture allows the signals from the entire array, from subsections, or even from a single pixel to be readout by a simple X-Y addressing technique — something a CCD can't do

Challenge to using capsule endoscopy for colonoscopy

There are challenges to using wireless capsule endoscopy for colonoscopy (Figure 1.3). Currently the capsule acquires images for 8 hours and has usually reached the right side of the colon before the battery expires. The capsule would have to run for 24–48 hours in order to perform a complete examination of the colon. The power problem could be addressed in several ways. Solutions to this difficulty might include: more batteries, batteries with a delay mode which are switched on when the capsule is in the ileum, external power transmission, or methods to move the capsule faster in the colon. Effective timed colon cleaning will be necessary. Deletion of identical frames would make it easier to examine the images since the capsule in the colon can remain stationary for prolonged periods. Wireless capsule colonoscopy has already generated images (Figure 1.4) from all areas of the colon and has imaged pathology, especially in the right side of the colon, but also in the rectum

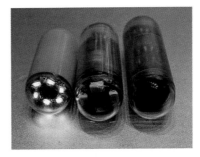

FIGURE 1.3 Three capsules with six, four, and two LEDs. The capsule with 6 LEDs is a commercial Given small bowel capsule, the one with 4 LEDs is an early colonic prototype, and the capsule with 2 LEDs is the first capsule to be used in a human.

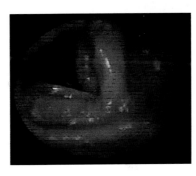

FIGURE 1.4 An early capsule image of the transverse colon in a human.

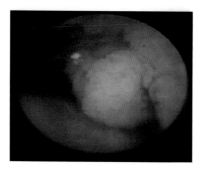

FIGURE 1.5 Large rectal villous adenoma.

(Figure 1.5).[10,11] Video 1.3 shows views of diverticula and a large seed in the descending colon taken with an experimental colonoscopy capsule.

Wireless laparoscopy is feasible (Figures 1.6, 1.7) but needs to develop and offer advantages over conventional laparoscopy. Wireless imaging of cardiac or vascular structures is conceivable, but would require substantial development and control strategies. The manufacture of an autonomous video capsule the size of a red blood cell, as described in Isaac Asimov's *The Fantastic Voyage* and made into a movie in 1966 by Richard Fleischer with Stephen Boyd, Raquel Welsh and Donald Pleasance, is some way in the future. Reduction in size by up to an order of magnitude is currently conceivable with available components. It would be relatively easy to halve the current diameter of the capsule.

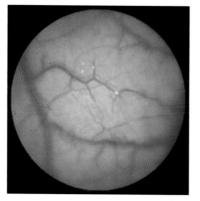

FIGURE 1.6 Serosal surface of live porcine stomach — capsule image acquired using transgastric route.

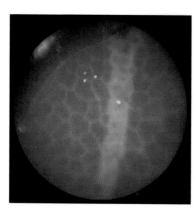

FIGURE 1.7 Surface of porcine liver showing septation — capsule image acquired live using transgastric route.

Attachment of capsule endoscopes to the GI tract

The capsule might be stitched or clipped to the wall of the stomach so that prolonged examination of bleeding ulcers or varices became possible (Figure 1.8). An on/off radio-controlled command might be helpful to conserve power. Long-term endoscopy with wireless endoscopes attached to the wall of the gut could improve management of bleeding and other disorders.

Tissue interactive diagnostic methods such as biopsy

At present the capsule does not take biopsies, aspirate fluid, or brush lesions for cytology. These common endoscopic maneuvers may be possible during capsule endoscopy. They require real-time viewing and will also require radio-controlled triggering and remote control capsule manipulation if they are to be used with precision. Biopsy using a spring loaded Crosby capsule (Figure 1.9) like device with an evacuated chamber would be feasible with existing capsule technology and patients seem able to retrieve capsules from stool using a net and a magnet almost all the time in preliminary patient studies. Brush cytology is another possibility and has been used in vivo.[12] Videos 1.4–1.6 show experimental brush, biopsy and radio-controlled release mechanisms which could be used in autonomous capsules (Figure 1.10). It may be possible to combine capsule technology with "optical biopsy."

Capsule coagulation

A prototype coagulation capsule has been built and tested which uses an exothermic chemical reaction to generate heat (Video 1.7) using the interaction of calcium oxide and water.

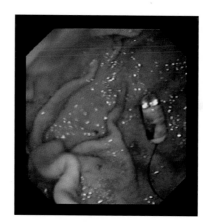

FIGURE 1.8 Flashing wireless capsule endoscopically sutured to porcine stomach in survival study.

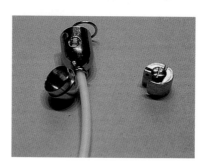

FIGURE 1.9 Watson small intestinal biopsy capsule.

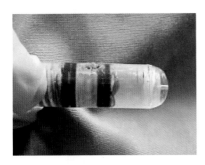

FIGURE 1.10 Spring loaded capsule cytology brush.

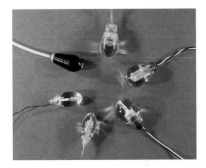

FIGURE 1.11 Six electrostimulation prototypes all using bipolar electrodes and ovoid in shape.

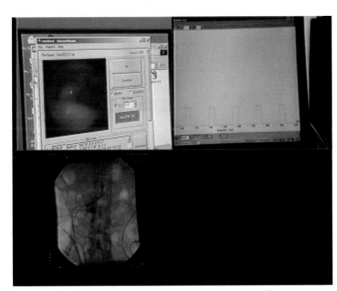

FIGURE 1.12 This illustration shows simultaneous imaging of an electrostimulation capsule in the small intestine of a human volunteer. The x-ray image shows the device in the proximal jejunum. The real-time viewer shows the capsule image acquired by the capsule. The oscilloscope trace indicates the pulse duration and current amplitude during the period of electrostimulation.

It seems probable that other thermal therapeutic applications will be added in the future.

Electrostimulation for propelling capsule endoscope

One way to manipulate a wireless capsule endoscope autonomously in the human gastrointestinal tract is to use electrostimulation to propel the device, for example with a pair of bipolar electrodes at either end of the capsule (Figure 1.11; Videos 1.8–1.11). This has been tested in man[13] (Video

1.14). Electrodes attached to an M2A capsule have been used to propel this device in the porcine (Videos 1.12, 1.13) and human small intestine (Figure 1.12; Videos 1.14, 1.15). A dumb-bell shaped capsule allows the imaging capsule to view the traction capsule (Figure 1.13; Video 1.12). A radio-controlled electrostimulation capsule has been developed (Video 1.15). Radio-commands can be sent from a transmitter and aerial (Figure 1.14) to the receiving traction capsule causing it to propel the video capsule (Figure 1.15) forwards (Video 1.16) or backwards (Video 1.17) in the human gastrointestinal tract (Figure 1.16).

Water-jet propulsion has also been used to propel this very lightweight (3.7 g) capsule in the gastrointestinal tract (Figure 1.17). The light weight of the capsule compared with the 1.5 kg of a colonoscope makes it possible to think of developing new types of very lightweight colonoscopes that can be passed on a wire through the anus into the colon and should require much less force on the wall of the colon to reach the cecum.

Olympus, in a recent news release (November 30, 2004), has announced the following developments in capsule endoscopy. These include wireless power supply system, capsule guidance system (Figures 1.18, 1.19), drug delivery system, body fluid sampling technology, self-propelled capsule, and ultrasound capsule. The details are shown in Table 1.2.

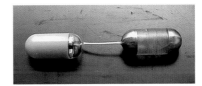

FIGURE 1.13 Dumb-bell arrangement of wireless capsule endoscope and electrostimulation capsule[14].

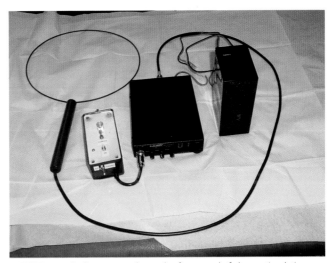

FIGURE 1.14 Radio command complex for control of electrostimulation capsule: circular radio antenna, command switching module, transmitter, and battery[15].

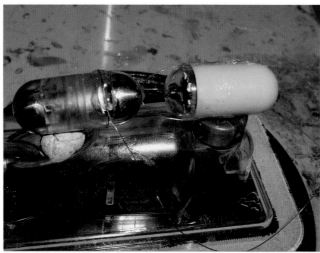

FIGURE 1.15 Electrostimulation capsule tethered to a small intestinal capsule as used in a human volunteer.

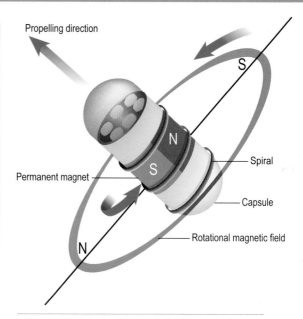

Propelling direction

S

Spiral

Permanent magnet

N

S

Capsule

Rotational magnetic field

N

FIGURE 1.18 Rotational magnetic field proposed for capsule propulsion (Olympus website).

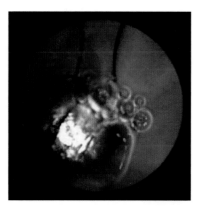

FIGURE 1.16
Electrostimulation propulsion capsule viewed by small bowel Given capsule in human small intestine.

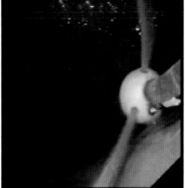
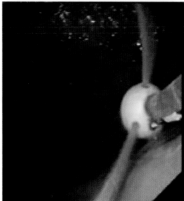

FIGURE 1.17 Water-jet propelled capsule endoscope.

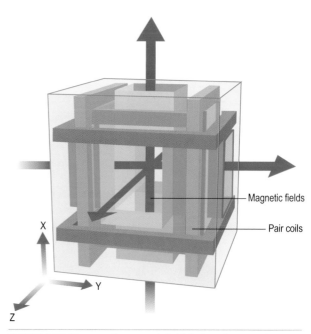

Magnetic fields

Pair coils

X

Y

Z

FIGURE 1.19 Diagram of a magnetic field designed to control a capsule endoscope (Olympus website).

Conclusions

Capsule video-enteroscopy has opened up a new world of diagnoses and possibilities to the gastroenterologist. It is a privilege to see images of small intestinal abnormalities at video-endoscopy such as an ulcerated Meckel's diverticulum or active bleeding from a tumour in the middle of the small intestine, which were not possible until recently. The development of wireless capsule endoscopy has changed video-endoscopy of the small intestine into a much less invasive and more complete examination. The increasing use of these resources and the comfort and ease with which some of these examinations can be performed make it likely that wireless capsule video imaging will have a substantial impact on the management of disease of the small intestine and other parts of the body.

It is hard and perhaps rather dull to write about history without bias. It is usually a mistake to try to predict the future because the chances of error are very high. "It is impossible to predict the future, and all attempts to do so in any detail look ludicrous within a very few years." These are the opening words of *The Profiles of the Future* by Arthur C Clarke, who wrote an amusing account of eminent scientists predicting that electric light, human flight, and space travel were impossible at the same time as Edison perfected the light bulb, the Wright brothers made their first motor powered flight, and Yuri Gagarin circled the earth in a sputnik. Einstein, who probably knew more than most about the potential impact of physics on the future of mankind, was goaded during an interview in 1929 on board the Belgoland into saying "I never think about the future; it comes soon enough."

Acknowledgments

I would like to acknowledge my debt to the Medical Physics Department at University College, London, and especially to Dr Tim Mills, principal physicist and my long-term colleague and friend. I thank Dr Feng Gong who wrote his PhD in part on this development, Dr Sandy Mosse who wrote his PhD in part on electrostimulation for moving the capsule remotely, as well as Paul Burke, Loren Schmitz, and Brian Kelleher. I would also like to thank my medical colleagues, especially Dr Mark Appleyard for his help with the demanding animal studies and the earliest clinical studies as well as his important contributions to the early publications on this method. Some of this work was included in his MD thesis. Dr Maria Mylonaki, Priv-Doz. Dr Annette Fritscher-Ravens, and Dr Keiichi Ikeda have continued the clinical studies and development and testing of new devices.

References

1. Iddan GJ, Swain CP. History and development of capsule endoscopy. Gastrointest Endosc Clin N Am 2004;14:1–9.

2. Meron GD. The development of the swallowable video capsule (M2A). Gastrointest Endosc 2000;52:817–9.

3. Gong F, Swain CP, Mills TN. An endorobot for gastrointestinal endoscopy. Gut 1994;35:S52.

4. Swain CP, Gong F, Mills TN. Wireless transmission of a colour television moving image from the stomach using a miniature CCD camera, light source and microwave transmitter. Gut 1996;39:A26.

5. Appleyard MN, Gong F, Mills TN, Mosse CA, Swain P. Endoscopy without air insufflation. Gastrointest Endosc 2000;51:AB260*7071.

6. Iddan G, Meron G, Glukovsky A, Swain P. Wireless capsule endoscopy. Nature 2000;405:417.

7. Gong F, Mills TN, Swain CP. Wireless endoscopy. Gastrointest Endosc 2000;51:725–9.

8. Appleyard M, Fireman F, Glukhovsky A, et al. A randomized comparison of push enteroscopy and wireless capsule endoscopy in detecting small intestinal lesions in an animal model. Gastroenterology 2000;119:1431–8.

9. Appleyard M, Glukhovsky A, Swain P. Wireless capsule diagnostic endoscopy for recurrent small-bowel bleeding. N Engl J Med 2001;34:232–3.

10. Mylonaki M, Fritscher-Ravens A, Swain P. Clinical studies of wireless capsule colonoscopy. Gut 2002;50:A42.

11. Swain P, Fritscher-Ravens A, Mylonaki M. Experimental and clinical studies of wireless capsule colonoscopy. Gastrointest Endosc 2004;59:103.

12. Swain P, Mosse C, Mills T, Green J, Ikeda K, Fritscher-Ravens A. Development of wireless capsule endoscope mechanisms for brush cytology, tissue fluid aspiration and biopsy. Gastrointest Endosc 2005;61:AB106.

13. Fritscher-Ravens A, Burke P, Mills T, Mosse C, Swain C. The development and testing of an electrically propelled capsule endoscope in man. Gastrointest Endosc 2003;57: AB84.

14. Fritscher-Ravens A, Swain P, Mosse S, Mills T. Dumb-bell wireless capsule endoscopy. Gastrointest Endosc 2005;61: AB164.

15. Swain P, Mills T, Kelleher B, et al. Radio-controlled movement of a robot endoscope in the human gastrointestinal tract. Gastrointest Endosc 2005;61:AB101.

CHAPTER **2**

How Does the Capsule Work?

Moti Frisch

KEY POINTS

1. The Given PillCam platform is an integrated wireless endoscopy system that allows noninvasive imaging of the intestine in its natural physiological state.

2. It consists of an ingestible camera with transmitter, a data recorder that receives and stores the images and a workstation for review of the video created from the images.

3. Two capsules are available and cleared for use, the PillCam Small Bowel capsule and the PillCam Esophageal capsule.

Introduction

Video capsule endoscopy (VCE) helps close a gap in the evaluation of the small bowel, which has been regarded as the "black box" of endoscopy. The invention of the PillCam™ SB capsule endoscope, a small, ingestible camera, established a minimally invasive method for imaging the gastrointestinal (GI) tract in its natural physiological state. A second version, the PillCam ESO capsule endoscope, was subsequently developed for imaging of the esophagus.

The disposable PillCam capsule endoscope glides through the digestive system and takes high quality color pictures of the inner GI tract. The pictures are immediately transmitted by radio via antennas attached to the patient's abdomen to an external, belt-worn data recorder/receiver. The data recorder picks up the images, allows for immediate real-time viewing of the captured images, and stores them for later review (see Figures 2.1, 2.2).

The pictures may be viewed in real-time by connecting the data to RAPIDAccess™, a special system for display of real-time pictures captured by the PillCam capsule endoscope.

Otherwise, the patient is free to move around, wearing the data recorder. When the test is over, the antennas and data recorder are removed from the patient and the pictures are transferred ("downloaded") from the data recorder to a computer workstation featuring the RAPID® application (RAPID standing for reviewing and processing image data). This process automatically prepares a RAPID video movie from the captured pictures and readies it for diagnostic review and evaluation. The capsule continues to pass through the digestive system until it is excreted naturally.

Once the RAPID video is ready in the RAPID Workstation, it can be viewed either on the RAPID Workstation using the RAPID Application or transferred to and viewed on any computer installed with the RAPID Reader application, which is a read-only (view-only) application for RAPID videos.

The main components of the Given Diagnostic System (GDS) are:

1. PillCam capsule endoscope
2. DataRecorder
3. RAPID Workstation with RAPID Application
4. RAPID Reader Application.

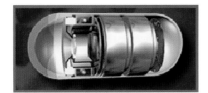

PillCam® Capsule

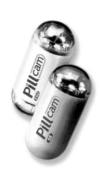

PillCam™ Capsule

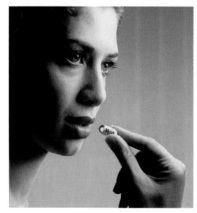

Ambulatory capsule ingestion

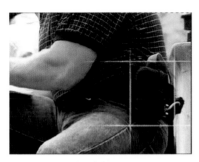

Ambulatory Data recorder™ on belt

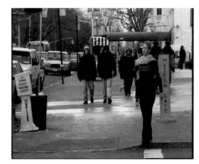

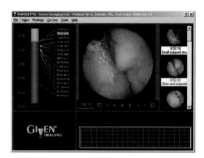

RAPID® Application

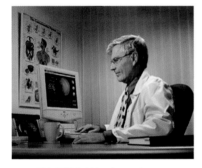

RAPID® Workstation

FIGURE 2.1 Capsule endoscopy. Courtesy of Given ® Imaging

Physiological endoscopy

Since the PillCam capsule endoscope is ingested naturally and is propelled in the GI tract by natural peristalsis (see Figure 2.3):

1. There is no insufflation of any part of the GI tract.
2. There is no effect on the pressure receptors in the intestinal wall due to insufflation and insertion of a long flexible tube (endoscope).
3. There is no rise in intraluminal pressure (up to 300 mmHg) common to conventional endoscopy, which may cause a decrease or even temporary arrest of blood flow to small vessels.

4. There are no effects on the intestinal wall related to the forceful insertion of the endoscope, in particular, no risk of perforation.
5. There is no sedation, common in conventional endoscopy; thus pharmacologically induced physiology changes during the examination, which may have an effect on the ability of the endoscope to detect vascular and inflammatory lesions, are avoided.
6. The GI tract propels the capsule by normal peristalsis toward excretion as if it were natural content.

Thus, the GI tract is visualized in its natural physiological state, representing a paradigm shift in the approach to endoscopic diagnosis (Figure 2.3).

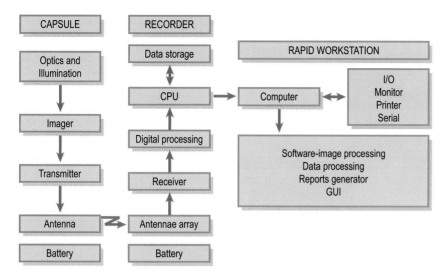

FIGURE 2.2 The Given Diagnostic System for capsule endoscopy. Courtesy of Given ® Imaging

PillCam capsule endoscope

The PillCam capsule endoscope is an ingestible cylindrical capsule incorporating a small video camera complete with light emitting diode (LED)-based illumination (3), optics (2), and a complementary metal oxide semiconductor (CMOS)-based imager (4), a small battery (5) as well as a wireless ASIC radio transmitter, all encapsulated in a biocompatible and inert plastic casing (6) (Figure 2.4).

The illuminating LEDs flash several times each second (depending on the type (3) of PillCam capsule endoscope) and illuminate through the transparent optical dome the inner intestinal wall. The illuminated image (1) passes through the lens (2) and is sensed by the imager (4), which translates it into electrical signals and transfers these signals to the transmitter (6) that transmits it through the antenna (7) outside the abdomen (see Figure 2.5).

One or both ends of the capsule, depending on its intended use for the small bowel or for the esophagus, is made of a transparent plastic dome through which the internal LEDs illuminate the wall of the GI tract and through which the video camera picks up the picture of the illuminated area of the gut wall.

The capsule is 26 mm long and 11 mm in diameter. The frequency of the imaging cycle (taking pictures and transmitting them outside the abdomen) depends on the type of capsule. The PillCam SB capsule, designed for small bowel examination, has one video head and takes pictures and transmits them outside the abdomen at a rate of 2 pictures per second. The PillCam ESO capsule, designed for examination of the esophagus, has 2 video heads, one at each end of the capsule, and takes pictures at a rate of 7 pictures per second for each head, altogether 14 pictures per second.

The shape of the transparent optical dome, as well as the material it is made of, keeps the dome from becoming smeared and obscured by gastrointestinal contents and from internal reflection of the illuminating light. The optical system is designed to assure a wide field of view and sharp images within the illuminated area of the gut.

The capsule is kept OFF by an internal magnetic switch as long as it is kept in its holder in close proximity of the magnet in its blister package. As soon as the capsule is removed from the vicinity of the magnet in the blister, the magnetic switch in the capsule closes and the capsule starts blinking as well as taking and transmitting images.

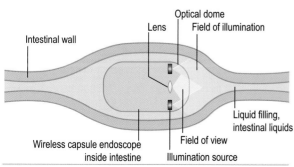

FIGURE 2.3 Physiological endoscopy. Courtesy of Given ® Imaging

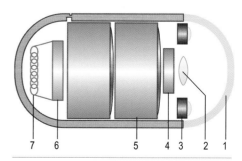

FIGURE 2.4 PillCam SB capsule endoscope. See text for explanation. Courtesy of Given ® Imaging

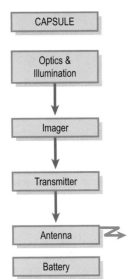

Transmission continues until battery depletion or until a preprogrammed switch-off, depending on the type of the capsule.

PillCam SB capsule endoscope

The PillCam SB capsule endoscope is designed for ambulatory examination of the entire length of the small bowel. According to the 2005 ICCE Consensus,[1] primary indications for small bowel capsule endoscopy include:

1. Obscure gastrointestinal bleeding
2. Investigation of suspected Crohn's disease
3. Surveillance of hereditary polyposis syndromes
4. Investigation of suspected small bowel tumor
5. Complicated celiac disease.

The PillCam SB capsule, with one video head imaging at 2 pictures per second, consists of the following elements, as illustrated in Figure 2.6:

(a) CMOS imager
(b) LED illuminators
(c) ASIC transmitter (RF IC)
(d) Antenna
(e) Battery pack

(f) Capsule case — high tensile force, two-dome shaped, encapsulating cylinder, made of biocompatible, pH-resistant plastic material using biocompatible adhesive.

While active, the capsule transmits images at a rate of 2 images per second. For each image, an illuminating light flash is applied with the illuminating LEDs. The transmission of images continues for as long as the battery power lasts.

The PillCam SB capsule images the small bowel up to the cecal valve for the majority of the patients. The typical number of pictures taken during an 8-hour SB capsule endoscopy procedure and stored in the DataRecorder is 56 700.

PillCam ESO capsule endoscope

The PillCam ESO capsule endoscope is designed for ambulatory examination of the entire length of the esophagus. According to the 2005 ICCE Consensus, primary indications for esophageal capsule endoscopy may include:

1. Screening patients with chronic reflux to detect Barrett's esophagus
2. Screening patients with suspected esophageal varices
3. Surveillance of patients with esophageal varices.

The capsule has two video heads that each take 7 pictures per second, totaling 14 pictures per second.

The PillCam ESO capsule endoscope consists of the following elements, as illustrated in Figure 2.7:

(a) 2 CMOS imagers
(b) 2 LED illuminator rings
(c) ASIC transmitter (RF IC)
(d) Antenna
(e) Battery pack
(f) Capsule-case — high tensile force, two-dome shaped, encapsulating cylinder, made of biocompatible, pH-resistant plastic material using biocompatible adhesive.

The opening and removal of the PillCam ESO capsule from the magnetic package activates it. While active, the capsule transmits images at a rate of 14 images per second, 7 images per second per imaging head, for a period of about 10 minutes, after which it continues transmitting at 4 images per second, 2 per video head. For each image, an illuminating light flash is applied with the illuminating LEDs.

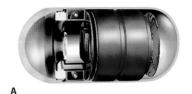

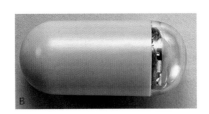

FIGURE 2.6 Illustration of the PillCam SB capsule endoscope. Courtesy of Given ® Imaging

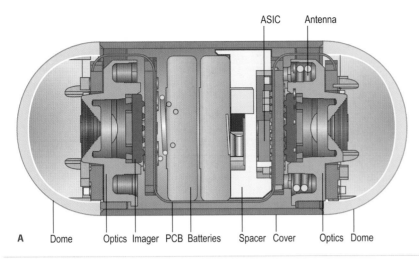

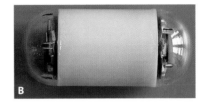

FIGURE 2.7 Illustration of the PillCam ESO video capsule. Courtesy of Given ® Imaging

The PillCam ESO capsule endoscope operates for 20 minutes, which assures imaging of the entire length of the esophagus for the majority of the patients. The typical number of pictures taken during a typical 20 minute esophageal capsule endoscopy procedure and stored in the DataRecorder is 7600. By the end of this period, the capsule stops transmitting.

Progression of the PillCam capsule endoscope in the GI tract to excretion

Depending on patient-specific factors, the capsule progresses through the GI tract, propelled by natural peristalsis that propels it towards excretion from the colon and from the GI tract. The capsule is usually excreted naturally. Typical passage times are shown in Table 2.1.[2,3]

Actual transit times vary from patient to patient, depending on patient-specific factors, underlying pathologies (e.g. tumors or strictures), or the presence of motility (peristalsis) disorders. In addition, prokinetics may affect the passage times.

The images transmitted by the capsule are time-stamped from capsule activation, allowing subsequent calculation of transit times and transit time analysis.

Capsule retention is rare[4] and details of this topic are addressed in the 2005 ICCE Consensus report.[1]

Table 2.1 PillCam capsule endoscope average transit times

Transit time type	Mean transit time
Gastric passage time	63 minutes[4]–80 minutes[5]
Duodenum-to-cecum transit time	90 minutes[5]–194 minutes[4]
Total GI (mouth-to-anus) transit time	24 hours[5]

Data recorder

The data recorder is a battery operated, external receiving/recording unit that receives the pictures captured and transmitted by the PillCam capsule endoscope. The data recorder consists of an antenna array to pick up the picture signal transmitted from the capsule endoscope, usually attached to the abdomen to assure proximity to the capsule, a receiver subsystem, and a small computer, complete with memory media, to accumulate the picture data from the capsule during the procedure (Figure 2.8).

Upon completion of the VCE procedure, the data recorder is returned to the physician and the data are transferred ("downloaded") to the RAPID Workstation for processing, display, and interpretation.

Naturally, the engineering implementation of the data recorder follows the advances in hardware developments of electronic components. Thus, the first version of the data recorder, the DR1, was based on a mini-disk permanently built into the data recorder. Following miniaturization of standard computer disks, the next version of the data recorder, the DR1.5, was based on a smaller size disk that was removable from the data recorder, thus allowing more portability, a higher turnaround time, and simultaneous processing of up to four disks from different procedures through the use of a special RAPID Booster USB disk bay. The current version of the data recorder, the DR2, while preserving the simple USB connectivity and parallel processing ability of the DR1.5, features some additional capabilities. The DR2 has a solid-state based disk that renders the data recorder less sensitive to mechanical shocks, uses less power, and allows the incorporation of the data recorder battery into the DR2 framework. Table 2.2 summarizes the different version main features of the data recorder.

The latest DR2 model data recorder features PillCam SB and PillCam ESO capsule support, reduced weight, integrated battery, integrated cradle for charging and downloading,

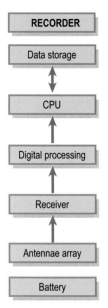

FIGURE 2.8 Data recorder operation scheme. Courtesy of Given ® Imaging

Table 2.2 Data recorder version vs. main features

	DR1	DR1.5	DR2
PillCam SB Supp.	+	+	+
Convent. Disk	+	+	
Secured Sensor Array Connector	+	+	+
Removable disk		+	
USB fast connection		+	+
PillCam ESO Supp.			+
Solid state disk			+
Integral battery			+

enhanced use and battery indicators, fast USB2 connections to the RAPID Workstation, and improved fast-connecting SensorArray connection mechanism (Figure 2.9).

Up to four separate cradle units may be connected in parallel to the RAPID Workstation, each via its own USB2 connector. Each cradle is separately connected to its own power outlet.

RAPID Workstation with RAPID Application

The RAPID Workstation and Application are used for off-line processing, storage, interpretation and analysis of the video data acquired from the Pillcam capsule endoscope. The RAPID Workstation performs the following tasks in the capsule endoscopy procedure cycle:

1. Initializing the data recorder before the VCE procedure
2. Downloading the stream of captured pictures from the data recorder and translating it into a standard video format
3. Image processing and extraction of clinically relevant data from the captured pictures using analytical algorithms
4. Video display and control during the reviewing process by the physician
5. Storage and management of patient videos prepared from downloaded data
6. Selection, annotation, and storage of selected pictures by the physician
7. Preparation of a Pillcam endoscopy report.

A schematic description of the RAPID Workstation is depicted in Figure 2.10. It is important to remember that the RAPID Workstation, despite advances in processing power of computer platforms, the development of sophisticated algorithms, and advances in image processing, is still only a tool in the hands of the physician who actually does the

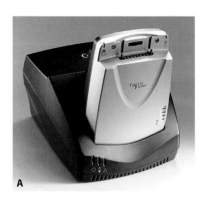

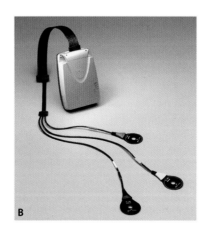

FIGURE 2.9 DataRecorder 2 kit with cradle and SensorArray. (a) DataRecorder in cradle; (b) DataRecorder with SensorArray connected. Courtesy of Given ® Imaging

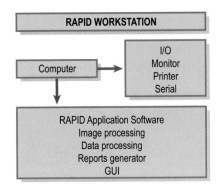

FIGURE 2.10 RAPID Workstation scheme (GUI, graphical user interface). Courtesy of Given ® Imaging

analysis and the diagnosis. Thus the (over time) naturally growing inventory of algorithms and features are aimed at conveniently displaying the captured image data from the digestive tract with sufficiently high quality. This allows:

1. Quick, error free, and diagnostically meaningful segmentation of the case video into the major anatomic locations of the GI tract (esophagus, stomach, small intestine, colon)
2. Quick and reliable detection of abnormalities and pathologies (if they exist) in the video stream together with their time and localization context

3. Effective display of diagnostically significant data extracted from the captured video stream for the evaluation of the physician.

The RAPID 4 has features designed to extract additional clinically significant data.

Table 2.3 depicts the progressive development of features for the RAPID Application.

The main screen of the RAPID Application (see Figure 2.11) allows for viewing the RAPID video while at the same time displaying a cursor on a time scale for temporal orientation in the video. Table 2.4 lists the main features.

The video controls are intuitive classical video controls, allowing for playing forward, backward, scrolling backward and forward, selecting and annotating suspicious images for storage and further analysis. Pull-down menus from the main screen provide for specific functions, such as data recorder initialization, downloading data from data recorders, and composing a summary report.

RAPID Reader

The RAPID Reader is a RAPID-like application that is designed to be installed on a variety of customer computers and allows for easy reading of RAPID videos. It is actually a RAPID without initialization and downloading capabilities.

Table 2.3 RAPID Application main features progress

RAPID Software Capabilities	2001 RAPID 1.3	2002 RAPID 1.4	2003 RAPID 2	2004 RAPID 3	2006 RAPID 4
Automatic Viewing Mode/speed	+	+	+	+	+
Localization		+	+	+	+
Suspected Blood Indicator (SBI)			+	+	+
Standard Reporting			+	+	+
Image Zoom Capability			+	+	+
HIPAA De-identification			+	+	+
HIPAA Security, CFR 21 Part 11				+	+
My GI Dictionary				+	+
Tissue Color Bar				+	+
PillCam ESO Capability				+	+
Full Screen Video Display				+	+
Password Support				+	+
Thumbnail Markings				+	+
DoubleView			+	+	+
QuadView				+	+
QuickView				+	+
RAPID Atlas					+
Circumference Scale					+

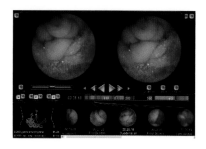

FIGURE 2.11 RAPID Application main screen. Courtesy of Given ® Imaging

In particular, it may be installed on portable laptops or home computers, thus lending to the VCE workflow of the physician significant portability and flexibility.

Capsule endoscopy procedure

The capsule endoscopy procedure involves ingesting the capsule endoscope, collecting the captured pictures in the belt-worn DataRecorder, returning the DataRecorder to the physician, and downloading the accumulated data to the RAPID Workstation and viewing the RAPID video.

Preparing the patient

Since capsule endoscopy is about direct visualization of the digestive tract mucosa, the digestive tract must be clean and free of content. Different parts of the digestive tract clean themselves in different times. For example, the esophagus is usually clean several seconds or minutes after ingestion (except in special rare cases). The stomach usually empties in less than 2 hours. Small bowel passage time, after which the small bowel is clean, is on the order of several hours.

Thus, an appropriate fasting period before the VCE procedure, depending on the type of capsule endoscopy, esophageal or small bowel, is usually appropriate to clean the respective part of the GI tract and allow unhampered direct visualization. A fast of about 12 hours before small bowel capsule endoscopy and 2 hours before esophageal capsule endoscopy is usually sufficient for the majority of patients. It is still a matter of discussion between physicians if there is sufficient benefit and no counterproductive effect in enhancing the fasting before small bowel capsule endoscopy by any kind of purgative prep or motility agent.

The prep instructions to the patient are usually given by the physician during a pre-procedure interview in which the eligibility of the patient for the VCE procedure is verified, usually patient consent is obtained, and fasting and other preparation instructions are given.

On the day of the ingestion, prior to the ingestion, the patient is outfitted with the procedure-specific SensorArray (ESO or SB), which is attached to his or her abdomen, and the RecorderBelt, which carries the initialized DataRecorder (Figure 2.12).

Table 2.4 RAPID Application features

Feature	Explanation/description
Autoview	Automatic viewing speed setting to equalize visual change rate
SBI	Automatic marking of images containing reddish features suspicious of bleeding
Localization	Rough localization and trace of the capsule in the GI tract
HIPAA compliance	Study de-identification capability and HIPAA Security, CFR 21 Part 11 compliance
ESO capsule capability	Support of ESO capsule procedures
Full Screen	Ability to view image on full screen
PW support	Support for multiuser, PW protected access to the RAPID Application
Thumbnail	Ability to add markings (arrows, circles) on thumbnails to highlight findings
Double/Quadview	Simultaneous display of 2 or 4 consecutive images for more effective viewing
Colorbar	Effective display of average image color for easy segmentation of video
Zoom	Displayed image magnified to maximum allowable size of screen
Report	Improved report capabilities
Dictionary	Built-in dictionary to assist in composing report
QuickView	Allows Fast preview of a small bowel video
RAPID Atlas	Enables comparison of case image to reference images
Circumference scale	Demonstrates a finding's circumferential involvement

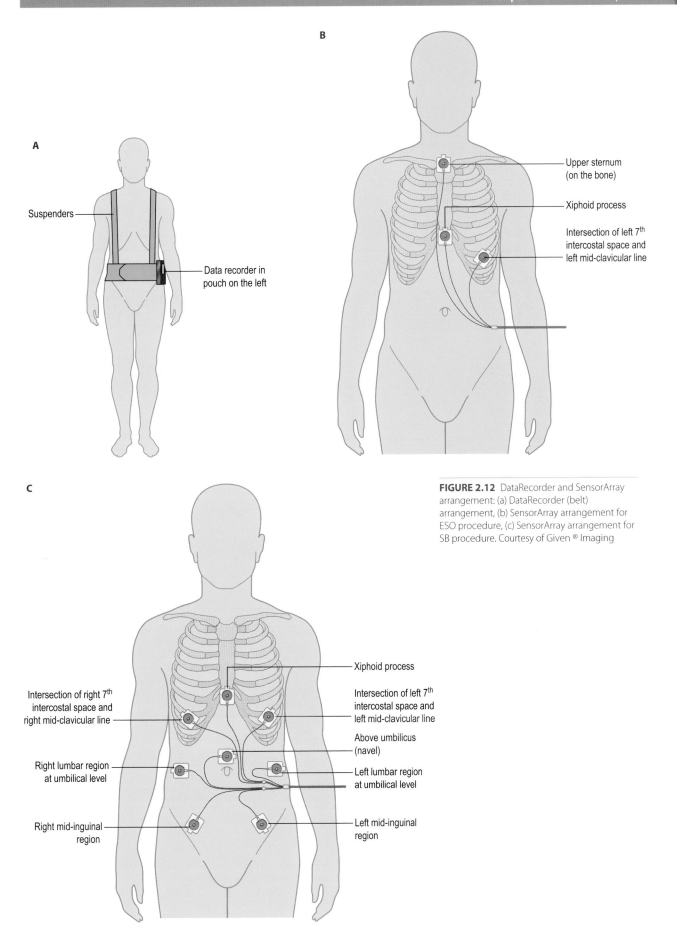

A

Suspenders

Data recorder in pouch on the left

B

Upper sternum (on the bone)

Xiphoid process

Intersection of left 7th intercostal space and left mid-clavicular line

C

Xiphoid process

Intersection of right 7th intercostal space and right mid-clavicular line

Intersection of left 7th intercostal space and left mid-clavicular line

Above umbilicus (navel)

Right lumbar region at umbilical level

Left lumbar region at umbilical level

Right mid-inguinal region

Left mid-inguinal region

FIGURE 2.12 DataRecorder and SensorArray arrangement: (a) DataRecorder (belt) arrangement, (b) SensorArray arrangement for ESO procedure, (c) SensorArray arrangement for SB procedure. Courtesy of Given ® Imaging

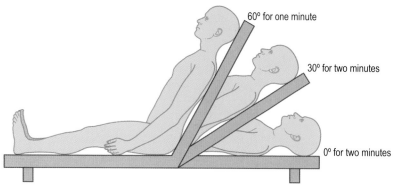

60° for one minute

30° for two minutes

0° for two minutes

FIGURE 2.13 ESO procedure reclining positions. Courtesy of Given ® Imaging

Capsule ingestion

The ingestion should take place only after verifying appropriate prep by the patient, at least 2 hours after last food intake for an ESO procedure and 10 hours after last food intake for a SB procedure.

The capsule endoscope is ingested in a natural way with some water. The specific details depend again on the type of the capsule endoscopy.

If a PillCam ESO capsule endoscope is ingested, the purpose is to slow down the progress of the capsule in the esophagus, especially in the vicinity of the lower esophageal sphincter (LES), and allow taking sufficiently numerous pictures for further analysis before the capsule passes on to the stomach. Therefore, the ingestion procedure for the ESO capsule endoscope is done in a series of reclining positions, starting in an almost flat ingestion position and going through gradually higher sitting positions until complete sitting during a period of several minutes (Figure 2.13).

All this should be done in a manner in which the patient is as inactive as possible in changing his position, thus avoiding adversely affecting capsule progress and dynamics in his esophagus. This type of ingestion is performed usually on a reclining bed that is changed by the attending nurse or physician and with a minimum amount of water, as tolerable to the patient.

After ingestion, the patient will generally wait in the physician's office until 20 minutes after ingestion, at which time the capsule will stop transmitting (and the DataRecorder blinking) and will return the SensorArray and DataRecorder. The DataRecorder will be downloaded according to the office workflow and the resulting video will be readied for reviewing by the physician.

If a PillCam SB capsule endoscope is ingested, the ingestion procedure is simple; after fitting the SensorArray (antennas) and DataRecorder (on belt) to the patient and after checking in the DataRecorder through the RAPID Workstation, the patient ingests the capsule, usually in a standing position. The purpose in this case is to have the capsule leave the stomach as soon as possible and start its journey along the small bowel and arrive at the cecum as early as possible to cover the complete small bowel. Some physicians think it is advisable for the patient to lie on the right side to facilitate the evacuation of the capsule from the stomach through the pylorus. Some others use motility agents prior to or during the procedure to speed up capsule progress and assure arrival at the cecum before the expiration of 8 hours of the PillCam SB operation time.

After about 8 hours, when the capsule stops transmitting (and the DataRecorder stops blinking), the patient returns the SensorArray and the DataRecorder to the physician's office for downloading and for preparation of a RAPID video for reviewing and analysis.

Conclusions

The Given PillCam platform is an integrated wireless endoscopy system consisting of an ingestible camera, data recorder, and workstation for review of images. The camera consists of a CMOS chip, LED light source, battery, and transmitter. The data recorder receives the transmitted images and stores them for later download. The computerized workstation initializes the data recorder and receives the downloaded images for review on proprietary software (RAPID). Two capsules are available and FDA approved for use. The small bowel capsule (PillCam SB) contains a single optical dome and obtains images at 2 per second for 8 hours. The esophageal capsule (PillCam ESO) has dual optical domes each obtaining images at 7 per second (total acquisition 14 per second).

References

1. 2005 ICCE Consensus. Endoscopy 2005;10:1065–1067.

2. Fireman Z, Kopelman Y, Fish L, Sternberg A, Scapa E, Mahaina E. Effect of oral purgatives on gastric and small bowel transit time in capsule endoscopy. Isr Med Assoc J 2004;6:521–3.

3. Dai N, Gubler C, Hengstler P, Meyenberger C, Bauerfeind P. Improved capsule endoscopy after bowel preparation. Gastrointest Endosc 2005;61:28–31

4. Gay G, Delvaux N, Rey J-F. The role of video capsule endoscopy in the diagnosis of digestive diseases: a review of current possibilities. Endoscopy 2004;36:913–920.

5. Blue Cross Shield Association. Wireless capsule endoscopy. Tec Assessment Program 2003;17:21.

CHAPTER 3

How to Set up the Suite and Perform Capsule Endoscopy

Douglas Morgan

KEY POINTS

1. Established indications for VCE include, OGIB, Crohn's Disease and abdominal SB imaging.

2. The safety of VCE is well established. Capsule retention helps identify the underlying disease aetiology in the majority of cases.

3. Endoscopic-guided VCE is appropriate for patients with known or suspected oesophageal or gastroduodenal pathology or dysmotility, which may interfere with the safe and efficient delivery of the capsule to the SB.

4. Definitive studies are needed to define the role of bowel preps and prokinetics.

Introduction

Video capsule endoscopy (VCE) uses an ingestible endoscope to acquire and transmit digital endoscopic images of the gastrointestinal tract in a wireless and noninvasive fashion. This chapter will review the performance of capsule endoscopy: indications, complications and considerations, patient preparation, and the procedure. The details of VCE technology and equipment are reviewed elsewhere. The discussion will focus upon the capsule endoscope developed by Given Imaging (Yoqneam, Israel), understanding that other manufacturers are developing similar devices. General references provide additional overviews in this evolving field.[1-5] VCE technology in its current form is ideally suited for visualization of the small bowel (SB). The technology will evolve to facilitate noninvasive visualization of the entire gastrointestinal tract. The current discussion focuses on the small bowel. Esophageal and pediatric VCE are discussed in separate chapters.

Indications

Established indications for VCE are obscure gastrointestinal hemorrhage (OGIB), Crohn's disease (CD), and abnormal imaging of the SB.[6] Evolving indications include celiac disease, indeterminate colitis, SB polyposis syndromes, and iron deficiency anemia. Examples of potential uses include malabsorption syndromes, AIDS, graft versus host disease, SB transplantation, and triage assessment of upper gastrointestinal hemorrhage (Table 3.1).

Obscure gastrointestinal bleeding

Obscure gastrointestinal hemorrhage is defined as gastrointestinal bleeding with a negative upper and lower endoscopy, which is often SB in origin. OGIB is divided into overt (melena, hematochezia) and occult subsets. The occult OGIB group is defined by either a positive fecal occult blood test (FOBT) or iron deficiency anemia (IDA). In published meta-analyses, VCE has been shown to have superior diagnostic yield compared with small bowel follow-through (SBFT) and push enteroscopy for OGIB.[7,8] The estimated number needed to treat (NNT) is 3 to yield one additional finding relative to these other exams.

The strength of indication for VCE varies with OGIB subset. VCE is clearly indicated for patients with overt OGIB. Studies suggest that the yield of VCE is significantly higher when the study is performed within 3–7 days of the bleeding event.[9] Whether the yield is further increased with scheduling of

Table 3.1 Indications for capsule endoscopy

Indication	Comments
Established indications	
OGIB, overt	Perform within 7 days of bleeding event
OGIB, IDA and FOBT+	Individualize. Await definitive studies
Crohn's disease Indeterminate colitis	Diagnosis and management
Suspected SB pathology	Abnormal imaging or clinical presentation
Polyposis syndromes	FAP, Spigelman stage III or IV PJS, biennial EGD and VCE
Emerging indications	
Celiac disease	Equivocal serology and biopsy Alarm symptoms for SB neoplasia
Melanoma	Stage IV staging evaluation
Malabsorption syndromes	AIDS
Upper GI hemorrhage	Determine need for emergent EGD
GVHD	
SB transplantation	

Notes: OGIB, obscure GI bleeding; IDA, iron deficiency anemia; FOBT, fecal occult blood test; SB, small bowel; FAP, familial polyposis syndrome; PJS, Peutz–Jeghers syndrome; EGD, esophagogastroduodenoscopy; GVHD, graft versus host disease.
Melanoma. Consider VCE in stage III disease in patients with anemia or GI symptoms.

the study at the time of hospital admission, immediately following a negative upper endoscopy, remains to be seen. The yield of VCE for patients who are FOBT positive or with IDA awaits definitive studies. Lastly, the utility of a second VCE exam for OGIB following an initial negative VCE study, which is a common practice with respect to upper and lower endoscopy, has not been defined.

Crohn's disease

Capsule endoscopy plays an important role in Crohn's disease (CD). VCE has been shown to be superior to SB barium evaluations and colonoscopy with ileoscopy in the diagnosis of CD.[10] In suspected CD, either in patients with possible SB disease or Crohn's colitis, VCE may provide vital information. One caveat: interpretation of mucosal irregularities in this setting can be challenging, since focal inflammation and ulcers can be nonspecific, as studies in healthy volunteers have shown.[11] The exam can also be helpful in indeterminate colitis. In established CD, VCE is an important tool to gauge the extent and severity of SB disease. This is very useful in determining the need to alter therapy for refractory CD. Many CD patients have concurrent IBS overlap wherein the disease activity is difficult to gauge. The cost of a VCE exam in this setting is modest relative to infused biologics.

Imaging abnormalities

Abnormal imaging of the SB wherein inflammation or neoplasia is suspected in the jejunum or ileum mandates evaluation, in the absence of contraindications. This may include barium studies or cross-sectional imaging with CT or MRI. VCE is considered a first tier imaging modality for the small intestine based upon the literature and data presented to the U.S. Food and Drug Administration (FDA).[12]

Suspected SB neoplasia is an indication for VCE, but the decision must be individualized based upon clinical presentation. Primary malignancies such as adenocarcinoma, carcinoid, lymphoma, or gastrointestinal stromal tumor (GIST) may be suggested based upon laboratory parameters or abdominal imaging. VCE may be indicated for the diagnosis of malignancies metastatic to the SB, either by local extension (ovarian, uterine, colon) or hematogenous spread (melanoma, breast, lung, renal). VCE is potentially useful in the staging evaluation of metastatic melanoma (stage IV), but studies are needed.

Novel uses

Indications for VCE are emerging beyond obscure bleeding, Crohn's disease, and abnormal small intestine imaging. Potential uses in celiac disease include equivocal diagnostic studies (positive serology with negative biopsy, or negative serology with ambiguous histology), positive serology but unable to perform an endoscopy, and lastly, known celiac disease with alarm symptoms concerning SB malignancy. The utility of VCE in celiac disease is discussed in detail elsewhere.

Guidelines are solidifying for the polyposis syndromes of the intestines.[13,14] For patients with FAP and advanced duodenal adenomas (Spigelman stage III or IV), VCE is recommended. Similarly, in Peutz–Jeghers syndrome, biennial upper endoscopy and VCE should be considered. Whether VCE will play a role in hereditary nonpolyposis colon cancer (HNPCC) is unclear.

A spectrum of studies are underway evaluating novel indications for SB VCE. These include SB transplantation, GVHD, malabsorption syndromes, and AIDS. Other intriguing uses include Emergency Department (ED) assessment of upper gastrointestinal hemorrhage to determine the need for emergent endoscopy.

Complications, contraindications, and considerations

Complications

The safety of VCE has been underscored by the worldwide use of the technology, with over a quarter of a million studies performed to date. Capsule retention in the SB is the most common serious complication. Capsule retention, or "non-natural" excretion, is defined by the documented capsule presence in the SB for greater than 2 weeks. It occurs in approximately 1 in 100–150 exams (0.75–1.0%). Retention is dependent upon the subject population, ranging from 0% in healthy volunteers to 1.5% in OGIB, and 5% in certain

Crohn's disease subsets.[11,15] Importantly, with retention, acute capsule impaction and small bowel obstruction does not occur. Physiologically, the capsule tumbles proximal to the luminal narrowing. (In contrast, there is a finite risk of acute obstruction with the patency capsule, which is discussed below.) If surgery is required for SB capsule retention, it may be arranged in a timely, but not urgent, manner. In general, surgery is recommended, as there are rare reports of capsule disintegration with perforation.[16] Lastly, it is important to emphasize that the true complication rate of VCE related to retention, as defined by unnecessary surgery, is significantly lower than 1%, since the retained capsule commonly diagnoses and localizes the underlying pathology.

Tracheal aspiration of the capsule during oropharyngeal transfer is a rare, but reported, complication of VCE.[17] While no deaths are reported, dyspnea, hypoxia, and the need for bronchoscopy are documented. Retention of the capsule in intestinal diverticula and Zenker's diverticula is also rare. Problems related to the technology — capsule failure, sensor array lead fracture, study file corruption, etc. — are uncommon. Studies which are incomplete or with poor visualization, as in the case of colonoscopy, should not be considered a complication, albeit an integral part of informed consent.

Contraindications and considerations (Table 3.2)

The expanding literature and widespread use of the technology suggest that there are few absolute contraindications to VCE.[18] The stated absolute contraindications include known gastrointestinal tract stricture, intestinal pseudo-obstruction, pregnancy, and implanted cardiac devices (pacemaker, defibrillator). The presence of significant co-morbidities which place the patient at high risk with general anesthesia

and/or abdominal surgery remains a strong contraindication in the event of capsule retention. Surgeons periodically request VCE in patients with SB obstruction or known SB strictures to visualize the involved region and localize the segment prior to surgery. This is a reasonable approach in selected cases.

VCE in patients with cardiac pacemakers has been shown to be safe.[19] Studies can be safely performed in subjects with implantable cardiac defibrillators (ICD). Patients with ICD devices should be monitored with inpatient telemetry during the VCE study. The use of telemetry for subjects with standard pacemakers is variable, but reasonable in subjects who are pacemaker dependent. In carefully selected subjects, VCE can be safely performed in pregnancy. In fact, VCE may be the optimal study in suspected Crohn's disease during pregnancy, to avoid radiation exposure and focus therapy, potentially improving outcomes for mother and child.

Considerations related to disorders of the upper gastrointestinal tract and the need for endoscopy guided VCE are discussed below. Morbid obesity may affect the ability of the sensor array to receive the capsule signal. Localization of the sensors on the subject's back, with inverted positioning, is a useful option.

Indications for patency capsule or barium exam

Capsule retention is the most common serious complication of VCE, as discussed previously. This usually occurs in the setting of an undiagnosed SB stricture. Crohn's disease, abdominal radiation or surgery history, NSAID use, or obstructive symptoms may warrant confirmation of SB luminal patency prior to VCE[15] (Table 3.3). Barium studies of the SB are helpful for significant strictures, but are of limited utility in the detection of mild to moderate luminal narrowing, which may cause capsule retention.

The patency capsule, or "dummy" capsule, has been developed to test the GI tract luminal patency prior to VCE.[20] The patency capsule (Agile®, Given Imaging, Yoqneam, Israel) consists of a radiofrequency tag within a lactose composition which dissolves after approximately 30 hours if retained in the luminal tract (Figure 3.1). The persistence of the patency capsule and tag is detected by a handheld scanner in the office or endoscopy setting. This capsule does not produce images. In contrast to VCE, the risk of acute intestinal obstruction with

Table 3.2 Capsule endoscopy: contraindications and considerations

Contraindication/ consideration	Comment
General High-risk for abdominal surgery or GA	Active co-morbidities
Morbid obesity	Alter sensor array placement
Pregnancy	Consider in selected patients
Dementia	Refusal to swallow capsule
Refusal of surgery if capsule retained	
Upper GI tract Oropharyngeal dysphagia	Aspiration risk
Esophageal disorders	Stricture, achalasia
Gastroduodenal pathology	See Table 3.4
Cardiovascular Pacemaker	Individualize telemetry
ICD	Telemetry monitoring

Notes: GA, general anesthesia; ICD, implantable cardiac defibrillator.

Table 3.3 Indications for patency capsule or small bowel barium study

Indication	Comments
Crohn's disease	Suspected SB stricture
Abdominal radiation history	Possible radiation stricture
Abdominal surgery history	Luminal anastomotic stricture, adhesions
NSAID use with obstructive symptoms	Risk for NSAID stricture or diaphragm
Obstructive symptoms	SB luminal narrowing

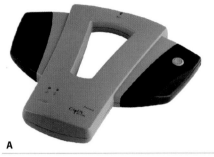
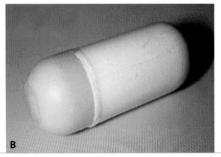
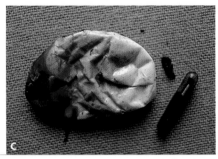

A **B** **C**

FIGURE 3.1 Patency capsule system. (a) Patency capsule scanner, for office use. (b) Intact patency capsule. (c) Disintegrated capsule, with empty shell and radiofrequency tag.

the patency capsule is finite.[21] With dissolution, the patency capsule becomes malleable and may mold into the stricture aperture to cause transient obstruction with abdominal pain or acute obstruction requiring expedited surgery. In the early experience, this may occur in up to 5% of patency capsule studies.[20]

The Capsule Endoscopy Unit

Capsule endoscopy is generally performed in the outpatient setting, but may be useful in certain inpatients (such as those with ongoing overt OGIB[9]). The equipment needed to perform VCE is relatively modest and does not require a large space commitment. The equipment includes a desktop computer, the recording device (worn on a belt), interface device between the recorder and the computer (to allow downloading of the study), data recorder battery charger, and printer. Additionally, storage space for past studies is useful, as the internal hard drive of the computer workstation will become filled. Studies may be stored on CD or DVD-ROM (and kept in binders) or on external drives or hospital mainframes. Whether studies should be stored indefinitely (or at all) is controversial, but each VCE unit should develop a policy and procedure.

VCE is generally performed in a physician's office but may be performed in an endoscopy unit. A specific room should be designated for VCE (although it may be used for other purposes). The room is furnished with a desk for the VCE workstation and an examining table. The patient will lie on the examining table to have the receiver leads placed on the abdomen. A razor should be available to shave any hair precluding good adhesion of the leads to the skin.

The efficient practice of VCE is enhanced by having a trained nurse or other assistant available. The assistant may enter the demographic information into the workstation, initialize the data recorder, apply the leads, and administer the capsule. The assistant is also useful for providing patient education and answering any questions the patient may have. At the end of the day, the assistant collects the recorder and belt, and downloads the study for review.

VCE may be performed on inpatients, even if the workstation is located elsewhere. The loading of demographic information into the workstation and initialization of the data recorder does not require the patient to be present. This may

be done in the outpatient clinic (or wherever the workstation is housed) and then the capsule, data recorder, leads, and belt are brought to the patient's hospital room where the leads are attached and the capsule is administered.

Informed consent should be obtained prior to administration of the capsule and documented in writing. The patient should be informed of the relevant risks, especially of capsule retention that may require surgery, and of alternatives (see below).

Capsule endoscopy procedure and patient preparation

Patient preparation

A good history is imperative, particularly for open endoscopy centers. Important aspects of the medical history include swallowing disorders, gastroparesis, other motility disorders, diabetes, abdominal surgery, and significant constipation. Specific inquiry regarding dysphagia and obstructive symptoms is central.

Specific instructions regarding medications are important.[4] Anticoagulation agents (e.g. warfarin) and anti-platelet agents (e.g. aspirin, clopidogrel) may and should be continued. Iron therapy should be stopped 3–5 days ahead of the procedure. Medications which affect gut motility, such as narcotics or anticholinergics, should be avoided if possible. As with standard endoscopic procedures requiring fasting, dosage adjustments may be required with some medications (e.g. insulin). Patients should be informed that their standard medications may be taken 2–4 hours after capsule ingestion.

The patient should fast for 12 hours prior to the procedure. The utility of a bowel prep the afternoon prior to the procedure is discussed below. Practical advice is helpful for patients. Loose clothing, particularly pants, is optimal. One-piece outfits such as dresses should be avoided.

Capsule endoscopy procedure

The equipment consists of the capsule, the sensor array and recorder, and the reading workstation, which are discussed elsewhere (Figure 3.2). The usual VCE exam begins between 7 and 8 a.m. with capsule ingestion, and ends the same day at 4 p.m. with the patient being disengaged from the data

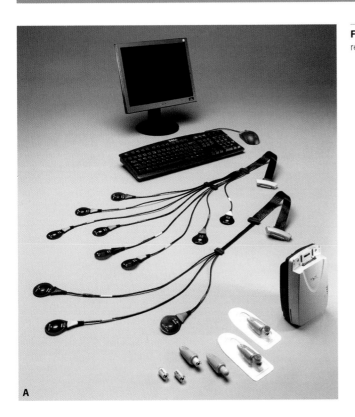

FIGURE 3.2 Capsule endoscopy components: capsule, sensor array and recorder, workstation.

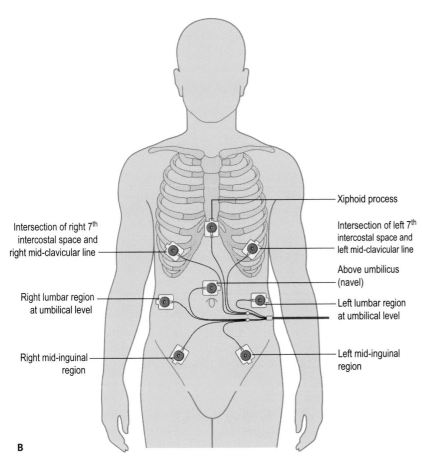

Xiphoid process

Intersection of right 7th intercostal space and right mid-clavicular line

Intersection of left 7th intercostal space and left mid-clavicular line

Above umbilicus (navel)

Right lumbar region at umbilical level

Left lumbar region at umbilical level

Right mid-inguinal region

Left mid-inguinal region

recorder. Initially, the 8-lead sensor array is fixed to the patient's abdomen. The capsule is activated by removal of the magnet, followed by confirmation of signal transmission to the data recorder. The patient should ingest the capsule with at least 8 ounces of water. Endoscopy centers often add simethicone (80 mg) either 20 minutes prior or at the time of ingestion. The vast majority of subjects swallow the capsule with ease.

During the daylong procedure, patients may return to home, work, or other activities. They may drink water 2 hours after ingestion. They may then take their medications and eat a light lunch 4 hours after ingestion. Patients should exercise care with the sensor array when changing clothes or in the bathroom. They are advised to avoid strenuous exercise or other activities which may dislodge the leads. They should avoid other patients undergoing capsule endoscopy as this may result in interference. Finally, while they may operate electronic equipment, they should avoid MRI scanners until capsule passage is confirmed.

Post procedure

The capsule facilitates physiologic endoscopy of the GI tract. The transit times are similar to a solid meal: esophagus, 2–10 seconds; stomach, 30–60 minutes; SB, 2–5 hours; colon, 10–40 hours. Most patients do not observe capsule passage. There is no risk of retention if the capsule is observed in the cecum during the study. An incomplete study is defined as one wherein the capsule fails to reach the cecum within the battery life. In these cases, an abdominal plain film is indicated if capsule passage is not clearly documented within 2 weeks. There is variability in the accuracy of patients' reports of capsule passage. Many centers routinely obtain an abdominal film if the capsule study is incomplete, regardless of patient report.

Endoscopy-guided capsule endoscopy

Endoscopy-guided capsule endoscopy (EGCE) may be needed for patients with known or suspected anatomic or motility disorders, or surgery, of the upper gastrointestinal tract.[18] A good history regarding swallowing disorders and abdominal surgery is important. Of note, prior gastric retention of the capsule does not imply underlying gastroparesis (Tables 3.4, 3.5).

There are three general techniques for endoscopy-guided capsule delivery: direct delivery, use of an overtube, and capsule ingestion with endoscopy ("swallow and follow"). The capsule may be directly delivered with a "cap" device or with accessories such as the Roth net® (US Endoscopy, Mentor, Ohio). US Endoscopy also manufactures the AdvanCE® device which utilizes a capsule holder to directly deliver the capsule to the small intestine. The holder is loaded onto a catheter-based system which passes through the endoscope channel. The flexibility of the Roth net® may make intubation of the esophagus difficult. In addition, there is a risk of capsule aspiration should the net release the capsule in passing the hypopharynx and upper esophageal sphincter. If endoscopic methods are used, the capsule should be delivered

Table 3.4 Indications for endoscopy-guided capsule endoscopy

Indication	Comment
Esophageal pathology	
Oropharyngeal dysphagia	Aspiration risk
Zenker's diverticulum	Known or suspected
Esophageal dysmotility	Achalasia, severe IEM
Suspected luminal narrowing	Web, ring, stricture
Psychologic factors	Inability to swallow
Gastroduodenal pathology	
Gastroparesis	Diabetes, narcotic-induced, etc
Gastric surgery Prior gastric retention of capsule	Individualize need
Gastrostomy	Safe delivery through tract

Notes: Gastric surgery: Billroth I, Billroth II, Roux-en-Y, etc. IEM, ineffective esophageal motility.

Table 3.5 Techniques for endoscopy-guided capsule endoscopy

Technique	Comments
Capsule delivery "cap" device	Minimizes capsule aspiration risk
Accessory device delivery	Use of snare, net, etc.
Overtube	Adequate internal diameter required
Ingestion followed by EGD	"Swallow and follow"
Gastrostomy introduction	Safe delivery through tract

to the second part of the duodenum to avoid possible gastric retention and also increase the probability of a complete SB exam by bypassing the stomach.

An overtube may be used to facilitate safe delivery into the upper esophagus. Typically, an accessory (net, snare, etc.) is used in conjunction with the overtube. The internal diameter of the flexed overtube must be sufficient to accommodate the capsule, which may affect patient comfort. Lastly, for patients with potential gastric retention, with disorders such as gastroparesis, the "swallow and follow" technique is an option. In this case, the patient swallows the capsule and immediately undergoes endoscopy for assured delivery of the capsule to the duodenum. Endoscopic accessories are typically used to advance the capsule from the stomach. Of note, the VCE can be performed with capsule delivery through a gastrostomy.

Improving diagnostic yield: bowel preparations and promotility agents

Bowel preparations

Visualization of the small intestine is adversely affected by air bubbles, food residue, and dark or bilious fluid. The goal of adding a bowel prep is to increase the sensitivity of the exam through improved visualization (Table 3.6). This is balanced against potential side effects, patient comfort, and cost. Some patients may decline VCE with the suggestion of a bowel preparation.

The standard preparation, as described above, is a 12 hour fast. Does the addition of a bowel prep enhance the visualization of the VCE study? The literature is in evolution, with the many studies in abstract form or underpowered. The studied preps include polyethylene glycol (PEG, 2 or 4 L) and sodium phosphate (90 mL), which are administered the afternoon prior to the procedure. The study by Viazis and colleagues, conducted in 80 total subjects, suggested that a 2 L PEG prep improved both the visualization (90% versus 60%) and diagnostic yield (65% versus 30%).[22] Improved visualization and diagnostic yield with the sodium phosphate prep is also suggested by published studies, but the irritant effects may lead to false positive results.[23,24] The 4 L PEG prep does not offer improved visualization when compared with 2 L, has increased side effects, and may adversely affect gastric and SB motility. Lastly, simethicone (80 mg) is often administered 20 minutes prior to the procedure, as noted above.

In conclusion, a bowel prep may improve the quality of visualization of the SB with VCE, but the recommendations are in evolution.[25,26] Optimal prep type, dosage, and timing remain to be defined. The reasons are twofold. The current literature consists of heterogeneous studies with respect to prep specifics, as well as endpoints. Secondly, the outcome difference with the addition of a prep may be small, requiring studies of higher power. At this juncture, most centers utilize one of two approaches: (1) 12 hour fast without a bowel preparation; (2) GoLytely 2 L, administered within 16 hours of the procedure.

Promotility agents

Slow gastric or SB transit may prevent the capsule from reaching the cecum within the battery life, decreasing the sensitivity of the VCE exam. This may occur in 5–10%

Table 3.6 Procedure adjuncts, bowel preps and prokinetics

Adjunct	Comments
Bowel preparations	
PEG 2 L	Prep of choice
PEG 4 L	May slow SB motility
Sodium phosphate 90 mL	May yield false positives
Promotility agents	
Metoclopramide, 10 mg	GTT decreased
Erythromycin, 200 mg	GTT decreased
Domperidone, 10 mg	Limited availability in some regions
Tegaserod, 6 mg	SBTT decreased

Notes: GTT, gastric transit time; SBTT, small bowel transit time; Tegaserod has been withdrawn from the market.

of exams, although it has been reported in up to 16% of early studies.[27] As is the case with bowel preps, the increase in percentage of complete studies to the cecum must be balanced by medication side effects and cost. In addition, if SB transit is too rapid, the sensitivity of the VCE exam may be adversely affected by the pathology "miss rate."

The promotility agents currently under study include metoclopramide, erythromycin, domperidone, and tegaserod. While the gastric (GTT) and small bowel (SBTT) transit times have been studied with sodium phosphate and PEG, they will not be considered promotility agents in the current discussion, as the literature is discordant. Studies suggest that gastric promotility agents consistently decrease GTT, but may or may not increase the percentage of complete studies.[28–30] In preliminary studies, tegaserod has been shown to decrease SBTT with improvement in diagnostic yield. The withdrawal of tegaserod from the market, will preclude its use in VCE. In addition, the need for gastric promotility agents may be obviated by routine use of the real-time viewer (see below).

In summary, the use of a pre-procedure promotility agent may improve the sensitivity of the VCE exam by insuring complete SB transit in the majority of exams. This may occur via decreased GTT or SBTT. The existing literature is again heterogeneous and the majority of studies are of limited power. Individualized use of promotility agents may be warranted. For example, incomplete exams are increased in the hospitalized and diabetic populations.

There may be a promotility agent threshold wherein VCE diagnostic yield is increased up to a point, but too rapid SB transit will then decrease the exam sensitivity by increasing the "miss rate." This threshold may vary in the individual patient, thereby hindering definitive studies and general recommendations. Other adjuncts, such as patient positioning in the right lateral decubitus position to decrease GTT, are unlikely to significantly increase diagnostic yield.

Conclusions

Firm recommendations regarding the use of bowel preparations and prokinetic agents are elusive.[25] The adjuncts may increase the diagnostic yield, but definitive evidence is lacking. Well-designed randomized controlled trials are warranted. The use of adjuncts must be balanced against patient acceptance and side effects, cost considerations, and effect upon the exam sensitivity ("miss rate").

Procedure adjuncts

Various adjuncts are available to improve the efficacy, efficiency, and availability of the VCE exam (Table 3.7). The real-time viewer (RTV) permits visualization of live capsule endoscopy images. The RTV is connected to the recorder during the study. The primary uses include confirmation of gastric transit to the duodenum and SB transit into the cecum. Potential future uses include assessment of the need for emergent upper endoscopy for upper gastrointestinal hemorrhage in the emergency room setting. Satellite systems are available to permit capsule ingestions at remote sites, with

Table 3.7 Procedure adjuncts

Device or accessory	Uses
Patency capsule	Document GI tract patency prior to VCE
AdvanCE®	Direct capsule delivery to the duodenum
Real-time viewer	Flat screen display of real-time images
Remote VCE	Satellite VCE with study transmission to a central location

study transmission to a central location. Capsule delivery devices are described above.

Conclusions

In summary, capsule endoscopy is a safe, well-tolerated exam, which provides for unique visualization of the small intestine. Small bowel indications are expanding beyond the current focus on OGIB and CD. The growing literature and extensive international experience underscore the diminishing number of contraindications, particularly in carefully selected patients. The development of the patency capsule, endoscopic delivery devices, and real-time viewer further enhance efficient application of the technology, and bode well for the future of "untethered endoscopy."[31]

References

1. Barkin JS, Lightdale CJ, eds. Small bowel enteroscopy. Gastrointest Endosc Clin N Am 2006; 16(2). April issue.

2. Lewis B. Capsule Endoscopy 2006: Results from the 2006 Consensus Conference. Endoscopy 2005; 37(10). October issue.

3. Keuchel M, Hagenmuller F, Fleischer D, eds. Atlas of video capsule endoscopy, First edition. Springer Medizin Verlag, Heidelberg, Germany, 2006.

4. Lewis B. Capsule endoscopy. In: Drossman D, ed. Handbook of gastroenterologic procedures, 4th edn. Lippincott, Williams & Wilkins, Baltimore MD, 2005: pp. 263–9.

5. Capsule Endoscopy scientific website, www.CapsuleEndoscopy.org

6. Cave D. Technology insight: current status of video capsule endoscopy. Nat Clin Pract Gastroenterol Hepatol 2006; 3:158.

7. Triester SL, Leighton JA, Leontiadis GI, et al. A meta-analysis of capsule endoscopy compared to other diagnostic modalities in patients with obscure gastrointestinal bleeding. Am J Gastroenterol 2005;100:2407.

8. Marmo R, Rotondano G, Piscopo R, et al. Meta-analysis: capsule enteroscopy vs. conventional modalities in diagnosis of small bowel diseases. Aliment Pharmacol Ther 2005;22:595.

9. Pennazio M, Santucci R, Rondonotti E, et al. Outcome of patients with obscure gastrointestinal bleeding after capsule endoscopy: report of 100 cases. Gastroenterology 2004;126:643.

10. Triester SL, Leighton JA, Leontiadis GI, et al. A meta-analysis of capsule endoscopy compared to other diagnostic modalities in patients with non-stricturing small bowel Crohn's disease. Am J Gastroenterol 2006;101:954.

11. Goldstein JL, Eisen GM, Lewis B, et al. Video capsule endoscopy to prospectively assess small bowel injury with celecoxib, naproxen plus omeprazole, and placebo. Clin Gastroenterol Hepatol 2005;3:133.

12. Federal Drug Administration. Meta-analysis report: performance evaluation of Given Diagnostic System in the diagnosis of small bowel diseases and disorders. FDA, 2003, version 2: pp. 1–36.

13. Burke CA, Santisi J, Church J, et al. The utility of capsule endoscopy small bowel surveillance in patients with polyposis. Am J Gastroenterol 2005;100:1498.

14. Schulmann K, Hollerbach S, Kraus K, et al. Feasibility and diagnostic utility of video capsule endoscopy for the detection of small bowel polyps in patients with hereditary polyposis syndromes. Am J Gastroenterol 2005;100:27.

15. Cave D, Legnani P, de Franchis R, Lewis B. ICCE Consensus for capsule retention. Endoscopy 2005;37:1065.

16. Gay G, Delvaux M, Laurent V, et al. Temporary intestinal occlusion induced by a patency capsule in a patient with Crohn's disease. Endoscopy 2005;37:174.

17. Buchkremer F, Hermann T, Stremmel W, et al. Mild respiratory distress after wireless capsule endoscopy. Gut 2004;53:472.

18. Storch I, Barkin JS. Contraindications to capsule endoscopy: do any still exist? Gastrointest Endosc Clin N Am 2006;16:329.

19. Leighton JA, Srivathsan K, Carey EJ, et al. Safety of wireless capsule endoscopy in patients with implantable cardiac defibrillators. Am J Gastroenterol 2005;100:1728.

20. Signorelli C, Rondonotti E, Villa F, et al. Use of the Given Patency System for the screening of patients at high risk for capsule retention. Dig Liver Dis 2006;38:326.

21. Gay G, Delvaux M, Laurent V, et al. Temporary intestinal occlusion induced by a "patency capsule" in a patient with Crohn's disease. Endoscopy 2005;37:174.

22. Viazis N, Sgouros S, Papaxoinis K, et al. Bowel preparation increases the diagnostic yield of capsule endoscopy: a prospective, randomized, controlled trial. Gastrointest Endosc 2004;60:534.

23. Niv Y, Niv G. Capsule endoscopy: role of bowel preparation successful visualization. Scand J Gastroenterol 2004;39:1005.

24. Dai N, Gubler C, Hengsteler P, et al. Improved capsule endoscopy after bowel preparation. Gastrointest Endosc 2005;61:28.

25. De Franchis R, Avgerinos A, Barkin J, et al. ICCE Consensus for small bowel preparation and prokinetics. Endoscopy 2005;37:1040.

26. Villa F, Signorelle C, Rondonotti E, et al. Preparations and prokinetics. Gastrointest Endosc Clin N Am 2006;16:211.

27. Rondonotti E, Herrerias JM, Pennazio M, et al. Complications, limitations and failures of capsule endoscopy: a review of 733 cases. Gastrointest Endosc 2005;62:712.

28. Selby W. Complete small bowel transit in patients: determining factors and improvement with metoclopramide. Gastrointest Endosc 2005;61:80.

29. Keuchel M, Voderholzer W, Schenk G, et al. Domperidone shortens gastric transit time of video capsule endoscope. Endoscopy 2003;35:A185.

30. Leung WK, Chan FK, Fung SS, et al. Effect of oral erythromycin on gastric and small bowel transit time of capsule endoscopy. World J Gastroenterol 2005;11:4865.

31. Faigel DO, Fennerty MB. "Cutting the cord" for capsule endoscopy. Gastroenterology 2002;123:1385.

CHAPTER **4**

Reading, Reporting, and Training

Douglas G Adler

KEY POINTS

1. Reading capsule endoscopy studies is a skill that requires time, effort, and practice in order to achieve proficiency.

2. Capsule studies should be read in a quiet environment without distractions in order to facilitate high yield rates.

3. Not all abnormalities seen on a capsule endoscopy are of equal importance and readers should distinguish between general abnormalities and definitive findings that may be the cause of the patient's illness.

4. At present, the gold standard for the diagnosis of GVHD is simultaneous upper and lower endoscopy with mucosal biopsies, but VCE has been found to be more sensitive and better tolerated than traditional endoscopy.

Introduction

Although on the surface reading capsule endoscopy studies seems like a simple and straightforward endeavor, the task is in reality both challenging and demanding. Endoscopists used to a mucosal-based view of the gastro-intestinal tract must familiarize themselves with a villus-based view (Figure 4.1). This chapter is presented to familiarize the reader with the specifics of reading capsule endoscopy studies and generating the procedure report from the study. In addition, attention will also be given to issues of training in capsule endoscopy with an eye on adequacy of training volume and the attainment of inter-reader reliability.

Reading capsule endoscopy

A typical capsule study generates over 57 000 images. In many cases all of these images will not need to be reviewed as the colonic portion of the study is often not evaluated (given that the exam was likely performed to evaluate the small bowel and the colon has not undergone a purge). Likewise, some readers will also skip the gastric portion of the study, a practice that this author does not agree with as relevant findings are often detected in this portion of the exam.

Before the specifics of reading are covered, some general statements are worth making. It should be stressed that viewing the video more slowly is preferable despite the fact that this will incur a significant time burden. As a rule, a faster frame rate will result in a lower study yield as small lesions or lesions that appear in only one or two frames can easily be missed. When reading capsule endoscopy, the images displayed must have the full attention of the reader and it is not feasible to view the study and perform any other activity simultaneously. The reading should be performed in a quiet place, preferably in low light. Outside distractions should be minimized or eliminated. Interruptions in viewing (looking up from the screen to answer the telephone or look at an electronic pager, etc.) should prompt the reader to "back-up" the video to a previously viewed segment upon the resumption of viewing as relevant lesions could be missed even if only brief segments of the video go unexamined. The decision of whether or not to read the entire video in one sitting or in multiple pieces is left to the viewer, but in either case the above guidelines should still apply.

The software available at the time of this writing (Rapid Reader 3.1.8.0, Given Imaging, Yoqneam, Israel) is significantly different from the first generation product marketed in 2000. The current reader allows viewing of

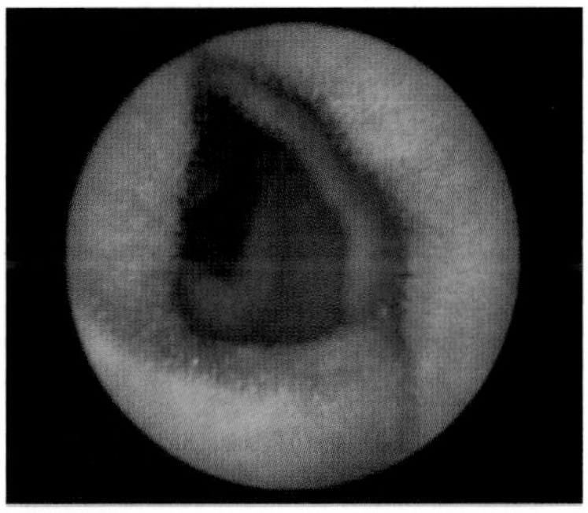

FIGURE 4.1 Wireless capsule endoscopy image of small intestine demonstrating "villus-based" view.

one, two, or four images simultaneously, as well as onscreen thumbnail views of selected images and the localization feature (Figure 4.2). The single view mode has a maximum frame rate of 25 frames per second (fps) while the two and four image views each have a maximum viewing rate of 40 fps. The two and four image modes offer the reader the opportunity to view the complete video in dramatically less time but are more difficult to read, especially the four image mode. The viewing mode and frame rate can be adjusted at any time during the viewing. The current software also allows for the creation of thumbnail images, as well as for a printed report that contains information including the indication for the study, the findings of the procedure, and a space for the reader to summarize the findings and make recommendations, as well as labeled thumbnail images in color.

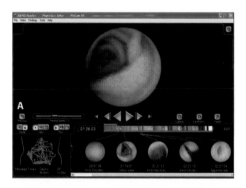

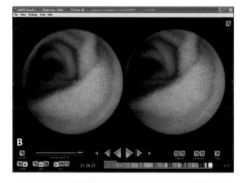

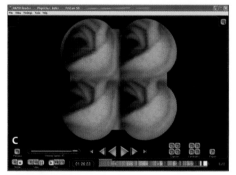

FIGURE 4.2 (a) Rapid Reader screen — single frame view. Note capsule image at center, localization feature at bottom left, timebar below large capsule image, and thumbnails along bottom of frame. (b) Rapid Reader screen — dual frame view. Note that not all features are visible in non-single frame view modes. (c) Rapid Reader screen — quad frame view.

Viewing times

Viewing times for reading capsule endoscopy vary widely between different examinations and readers. In one study of 20 studies viewed by two different readers, the average viewing time was 60.1 minutes (range: 28–93 minutes).[1] These viewings did not include the colonic portion of the study. Other authors have reported similar lengths of time to review capsule studies; Lewis et al averaged 56 minutes to review only the small bowel portion of the study in 20 patients, whereas Ell et al reported an average of 50 minutes to review the small bowel portion of 32 studies.[2,3] Although in several cases these times were based on first generation software where only one frame could be viewed at a time, these data all illustrate the fact that capsule endoscopy is a time-intensive procedure. Soon after the advent of capsule endoscopy, there were concerns that such long read times would render the technique impractical and uneconomical, although it was foreseen (correctly) that subsequent versions of the software would allow more rapid evaluation of the data.[4] The dual and quad image views allow for a significantly shorter read time. It is not known if using the dual and quad image views results in a higher or lower yield rate for capsule endoscopy.

Thumbnails and landmarks

All versions of the Rapid Reader software allow for the creation of "thumbnail" images. This refers to the specific ability on the part of the operator to capture relevant images, label them appropriately (both with text and with visual aides such as arrows to or circles around relevant findings), and set them aside for possible incorporation into the report generated at the end of the study.

When viewing the capsule video, the reader should take advantage of the ability to thumbnail and bookmark certain landmarks. Although often only a small number of images from the esophagus will be apparent, the transition to the gastric portion of the video will be abrupt and difficult to miss. Likewise, other transitions are readily apparent including the first duodenal image, the passage through the ileocecal valve, and the first image of the cecum (which is often full of stool unless the patient has undergone a prior purge). All of these transitions can and should be bookmarked and the current version of the Rapid Reader software has pre-labeled thumbnail image slots that can be selected for these transitions. The value of these transitions is that, by performing elementary mathematics, useful data such as the gastric emptying time and small bowel transit time can be ascertained. These times are displayed as part of the localization feature on screen (see below). The added value of creating these bookmarks is that if the data are viewed at a later date the reader can jump to the relevant portion of the video without having to scan many images to find the desired anatomy.

Localization system

Although not available on the initial version of the Rapid Reader software, subsequent versions have incorporated a two-dimensional image locator system. The capsule's location at any given time is estimated from the RF signal level measurements obtained by the eight antennae located on the patient's abdomen. The antenna lead closest to the capsule at any given time receives the strongest signal.[5]

On the bottom left-hand corner of the reader, a simple rendition of the patient's abdomen is drawn and the capsule's location within the abdomen at the time of the current image is displayed (Figure 4.3). In addition, the capsule's passage through the abdomen is indicated by a solid line that trails the capsule, which itself is represented as a bright white dot with a dark center. As one might expect, this line often follows a tortuous course consistent with the small bowel. The line is color-coded and is linked to the thumbnail images showing points of major transition. The line is dark blue during the gastric transit, light blue/aqua in the small bowel, and yellow/tan once the cecum is reached. The line is gray in segments of the video the reader has yet to see. In individuals without a prior history of abdominal surgery, a crude rule of thumb is often very helpful; when the capsule is in the small bowel located towards the left upper abdomen, this likely represents jejunum. Similarly, when the capsule is located in the right lower quadrant, this likely represents ileum. This information can be useful when capsule endoscopy is being performed prior to push enteroscopy as the level of a particular lesion can be estimated based on the data obtained from the localization feature.

The specific points of transfer (first gastric image, first duodenal image, and first cecal image) are represented on the multicolored line as discreet and bright dots. The first gastric image is tagged with a bright dark blue dot; the first duodenal image is tagged with a bright light blue dot; and the first cecal image is tagged with a yellow/tan dot. The first ileocecal valve view can also be thumbnailed.

The localization module has been clinically assessed in a group of healthy volunteers who underwent capsule endoscopy combined with serial sets of fluoroscopic images every 1.5 hours for the first 6 hours of the study. Data on capsule location at fluoroscopy were compared to data generated based on signal strength as recorded by the skin sensors. Sixty-two percent of samples were accurate to within 4 cm, and 87% of samples were accurate to within 6 cm.[5] Although limited, these data suggest that the localization feature is reliable enough to at least guide endoscopic investigations for lesions

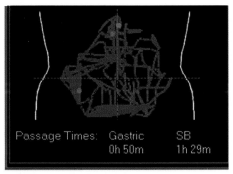

FIGURE 4.3 Representative image of the localization feature with all gut segments, transition points, and passage times demarcated.

seen at capsule endoscopy. It should also be pointed out that many (if not most) push enteroscopy examinations are not performed under fluoroscopic guidance, arguing further that a general localization of a suspected lesion should be adequate to guide the endoscopist to the target at push enteroscopy.

The localization feature thus can give the reader both a snapshot of the capsule's progress during the time the study is being read and an overall roadmap of the capsule's trajectory once the study has been completed. In addition, watching the generation of the line depicting the motion of the capsule while reading the study can also give information about areas of possible stricture as the capsule will often experience significant delay at these sites, and this can be correlated to areas of stricture, inflammation, or neoplasia seen on the corresponding capsule endoscopy images.

Suspected blood indicator

Recent versions of the Rapid Reader software package have included a suspected blood indicator (SBI) feature. This, added in an attempt to possibly decrease the amount of time required to read capsule endoscopy studies, automatically "tags" images with a high degree of red color visible, on the assumption that these images may in fact depict blood or lesions that could be the cause of bleeding (ulcers, angioectasia, tumors, etc.). The SBI feature is optional and the reader may elect to not use the function at all, to evaluate the images selected by the SBI prior to viewing the entire video, or to use the SBI as a "double check" of his or her own interpretation of the study after the entire video has been viewed and to make sure that all areas possibly containing blood have at least been evaluated. The personal preference of the author is to use the SBI only after the entire video has been viewed in an attempt to avoid reader bias.

Although it has been available for some time now, there are few published data on the value or usefulness of the SBI. To date, one abstract and two published studies have formally evaluated the SBI. Liangpunsakul et al[6] reported results obtained when the SBI was specifically evaluated in 24 patients, 18 of whom had documented iron deficiency anemia, and 6 of whom had chronic abdominal pain. Preparation only involved an overnight fast for the patients. The studies were viewed by gastroenterologists and the findings of the physicians were compared to those of the SBI. In this study, the overall results were mixed. When looking at all lesions, the sensitivity, specificity, positive predictive value, and negative predictive value of the SBI were 25.7%, 85%, 90%, and 17.3% respectively, with an overall accuracy of 35%. Although these overall findings were somewhat less than encouraging, the SBI performed somewhat better when specific types of lesions were analyzed. For example, sensitivity of active small bowel bleeding was markedly higher at 81% and the overall accuracy for the detection of active small bowel bleeding in this study was 83%. Still, it should be recognized that most patients do not have active bleeding at the time of the study.

Another similar but larger study was performed by D'Halluin et al, who evaluated the usefulness of the SBI in a multi-center study of 156 capsule studies.[7] This study was limited to patients with a history of gastrointestinal bleeding who had undergone prior unrevealing upper endoscopy and colonoscopy with ileoscopy. In addition, patients in this study did undergo a purge with 2 L of polyethylene glycol solution prior to swallowing the capsule. Seventy-three of these studies contained at least one abnormal image. The overall sensitivity, specificity, positive predictive value, and negative predictive value of the SBI in this study were 45%, 72%, 52%, and 67%, respectively. When specific types of lesions were evaluated, the SBI again performed best with regards to its ability to detect actively bleeding areas/blood in the lumen and less well when areas not actively bleeding, but with the potential to bleed in the future, were evaluated. There was a high degree of inter-center reliability with regards to the usefulness of the SBI. Overall, these authors did not feel that the SBI markedly assisted in the interpretation of capsule endoscopy studies. In addition, they recommended that the SBI not be used as a tool to initially assess capsule studies but felt that the value of the feature was its ability to give a second opinion to the reader regarding certain images.

Definitive findings versus abnormalities

The indication for performing a capsule endoscopy will often shape the expectations of the reader when reviewing the study; i.e. in a patient with anemia, the reader will likely be looking for ulcers, angioectasia, or masses, while in a patient with suspected Crohn's disease the reader may be looking for linear ulcerations. Such biases are to be expected and may not be unhelpful. Indeed, clear images of these types of findings very often represent definitive findings. However, when viewing capsule endoscopy studies, for any indication, the reader will inevitably encounter mucosal abnormalities of an undetermined nature (Figure 4.4). When encountering these abnormalities, which are often visible in a limited number of frames and may be blurred by motion artifact, the reader must avoid the temptation to label them as definitive findings. Many early published studies of capsule endoscopy with very high yield rates have not segregated their findings into definitive vs. non-definitive findings. Still, these small or indeterminate lesions may represent abnormalities and should be commented upon in the final report.

Reporting of findings from capsule endoscopy studies

All versions of the Rapid Reader software have allowed users to generate a printed report of the findings of the study to facilitate record keeping and communication between physicians. Procedure reports can be saved electronically, printed, or emailed to referring physicians.

The current version of the software allows the generation of a report that contains the following data as text:

* Demographic data on the patient including:
  — Medical record number
  — Date of the procedure (not the date the study is read)

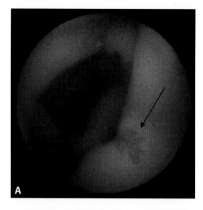

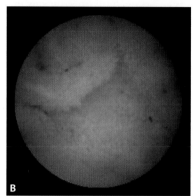

FIGURE 4.4 (a) A well-visualized angioectasia — a definitive finding. (b) A red spot without clear features — a non-definitive abnormality.

  — Gender
  — Birth date
* Reason for referral
* Specific data regarding the capsule procedure (patient body habitus, size, weight, etc.)
* Findings of the procedure
* Summary and recommendations.

The information for the referral, findings, and summary and recommendations section can be entered as free text at any time during the viewing and reporting phase of the study. The current software also includes a small dictionary of commonly used terms that can be selected from when describing findings.

In addition to text, the operator has the ability to append full color images, selected and labeled during the reading phase of the study, to the report. Some or all of the selected images may be chosen, and in addition to a text label, the images are accompanied by a small version of the localization feature. In this manner, the reported images can quickly convey a finding as seen during the study, the reader's impression of what the finding likely represents, as well as the location of the finding within the patient's abdomen.

In some cases, the recording of more than just still images is warranted or may be of special use to physicians. In these cases, multiple consecutive frames of the study may be more helpful and the software allows the recording of short video segments for exactly this purpose. While these video segments cannot be incorporated into any printed report they can be saved electronically and sent to referring physicians. This can be an especially helpful feature when requesting a second opinion regarding a finding if only a small section of the entire study is under consideration.

Training physicians to perform and interpret capsule endoscopy

Training in capsule endoscopy can be achieved by several different routes. Currently, many GI trainees receive direct training in capsule endoscopy as part of their core GI fellowship endoscopy training. For practitioners who completed training prior to the advent of capsule endoscopy, routes to learning capsule endoscopy include mentorship by an experienced capsule endoscopist with supervisory reading of capsule studies, participation in a capsule endoscopy course, or both. This author discourages individuals from attempting to teach themselves to read capsule endoscopy studies.

As of this writing, there are no universally agreed upon criteria for training physicians to perform and interpret capsule endoscopy. In addition, there are no universally agreed upon benchmarks for competence to read capsule endoscopy studies independently. The difficulty in this matter stems from the fact that capsule endoscopy is different than all other endoscopic procedures, where direct hands-on manipulation of an endoscope is called for. With capsule endoscopy the issue of *technical* competence is essentially moot, and thus the emphasis must be on *interpretive* competence. Physicians must be able to reliably detect and correctly diagnose abnormalities based on their appearance at capsule endoscopy, while at the same time recognizing normal anatomy or variations of normal anatomy that do not, in fact, represent diagnostic abnormalities.

There are few published data regarding the learning curve for capsule endoscopy. In the context of a prospective comparison between capsule endoscopy and push enteroscopy in patients with gastrointestinal bleeding of obscure origin, Adler et al also compared the accuracy of a senior therapeutic endoscopist with significant experience in both capsule endoscopy and push enteroscopy to a fourth year "advanced" endoscopy fellow who had performed approximately 30 push enteroscopy examinations and had reviewed approximately 15 capsule endoscopy examinations prior to the study.[1] In this study, the senior endoscopist performed sequential unblinded capsule endoscopy and push enteroscopy on 20 patients, and a blinded reader (the advanced endoscopy fellow) read the capsule studies only. When the results of the capsule interpretation were compared, there was complete agreement in 18/20 (90%) of capsule studies (kappa statistic 0.69). In one patient, each reader saw a finding the other did not see and in one patient the unblinded reviewer saw a finding the blinded reader did not. None of these findings were felt to represent definitive causes of gastrointestinal bleeding. This study suggested that the learning curve for reading capsule endoscopy among physicians with some degree of endoscopic experience was short. Another report, available in abstract form only, focusing on inter-reader reliability in capsule endoscopy, evaluated 24 patients and found a high degree of inter-reader reliability with disagreement only on minor findings of unclear clinical significance.[8] Another study, also available only in abstract form, demonstrated high inter-reader reliability when comparing 72 capsule endoscopy studies. These authors had an overall agreement of 90% (with a kappa statistic of 0.787) between experienced capsule endoscopists.[9]

One study assessing the potential viability of non-physician readers compared the accuracy of a gastroenterologist to an experienced endoscopy nurse who had received training in capsule endoscopy.[10] In this study of 20 patients, the physician detected 27 significant lesions, while the nurse detected 28 significant lesions. Twenty-five of the 27 lesions seen by the physician were seen by the nurse (93% sensitivity, 95% CI = 74–99%). The physician detected 25 of the 28 significant lesions seen by the nurse. Based on this study, it can be argued that perhaps experience of looking at endoscopic images (as this nurse had) may be enough to allow non-physicians to function either as capsule endoscopy pre-readers or even possibly as independent readers.

In an attempt to assist physicians interested in either performing capsule endoscopy or choosing a physician to perform capsule endoscopy, the American Society of Gastrointestinal Endoscopy recently published a guideline for credentialing and granting privileges for capsule endoscopy.[11] This consensus statement recommends the following training guidelines before competency can be assessed:

- Completion of a GI fellowship training program (or equivalent)
- Competence in performing upper endoscopy, colonoscopy, and push enteroscopy
- Familiarity with capsule endoscopy hardware and software systems
- One of the following two options:
  — Formal training in capsule endoscopy in the context of a gastroenterology fellowship
  — Completion of a hands-on course with at least 8 hours CME credit which has been endorsed by a national or international GI or surgical society and review of first 10 capsule studies by a credentialed capsule endoscopist.

In addition, this guideline emphasizes that practitioners must understand the indications, risks, and potential complications of capsule endoscopy and be able to document the findings of capsule endoscopy and communicate them with referring physicians. The European Society of Gastrointestinal Endoscopy Guideline on Capsule Endoscopy does not make recommendations regarding training or credentialing, although this document is more focused on indications of capsule endoscopy and the yield of the test in different clinical situations.[12]

Acknowledgment

The author thanks Dr Waqar Qureshi for his assistance in the creation of the figures for the manuscript.

References

1. Adler DG, Knipschield M, Gostout C. A prospective comparison of capsule endoscopy and push enteroscopy in patients with GI bleeding of obscure origin. Gastrointest Endosc 2004;59:492–8.

2. Lewis BS, Swain P. Capsule endoscopy in the evaluation of patients with suspected small intestinal bleeding: Results of a pilot study. Gastrointest Endosc 2002;56:349–53.

3. Ell C, Remke S, May A, Helou L, Henrich R, Mayer G. The first prospective controlled trial comparing wireless capsule endoscopy with push enteroscopy in chronic gastrointestinal bleeding. Endoscopy 2002;34:685–9.

4. Fleischer DE. Capsule endoscopy: the voyage is fantastic — will it change what we do? Gastrointest Endosc 2002;56:452–6.

5. Fischer D, Schreiber R, Levi D, Eliakim R. Capsule endoscopy: the localization system. Gastrointest Endosc Clin N Am 2004;14:25–31.

6. Liangpunsakul S, Mays L, Rex DK. Performance of Given suspected blood indicator. Am J Gastroenterol 2003;98:2676–8.

7. D'Halluin PN, Delvaux M, Lapalus MG, et al. Does the "Suspected Blood Indicator" improve the detection of bleeding lesions by capsule endoscopy? Gastrointest Endosc 2005;61:243–9.

8. Sigmundsson HK, Das A, Isenberg G. Capsule endoscopy (CE): interobserver comparison of interpretation [abstract]. Gastrointest Endosc 2003;57:AB165.

9. Mergener K, Enns R. Interobserver variability for reading capsule endoscopy examinations. Abstract 489. Gastrointest Endosc 2003;57:AB10.

10. Levinthal GN, Burke CA, Santisi JM. The accuracy of an endoscopy nurse in interpreting capsule endoscopy. Am J Gastroenterol 2003;98:2669–71.

11. Faigel DO, Baron TH, Adler DG, et al. ASGE guideline: Guidelines for credentialing and granting privileges for capsule endoscopy. Gastrointest Endosc 2005;61:503–5.

12. Rey JF, Gay G, Kruse A, Lambert R. ESGE Guidelines Committee. European Society of Gastrointestinal Endoscopy guideline for video capsule endoscopy. Endoscopy 2004;36:656–8.

The Role of Surgery in Capsule Endoscopy

Calvin W Lee and David R Cave

KEY POINTS

1. About 20–40% of video capsule endoscopy (VCE) procedures detect lesions amenable to further therapy, and 10–20% undergo surgical therapy.

2. Localization of abnormalities in the small bowel by video capsule endoscopy (VCE) is imprecise, and intraoperative endoscopy or double balloon endoscopy is often helpful to target surgical intervention.

3. It is anticipated that VCE will allow earlier detection of small bowel tumors.

4. VCE-guided laparoscopic surgery has been reported.

5. The risk of capsule retention varies with the patient population, is highest in patients with known Crohn's disease, and may require endoscopic or surgical retrieval.

6. VCE findings are expected to increase the number of surgical interventions for small bowel pathology, but it is difficult to assess the impact of VCE on surgical outcomes. Nevertheless, a complete road map of lesions should help the surgeon determine the operation to perform and allow for a more targeted surgical exploration.

Introduction

Surgical intervention was the method of last resort for the diagnosis and treatment of many lesions in the small intestine, particularly those patients presenting with obscure bleeding or abdominal pain suggestive of intermittent or partial small bowel obstruction. Such intervention was almost invariably met with a lack of enthusiasm on the part of both the surgeon and the gastroenterologist because the procedure was often a fishing expedition, which might involve intraoperative endoscopy, which in turn was limited by inadequate scope design, interpretive difficulties, long procedural time, and risk of complications. This situation has been improved by the development and deployment of video capsule endoscopy (VCE). This tiny device now provides a new and effective tool for the noninvasive diagnosis of small bowel pathology.

Despite the availability of VCE for five years since its FDA approval in August 2001, there is a lack of published data on how VCE has changed the role of surgery in the investigation and management of small bowel disease. The objective of this chapter is to examine the new role of surgery in the management of small bowel pathology in the era of VCE. We believe that VCE can be used to direct surgical intervention with considerably greater precision than in the past, often with an intervening step using either push or double balloon endoscopy. Indeed, the possibility of initially localizing small bowel lesions by VCE and then tattooing them endoscopically allows much greater use of laparoscopy than in the past and opens up the possibility of laparoscopically guided intraoperative endoscopy.

Technology review

The only available video capsules at present are the PillCam SB and the PillCam ESO (Given Imaging, Yoqneam, Israel) for the small bowel and the esophagus respectively. The latter will not be further discussed in this chapter. The small bowel capsule is 11×26 mm and has a CMOS chip with illumination from 6 light emitting diodes. The two non-toxic silver oxide batteries last about 8 hours. Image data are transmitted to a 5 GB recorder. Approximately 55 000 images are transmitted over 8 hours, i.e. two images per second.

Localization and suspected blood indicator (SBI) software

The goal of noninvasive imaging of the small bowel is to identify and locate lesions amenable to subsequent therapy, including surgery. Capsule endoscopy is a sensitive and accurate method of detecting mucosal lesions of the small bowel. However, localization of detected lesions is imprecise. The small bowel lacks landmarks to allow for visual localization. Progression of the capsule endoscope through the small bowel is not uniform, and it may move both antegrade and retrograde,[1] which may confound localization techniques based solely on transit time. Assuming that the capsule study is complete and the cecum is reached within the 8 hour recording time, many investigators divide the total time spent in the small bowel into halves or thirds, and thus label lesions as being in the proximal, mid, or distal small bowel.

Lewis generalizes that a lesion seen in the first 1 hour past the pylorus is in reach of a 2.5 m push enteroscope, assuming a total small bowel transit time of 4 hours and normal motility, but lesions beyond the 2 hour mark require double balloon endoscopy or surgery.[2] Sachdev and Cave are more conservative, demonstrating in their series that lesions 30 minutes beyond the pylorus cannot be reached with a push enteroscope.[3]

The capsule locator available on the imaging software uses an array of sensor leads to produce a two-dimensional trace of a capsule endoscope's path in the abdomen.[4] Identification of the duodenum, the ligament of Treitz, and the cecum is possible with a combination of visual appearance and the localization software.[2] A combination of the fixed landmarks, total transit time, time to lesion, time from lesion to cecum, and localization software may be used by experienced readers to localize lesions in the proximal, mid, or distal small bowel. These designations allow the surgeon some approximate location, but further localizing measures, such as tattooing by means of push enteroscopy or double balloon endoscopy (DBE), or precise localization by intraoperative endoscopy, are often necessary. Even during exploratory laparoscopy or laparotomy, up to 70% of mucosal lesions are neither palpable nor visible on the serosal surface.[5]

VCE has been used to guide the initial insertion route of double balloon endoscopy. Gay chose a time index of 75% of the total time from ingestion to cecal visualization as the cutoff to determine the route of double balloon endoscopy for biopsy or treatment of visualized lesions.[6] When patients with lesions in the first three quarters of the timeframe initially underwent oral DBE and patients with lesions in the last quarter of the timeframe initially underwent anal DBE, only 12% of the cases required DBE by both oral and anal route.

The 8 hour recording time of the capsule endoscopy results in many images, requiring long review time. A more efficient means of reviewing images for active bleeding is desirable, and the Given Suspected Blood Imager (SBI) is a tool developed to accomplish this (Given Imaging, Yoqneam, Israel). Parallel to the timeline of the capsule is a bar which tags certain images as potentially containing red blood. This can be useful in cases of active bleeding where long segments of the small bowel are colored bright red or there is a well-demarcated transition between the color of normal bowel and that of red blood. Sensitivity and specificity of the SBI for actively bleeding lesions was about 80% in a small study of 24 patients referred for VCE.[7] A larger study with more lesions distributed more evenly amongst patients referred for OGIB (obscure gastrointestinal bleeding) only achieved similar sensitivity for blood in the lumen.[8] However, for the more subtle but clinically relevant red colored mucosal lesions, such as arteriovenous malformations or erosions, sensitivity was only 43% and specificity 64%. In a significant number of cases, the SBI will miss lesions and also generate a fair number of false alarms, such that detailed review of the entire video is essential.

Patency device

Capsule retention occurs in about 1% of all capsule endoscopy procedures, usually in the context of a stricture, adhesion, or mass.[9] Barium small bowel follow-throughs or other imaging modalities prior to capsule endoscopy are poorly sensitive to potential sites of capsule retention. Surgery is occasionally required for capsule retrieval and/or treatment of the underlying lesion. To reduce the risk of unanticipated capsule retention, a "patency capsule" has been developed.[10] The device is an 11×26 mm collapsible plastic shell containing lactose, barium, and a transponder. Plugs at one or both ends dissolve in the presence of moisture over time. The device disintegrates slowly over 48 hours, allowing passage of capsule fragments and resolution of the temporary capsule retention.

Three studies totaling 78 patients with known or suspected strictures, mostly from Crohn's disease, underwent exam with the older, one plug design.[10-12] Five patients developed symptomatic small bowel obstruction requiring hospitalization: three of these underwent emergency surgery, and two resolved with medical management. In a case report, Gay hypothesized that the capsule was retained at the stricture and began dissolving.[13] When it reached the size of the stricture lumen, it was propelled into the stricture by peristalsis, but then became impacted and completely occluded the lumen. Thus, the patency capsule does reduce the risk of unanticipated capsule retention, but does not completely eliminate the need for surgical retrieval. One could argue that in these high-risk patients, the patency capsule performed as designed in most patients, as there were a significant number of patients who had painful passage of an intact or disintegrated capsule. On the other hand, the small but significant risk of surgery for patency capsule retention may have limited the utility of the older, one plug patency capsule design. The performance of the newer two plug design recently approved for use by the FDA in the United States has not yet been revealed in published studies (Given Imaging, Yoqneam, Israel).

Current role

Obscure gastrointestinal bleeding

Obscure gastrointestinal bleeding is the most established indication for capsule endoscopy. Capsule endoscopy is usually utilized after standard endoscopic techniques of upper endoscopy, colonoscopy with intubation of the terminal ileum, and push enteroscopy do not reveal an obvious source of bleeding.[14] Visible lesions within the small bowel include angioectasias, ulcers/erosions, neoplasms, diverticula, and varices (Figure 5.1).[15] Such lesions are potentially amenable

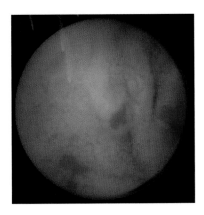

to surgical resection in cases of severe bleeding, chronic bleeding with significant transfusion requirements, or neoplastic bleeding. Double balloon endoscopy, a recently developed technique that allows endoscopy of the entire small bowel, can be used to tattoo, biopsy, and resect mucosal lesions and deliver injections, electrocautery, and argon plasma coagulation for hemostasis, but has very limited availability and involves significant investment of time, personnel, and expertise.[16] Its role in the workup and treatment of OGIB is

currently being defined.[16–18] Currently, laparoscopic-guided or standard intraoperative endoscopy (IOE) is often useful for precise localization of the lesion prior to resection, as many lesions are not visible or palpable from the serosal surface of the bowel.[19] DBE may replace IOE in the future in this role (Figure 5.2).[20] Laparoscopy alone may be useful in making the diagnosis, as well as performing treatment via mini-laparotomy.[21]

Numerous reports have described VCE findings during workup for obscure GI bleeding which is ultimately managed surgically (Figure 5.3). About 20–40% of VCE studies detect lesions amenable to further therapy, and 10–20% undergo surgical therapy (Table 5.1).

There is also a growing literature on lesions detected by VCE for OGIB that are ultimately treated by double balloon endoscopy.[32–34] The comparative studies showed that VCE had higher diagnostic yield compared to DBE[32,34] and VCE visualized the entire small bowel more often than DBE. These data led the authors to conclude that VCE is superior to DBE as a diagnostic test and should be done first, followed by DBE for biopsy/therapeutic purposes if VCE results warrant.

Information obtained by VCE may allow for more focused intraoperative endoscopy and improved clinical outcomes. The single study which reported outcomes in meaningful

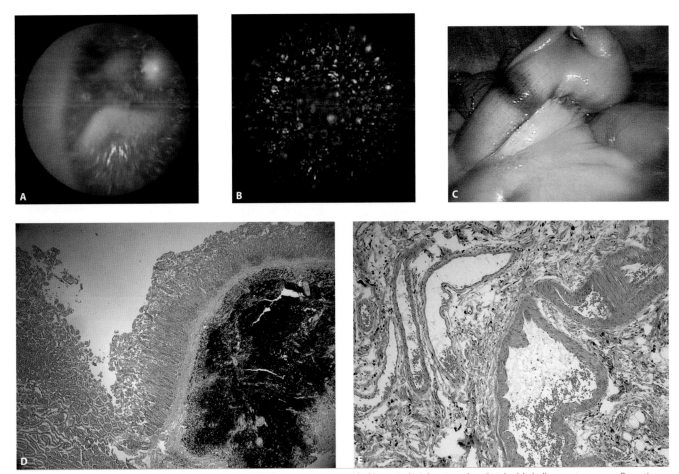

FIGURE 5.2 (a) Active bleeding in the jejunum seen by VCE. The surgeon was guided by an India ink tattoo placed at double balloon enteroscopy. Resection of the jejunum revealed a submucosal angioectasia. (b) Melena. (c) Tattoo of the serosal surface of the jejunum placed endoscopically. (d) Microscopic image of tattoo in the submucosa. (e) Microscopic image of angioectasia in the submucosa.

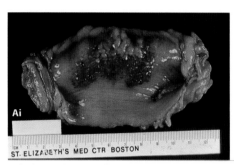
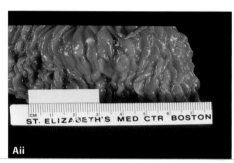
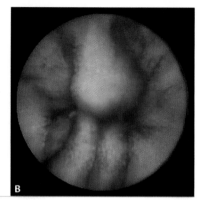

FIGURE 5.3 (a) Surgical resection of a large serosal hemangioma that had eroded through the jejuna wall into the lumen to cause massive intermittent bleeding (b).

Table 5.1 Small bowel surgery prompted by VCE findings

Authors	Year	#	#	%	Diagnosis	Surgical notes	Outcomes
Katz et al[22]	2003	267	31	12	Tumor (15)	Laparoscopy 7/15	31/31 resolved (4 mo. followup)
					Angioectasia (6)	Laparoscopy 1/6	
					Ulcers (5)	Laparoscopy 4/5	
					Capsule retention (3)	Laparoscopy 0/3	
Wolff et al[23]	2003	154	21	14	Strictures — NSAID (4)	Surgical resection (12)	
					Tumor (3)	Laparoscopic localization (3)	
					Fragile intestinal mucosal syndrome (2)	IOE localization (9)	
					Angioectasia (2)	2 negative explorations	
					Dieulafoy		
					Crohn's disease		
Pennazio et al[24]	2004	100	8	8	Stricture — Crohn's disease with capsule retention (3)		7/8 resolved
					Tumor (3)	IOE (1)	
					Angioectasia	IOE	
					Dieulafoy		
					Crohn's erosions		
Neu et al[25]	2005	56	9	17	Angioectasia/ulcers (6)	4/6 resected, 2/6 APC	4 angioectasia rebled
					Tumor (3)		2 postop deaths
Hartmann et al[26]	2005	47	47	100	Angioectasia (22)	All patients underwent VCE and IOE	35/46 resolved
					Ulcers (5)	Angioectasias resected or APC	12/46 rebled (mostly angioectasias)
					Tumor (3)	All other lesions resected (13)	
					Bleeding without source (2)	False positive (blood) (2)	
					Diverticulum	False negative (angioectasia)	
					Meckel's diverticulum		
					Varices		
Delvaux et al[27]	2004	44	5	11	Tumor (4)	False negative (hemangioma)	
					Stenosis — ischemic		

Table 5.1 Small bowel surgery prompted by VCE findings—cont'd

Authors	Year	#	#	%	Diagnosis	Surgical notes	Outcomes
Mata et al[28]	2004	42	3	7	Tumor (2) Stricture — Crohn's disease with capsule retention		
Taller et al[29]	2005	28	21	75	Angioectasia (12) Tumor/stricture (8)	Diagnostic laparoscopy (DL) planned for all DL successful 13/21 (8 failed — adhesions) Open exploration and IOE 19/21 (DL diagnostic and therapeutic — 2/21) 1 negative exploration	No perioperative complications
Kim et al[30]	2005	24	12	50	Active bleeding (7) Stricture — Crohn's disease, with capsule retention (2) Stricture — TB Tumor Peritonitis	IOE necessary in 5 Laparoscopy sufficient in 4 Palpation of retained capsule in 3	
Rastogi et al[31]	2004	18	2	11	Angioectasia Ulcer — anastomotic	Ex lap/IOE	2/2 resolved

Notes: IOE, intraoperative endoscopy; APC, argon plasma coagulation; VCE, video capsule endoscopy; DL, diagnostic laparoscopy; Ex lap, exploratory laparotomy.

comparison groups is a retrospective review of 16 patients who underwent VCE before intraoperative enteroscopy and 47 patients who underwent intraoperative enteroscopy before VCE.[35] Patients with VCE before intraoperative enteroscopy had increased diagnostic/therapeutic yield of intraoperative enteroscopy (87% vs. 53%), more confirmed diagnosis (100% vs. 69%), fewer negative evaluations (12.5% vs. 45%), fewer negative intraoperative enteroscopies (13% vs. 47%), fewer empiric colectomies (0% vs. 12.7%), and fewer postoperative complications (not statistically significant). While this study is strengthened by statistical comparisons between two groups, as opposed to merely descriptive numbers, we note its retrospective design and await the full published report for details on the circumstances of the workup.

VCE-guided IOE and laparoscopic surgery for OGIB

Several descriptive reports demonstrate the feasibility of VCE-guided, intraoperative enteroscopy and laparoscopic management of obscure GI bleeding. In a published report, 24 actively bleeding patients underwent VCE, with positive findings in 12 prompting surgery.[30] Indications for surgery were fresh bleeding during or after VCE (7), tumor (1), peritonitis during VCE (1), and capsule retention with bleeding (3). All received diagnostic laparoscopy, and if that failed to localize a lesion, intraoperative enteroscopy was done via mini-laparotomy guided by VCE results. VCE-guided laparoscopy was sufficient in four patients (2 tumors, 1 Meckel's diverticulum, 1 ischemic necrosis). Palpation of

a retained capsule localized three other lesions (2 Crohn's strictures, 1 TB stricture). Intraoperative endoscopic localization was necessary in five patients for mucosal lesions (2 capillary hemangiomas, 2 angiodysplasias, 1 submucosal hemorrhage). In the largest series reported, 31 of 267 patients (11.6%) who underwent VCE for severe, chronic obscure GI bleeding had findings prompting surgical management.[22] Limited intraoperative endoscopy guided by capsule endoscopy results was utilized in 9 (29%) patients. Fifteen patients had tumors: seven (47%) of these were managed laparoscopically and eight required laparotomy. Six patients had angioectasia: one (17%) of these had laparoscopy. Five patients had ulcers: four (80%) had laparoscopy. Three patients had capsule retention: all underwent open retrieval. No patient rebled during an average of 4 months' follow-up. The abstract did not report conversion rate from laparoscopy to open exploration or factors which guided the decision to operate laparoscopically. In another abstract, VCE findings prompted surgery in 21 of 28 patients evaluated for obscure GI bleeding and/or chronic abdominal pain.[29] Diagnostic laparoscopy was planned for all, but eight patients required conversion to open exploration due to adhesions from prior surgery. Two patients had obvious small bowel tumors seen by VCE and diagnostic laparoscopy; these were resected without further IOE/open exploration. The remaining 19 patients underwent open exploratory laparotomy with intraoperative enteroscopy via enterotomy, leading to resections for tumor or stricture in six (32%) and oversew or resection for angioectasias in 12

(64%). One patient had a negative exploration. There were no perioperative complications.

Miscellaneous OGIB topics

VCE utilization is expected to improve the yield of empiric colectomies for presumed diverticular bleeding. De la Mora documented a statistically significant reduction in empiric colectomies when VCE was used before intraoperative enteroscopy.[35] Capsule endoscopy findings of blood in the upper GI tract in a patient with one week of active gastrointestinal bleeding canceled plans for an empiric subtotal hemicolectomy.[36] Conversely, a lack of a small bowel lesion can lead surgeons to recommend colonic surgery with greater confidence.[19,37]

False negative and false positive VCE studies have an impact on surgical utilization as well. A same day or subsequent day comparison of VCE with the gold standard intraoperative endoscopy has not been done, likely due to logistical difficulties involving the time of capsule transit, excretion, and image review. An estimate of the false negative and false positive rate of VCE comes from a prospective, blinded comparison with IOE in 47 patients, which had two false positives (FPR 4.3%) manifest as active bleeding on VCE that was not present on DBE less than 1 week later and one false negative (missed angioectasias, FNR 2.1%).[26] Other large trials of VCE occasionally report a false negative or false positive based on comparison with endoscopic or surgical findings.[24] De Leusse reported a false positive diagnosis of a possible small bowel tumor which was not seen on subsequent push enteroscopy or intraoperative endoscopy.[38] Also reported was a Dieulafoy's lesion missed on VCE, which required intraoperative enteroscopy to make the diagnosis. The transient nature of bleeding vascular lesions complicates the determination of false negative and false positive studies.

False positive findings on VCE are more likely to prompt unnecessary morbidity, due to the subsequent invasive procedures including intraoperative endoscopy. The impact of false negative VCE exams is more difficult to quantitate. A small study from Hong Kong demonstrated that 18 of 49 patients undergoing VCE for obscure GI bleeding had negative exams, but only 1 of the 18 had rebleeding after a mean followup of 1 year, resulting in a negative predictive value of 94%.[39] The bleeding site remained unidentified despite subsequent laparotomy and intraoperative endoscopy in that

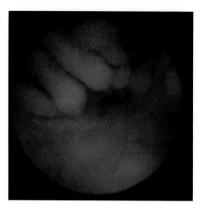

FIGURE 5.4 A 28-year-old white male had four episodes of abdominal pain and hematochezia requiring blood transfusion. VCE demonstrated a papillary structure in the distal ileum. Resection showed prolific lymphoid hyperplasia that was probably the focus of recurrent intussusception.

patient. The authors concluded that patients with a negative VCE did not routinely require subsequent invasive testing.

Tumors

Small bowel tumors are generally rare, but they represent a significant portion of surgically resectable lesions in the small bowel. The number of small bowel tumors diagnosed prior to surgical intervention is anticipated to rise because of increased utilization of capsule endoscopy. In a meta-analysis of 24 studies of 530 patients with a total of 1349 lesions, 86 (6.4%) were intestinal neoplasms.[40] Large studies estimate the prevalence of small bowel tumors to range from 3.8%[41] to 8.9%.[42]

A significant percentage of small bowel tumors are diagnosed in patients younger than 50 years of age (Figure 5.4). Before the availability of VCE, early surgical exploration for younger patients with obscure gastrointestinal bleeding was recommended to search for small bowel tumors.[42–44] VCE diminishes the need for such unguided exploratory surgery.

Historically, small bowel tumors have been difficult to diagnose. Small bowel tumors may present with occult GI bleeding, abdominal discomfort, weight loss, or diarrhea (Figure 5.5). Standard workup may include conventional upper endoscopy and colonoscopy, which are unable to examine most of the small intestine, and small bowel followthrough, which is poorly sensitive for small bowel tumors.[45] Enteroclysis is more sensitive,[46] but it may be difficult to

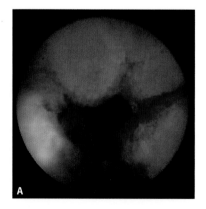

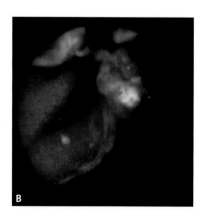

FIGURE 5.5 (a) A 60-year-old white male had one episode of hematochezia requiring 6 units of blood. VCE showed a hemorrhagic mass in the jejunum. Conventional workup was unrevealing. Laparotomy revealed a single metastasis in the jejunum from a melanoma resected from his chest wall 2 years previously. (b) Bleeding from melanoma.

obtain an optimal study due to the need for sedation and technical challenges in performing and interpreting the test.[47] CT enteroclysis, a combination of traditional enteroclysis and thin-slice CT imaging, approaches the sensitivity of VCE for small bowel mass lesions, but is less comfortable for the patient and generally does not detect flat mucosal lesions.[48]

VCE may be utilized in the workup of symptoms which could be due to lesions in the small bowel when conventional radiological and endoscopic exams are unable to identify an etiology.[49] Multiple studies have suggested that VCE is superior to push enteroscopy in the detection of small bowel lesions. One such study utilized a canine model of surgically implanted small beads (3–6 mm) throughout the small intestine.[50] Appleyard demonstrated that VCE was more sensitive than push enteroscopy (64% vs. 37%) in detecting small bowel mass lesions due to its ability to detect lesions beyond the range of a push enteroscope. However, within the range of the push enteroscope, push enteroscopy was superior (sensitivity 94% vs. 79%). Several authors view push enteroscopy and VCE as complementary exams in detecting small bowel tumors.[41,49] The advantages of VCE in the diagnosis of small bowel tumors are illustrated by a case series of 86 patients with known tumors.[51] Despite a thorough workup, which could include CT scan, enteroclysis, bleeding scan, angiography, upper endoscopy, and colonoscopy, no etiology could be found prior to the VCE exam. Each patient had an average of 4.6 negative studies.

The goal and extent of surgical resection, as well as the option of additional treatment modalities, depend on the pathology and location of the tumor.[52] The endoluminal appearance of VCE is not sufficient to characterize a mass lesion as benign or malignant, so further studies are desirable prior to surgery. Masses appreciated by capsule endoscopy or other diagnostic exams may be tattooed, biopsied, or resected by push enteroscopy or double balloon endoscopy[53] to determine the need for further surgical therapy. When a tumor is not within reach of a push enteroscope and double balloon endoscopy is not available, CT enteroclysis may be attempted to further localize the lesion. Patients who are surgical candidates are then taken to the operating room for laparoscopy or laparotomy. Intraoperative endoscopy may be useful, as some neoplasms may be difficult to palpate due to size, softness, or difficult exposure (Figure 5.6).

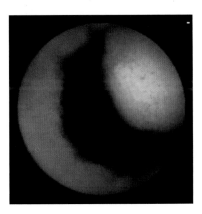

FIGURE 5.6 A 38-year-old white female had three episodes of hematochezia requiring transfusion. VCE showed a medium sized sessile polyp. Resection of the tumor, guided by intraoperative enteroscopy since the tumor was not palpable, showed a multicentric carcinoid.

As the treatment of small bowel tumors is primarily surgical, it is hoped that VCE will contribute to earlier diagnosis and better prognosis. Multiple studies have documented a relatively long duration between symptom onset and diagnosis, due primarily to the vague gastrointestinal symptoms at presentation.[54,55] The frequency of preoperative diagnosis has historically been low.[52] Prognostic factors are generally limited to tumor stage and curative resection.[55,56]

VCE and hereditary polyposis syndromes

VCE is safe and effective in documenting extent and size of polyps in hereditary polyposis syndromes, thus altering surgical management. VCE is recommended to replace radiological imaging for routine surveillance or diagnostic workup of abdominal symptoms in patients with Peutz–Jeghers syndrome due to superior sensitivity to polyps requiring surgical resection in two case series.[57,58] Burke has suggested preoperative VCE screening of all patients with familial adenomatous polyposis syndrome (FAP) planned for duodenectomy, as it could theoretically detect distal polyps that require more extensive resection.[57] However both Burke and Schulmann agree that the significance of small intestinal polyps in FAP is not currently known and requires further study.[57,58]

Crohn's disease

VCE can alter the surgical management of Crohn's disease in several ways. Diagnostically, VCE has identified Crohn's disease presenting as GI bleeding, thereby avoiding the next step of intraoperative endoscopy.[59] VCE is as good as ileocolonoscopy for detecting Crohn's lesions at the terminal ileum and superior to CT enteroclysis for small bowel lesions.[60] It is therefore hoped that the early application of VCE will shorten the time interval between the initial symptoms and the diagnosis of Crohn's disease, resulting in earlier treatment that reduces disease activity and complications which contribute to a high rate of surgery within the first three years post diagnosis.[61,62] VCE is also useful in distinguishing Crohn's disease from ulcerative colitis in patients with a working diagnosis of ulcerative or indeterminate colitis for which surgery is being considered. In a group of 22 patients with colitis evaluated for small bowel involvement consistent with Crohn's disease, 9 had VCE findings diagnostic of Crohn's disease, and 8 improved with increased medical therapy without surgery.[63]

Patients with Crohn's disease may have inflammatory strictures or scarred, non-inflammatory strictures (Figure 5.7). A suspected or known stricture in the setting of Crohn's disease is a relative contraindication to capsule endoscopy. Patients who are willing to undergo surgery for capsule retention may be reasonable candidates for the exam. Indeed, some authors state that capsule retention is clinically useful diagnostically and prompts effective therapy for strictures,[1] although there is less enthusiasm for patients with Crohn's disease, due to their high risk of postoperative recurrence of disease and subsequent complications. It is well documented that radiological imaging may miss clinically relevant strictures prior

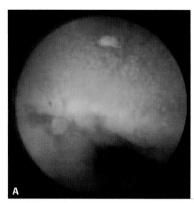
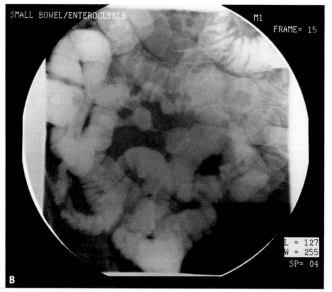

FIGURE 5.7 (a) Capsule retained for 24 hours in a 78-year-old white female with transfusion-dependent Crohn's disease that had been previously undiagnosed, despite several previous workups over a 10 year period. She subsequently underwent a 20 cm resection of terminal ileum and resection of the stricture. (b) Enteroclysis showing a string sign and irregular terminal ileum.

to capsule endoscopy, but most authors recommend imaging as a precaution in patients with Crohn's disease with known or suspected strictures.[60,64,65]

In general, it is preferable to avoid surgery in patients with Crohn's disease. For patients who have capsule retention, surgery may be unavoidable but is rarely urgent. Chang reported two cases of capsule retention in patients with known Crohn's disease which required surgical retrieval.[66] The authors discussed the need for proper planning and workup to deal with all lesions in Crohn's patients that may be encountered during surgery for capsule retention, such as bleeding, multiple strictures, tumor, perforation, and fistulas. Imaging to ensure that the capsule is still retained immediately prior to surgery and possible need for intraoperative fluoroscopy to locate the capsule was emphasized. Laparoscopy for Crohn's disease is preferred when possible. General principles for Crohn's surgery should be followed, including avoiding enterotomy in an area of diseased bowel unless stricturoplasty or resection is necessary. Enterotomy in an area of normal bowel allows a passageway through which the capsule may be retrieved by milking the capsule proximally.

VCE may not be useful in predicting postoperative recurrence of Crohn's disease. Unresected small bowel lesions detected by intraoperative endoscopy at the time of surgery for Crohn's disease had no predictive value for postoperative recurrence in small studies.[67,68] By extension, it is unlikely that lesions detected by VCE prior to surgery in Crohn's patients will have any prognostic value. In another study, VCE was safely used within 6 months following ileocolonic resection in Crohn's disease without any episodes of capsule retention in all 32 patients studied.[69] However, ileocolonoscopy was superior to VCE in detecting Crohn's recurrence at the neo-terminal ileum (90% vs. 60–70%).

NSAIDs and radiation

NSAIDs may cause intestinal diaphragms which are thin, concentric rings of tissue which may result in symptomatic or asymptomatic strictures (Figure 5.8).[70] Radiological studies and even exploratory laparoscopy/laparotomy will often miss these lesions, as they may not be palpable and easily collapse on gross examination of a resected specimen when it is opened.[71] Capsule endoscopy, double balloon, or intraoperative endoscopy are useful for diagnosis. Multiple diaphragms are also generally the rule, so intraoperative or double balloon endoscopy may be helpful in defining the symptomatic lesion and avoiding missed lesions.

In an illustrative case series, seven patients with NSAID-induced enteropathy presented with obscure GI bleeding or obstructive symptoms and underwent extensive workup.[72] VCE made the diagnosis in six patients, all of which developed transient capsule retention above the diaphragms. Resection is possible if diaphragms are clustered together in a short segment, otherwise stricturoplasty is a treatment option for more diffuse cases.

Three cases of radiation-induced strictures diagnosed by capsule endoscopy resulting in asymptomatic capsule retention are reported in the literature. Surgical treatment was done in all three cases.[73,74]

Capsule retention

Capsule retention has been defined by the 2005 ICCE consensus statement as a capsule endoscope retained in the gastrointestinal system: (1) for greater than two weeks or (2) any length of time that requires directed therapy for removal.[9] Retention was distinguished from regional transit

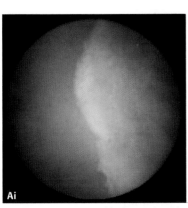 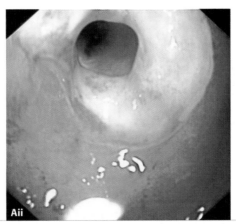 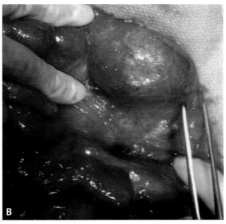

FIGURE 5.8 A 17-year-old white male with abdominal pain, weight loss, and anemia had an NSAID ulcerated stricture (a) above a pre-existing congenital long stricture as demonstrated at the tip of the forceps (b).

abnormalities, which describe non-progression of a capsule for greater than 60 minutes in a segment of bowel. The risk of capsule retention varies with the patient population. Patients with known Crohn's disease have a capsule retention rate of about 5% (4/80 cases), compared with 1.5% for patients with obscure GI bleeding or suspected Crohn's disease (15/1089 and 1/71 respectively). Other known risk factors include symptoms suggestive of intermittent or ongoing obstruction and prior or current chronic NSAID use. Prior small bowel resection or other intra-abdominal surgery, abdominal/pelvic radiation therapy, and a remote history of small bowel obstruction may be risk factors for strictures and adhesions, but are not indicators of probable retention.[9,75]

There is no way to completely eliminate the risk of capsule retention. As mentioned previously, radiological exams often miss clinically relevant strictures. The 2002 American Society for Gastrointestinal Endoscopy (ASGE) technical review of VCE recommended consideration of barium small bowel follow-through (SBFT) exam before VCE[76] and some authors routinely obtain this in patients who have risk factors,[77] but the test is poorly sensitive, and the updated 2006 ASGE technical review is silent on this issue.[78] While CT enteroclysis is superior to SBFT in detecting strictures, capsule retention still occurred in 2 of 40 patients who did not have visible strictures on CT enteroclysis prior to VCE.[60] We generally do not obtain radiologic exams prior to VCE unless they are indicated for symptoms or other clinical reasons. The clinical utility of the newer two-plug patency capsule has yet to be determined.

There has been one report of acute jejunal obstruction caused by occlusion of a Crohn's stricture which was subsequently treated surgically.[79] Furthermore, one patient had intestinal perforation due to capsule retention of over 2 months' duration.[80] Capsule retention has occurred in patients without intestinal pathology at the ileocecal valve requiring surgical retrieval[81] and in the duodenum at an area of acute angulation.[82] The longest documented duration of asymptomatic capsule retention is 3 years.[83] The longest duration of retention in a patient with Crohn's disease before elective surgery was 7 months.[84]

Treatment has been primarily surgical via enterotomy, although occasionally the capsule is within reach of standard endoscopes. The ability to intervene on the underlying small bowel pathology which caused the capsule retention is an advantage of surgery. Double balloon endoscopy has been utilized to retrieve foreign objects, including retained capsule endoscopes,[85] however one might be hesitant to proceed with this intervention in the setting of small bowel obstruction.

Influence of prior surgery

Capsule endoscopy is usually safe and effective following small bowel resection in the setting of no obvious obstruction,[86] but intra-abdominal surgery may be a risk factor for capsule retention. Several studies and case reports have shown capsule retention in the setting of prior surgery (Figure 5.9).[83,87,88] To our knowledge, no one has calculated the relative risk of the post-surgical state, but it would be important to separate the contribution of the surgery from the underlying condition (e.g. Crohn's disease).

VCE is able to detect peri-anastomotic ulcerations/strictures, as demonstrated by a two patient case series in which VCE done for obscure GI bleeding led to capsule retention above ulcerated strictures, which were subsequently resected and primarily re-anastomosed.[89]

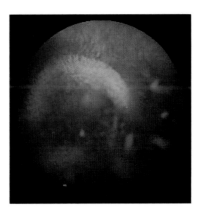

FIGURE 5.9 Capsule retained at a stricture at a previous small bowel surgical anastomosis that had been missed on an extensive radiological workup and on two previous laparotomies. The surgeon was able to locate the stricture by palpation of the capsule, resect the stricture, and

Endoscopic placement of the capsule endoscope in the efferent loop is necessary in the setting of prior reconstructive gastric surgery, such as Billroth II or Whipple's operation. Hellmig reports such a strategy in a patient with pancreatic cancer status post pylorus-preserving Whipple's operation who developed overt transfusion-dependent chronic obscure GI bleed.[90] Contrast injection during Esophagastroduodenoscopy (EGD) facilitated identification of the efferent loop, which was marked with a hemoclip. Subsequently, the capsule endoscope was delivered into the correct loop by snaring of a swallowed capsule and endoscopic advancement. Of note, there are now specialized VCE delivery systems commercially available (US Endoscopy, Mentor, Ohio).

VCE has successfully been used post small bowel transplant for monitoring of the graft.[91]

Laparoscopy vs. laparotomy

Laparoscopic surgery has been used to facilitate IOE and small bowel resection via mini-laparotomy. Localized small bowel pathology including tumors,[92-95] ulcers,[96] vascular malformations,[97] Meckel's diverticula,[98] and strictures[99] have been successfully treated in this fashion. Laparoscopic small bowel resections done by experienced surgeons may result in improved cosmesis, less postoperative pain, reduced duration of ileus, shorter hospital stay, decreased atelectasis/pneumonia, lower wound complication rate, and fewer adhesions compared with laparotomy,[100] but no comparative studies have been published.

Laparoscopic surgery in patients with Crohn's disease has been shown in various studies to reduce hospital length of stay,[101,102] costs incurred,[101-103] and morbidity.[102,103] Casillas and Delaney usually attempt a laparoscopic approach initially, with low threshold for converting to open exploration, but they emphasize the need for adequate training and experience with this procedure. They prefer the laparoscopic approach to minimize the effect of repeated surgeries, since many patients with Crohn's disease will require multiple procedures over their lifetime.[104]

Intraoperative endoscopy

The techniques of intraoperative enteroscopy have been widely discussed.[105,106] None has proved ideal and the procedure is potentially hazardous with currently available endoscopes. This is due in part to the lack of ideal endoscopes. The inherent limitation of conventional endoscopes is that when they are curled up, the rolls have a radius of curvature of about 12 cm, which is longer than the length of the mesentery in most people. Hence as the scope is inserted into the small intestine, there is progressive stretching of the mesentery which imperils the integrity of the mesenteric vessels and the mucosa of the small bowel.[107] Thus most endoscopists favor the creation of a mid small bowel enterotomy so that a conventional endoscope or colonoscope can be passed proximally and distally. It is often difficult to maintain sterility in the operative field due to spillage of intestinal fluid. The endoscopes themselves are not sterile and need to be contained within sterile plastic sheets or bags. Insertion of colonoscopes via the rectum or push enteroscopy via the mouth with manipulation by the surgeon does not often allow complete examination of the entire small bowel. The Sonde enteroscope allows for atraumatic evaluation of the small bowel at laparotomy but suffers from a lack of rigidity, making it sometimes difficult for the surgeon to pass it around the duodenal loop.[105] This endoscope has a radius of curvature of about 4 cm which allows it to be passed through the entire small intestine without stretching the mesentery. Inflation of the balloon at the tip allows the surgeon to get traction on the scope once it is past the ligament of Treitz.[108] It has proved possible to perform intraoperative enteroscopy at laparoscopy but this is rare.[30,108] Success at detecting lesions by intraoperative enteroscopy in patients with obscure GI bleeding varies from 52% to 90% with some mortality, morbidity, and recurrence of bleeding. The combination of VCE followed by intraoperative enteroscopy leads to excellent results with a sensitivity and specificity of VCE compared to intraoperative enteroscopy of 95% and 97% respectively.[26]

Limitations of surgery

Surgery is usually definitive. However, there are several limitations which may have an impact on surgical outcomes. The procedures are invasive, and patients may not be good candidates due to comorbidities. Surgeons and anesthesiologists have variable skill and experience. The difficulties with patients with prior intra-abdominal surgeries have been discussed, as anatomy and adhesions may make the operations technically challenging. Multiple pathologies may be encountered, forcing the surgeon to choose the most likely culprit lesion or make a decision to resect all abnormalities, which leads to prolonged operating time and increased risk of complications. Underlying conditions, such as Crohn's disease, may make recurrence and complications from surgery more likely. Surgery is less effective in managing diffuse and recurrent processes, such as angioectasias. The less invasive double balloon endoscopy is able to circumvent some of these limitations.

Conclusions

VCE is an essential component of the workup for obscure GI bleeding and is an important noninvasive tool in diagnosing small bowel tumors and stenoses. Patients with obstructive symptoms or suspected/known strictures should have pre-VCE imaging. The safety and efficacy of the newer two-plug patency capsule has not been reported in published studies, but if it is superior to the older one-plug version, it may have clinical utility. Capsule retention may necessitate retrieval by endoscopic or surgical means. Localization of small bowel lesions by VCE is relatively imprecise. Double balloon endoscopy holds great promise both diagnostically and therapeutically, and despite technical challenges, is less invasive than intraoperative endoscopy. Intraoperative endoscopy is still the gold standard endoscopic test and continues to be useful.

While VCE findings are expected to prompt more surgical interventions for small bowel pathology, it is difficult to assess the impact of VCE on surgical outcomes. To our knowledge, there are no published studies comparing mortality and morbidity based on whether or not VCE was part of the diagnostic workup. Reasons for this include: (1) the variety of possible etiologies, each with heterogeneous prognosis, (2) the lack of standardized approaches in the diagnostic workup, (3) the large variety of surgical and endoscopic techniques which may be employed with variable efficacy,[109] and (4) the relative infrequency of surgical interventions for small bowel pathology. Nevertheless, a complete road map of lesions a surgeon will encounter, especially with lesions precisely localized with ink or diagnosed by biopsy utilizing push enteroscopy or double balloon endoscopy when possible, should help the surgeon decide which operation to perform as well as allow for a more limited surgical exploration.

References

1. Swain P. Wireless capsule endoscopy and Crohn's disease. Gut 2005;54:323–6.

2. Lewis B. How to read wireless capsule endoscopic images: tips of the trade. Gastrointest Endosc Clin N Am 2004;14:11–6.

3. Sachdev R, Cave D. Relationship of time by capsule endoscopy to depth of insertion of push enteroscopy. Am J Gastroenterol 2006;99(suppl):S298.

4. Cave DR. Reading wireless video capsule endoscopy. Gastrointest Endosc Clin N Am 2004;14:17–24.

5. Dulai GS. Diagnostic yield of capsule endoscopy in patients with recurrent, overt GI bleeding of obscure origin. J Investig Med 2003;51(Suppl 2):S387.

6. Gay G, Delvaux M, Fassler I. Outcome of capsule endoscopy in determining indication and route for push-and-pull enteroscopy. Endoscopy 2006;38:49–58.

7. Liangpunsakul S, Mays L, Rex DK. Performance of Given suspected blood indicator. Am J Gastroenterol 2003;98:2676–8.

8. D'Halluin PN, Delvaux M, Lapalus MG, et al. Does the "Suspected Blood Indicator" improve the detection of bleeding lesions by capsule endoscopy? Gastrointest Endosc 2005;61:243–9.

9. Cave D, Legnani P, de Franchis R, Lewis BS. ICCE consensus for capsule retention. Endoscopy 2005;37:1065–7.

10. Spada C, Spera G, Riccioni M, et al. A novel diagnostic tool for detecting functional patency of the small bowel: the Given patency capsule. Endoscopy 2005;37:793–800.

11. Boivin ML, Lochs H, Voderholzer WA. Does passage of a patency capsule indicate small-bowel patency? A prospective clinical trial. Endoscopy 2005;37:808–15.

12. Delvaux M, Ben Soussan E, Laurent V, Lerebours E, Gay G. Clinical evaluation of the use of the M2A patency capsule system before a capsule endoscopy procedure, in patients with known or suspected intestinal stenosis. Endoscopy 2005;37:801–7.

13. Gay G, Delvaux M, Laurent V, Reibel N, Regent D, Grosdidier G, Roche JF. Temporary intestinal occlusion induced by a "patency capsule" in a patient with Crohn's disease. Endoscopy 2005;37:174–7.

14. Tang SJ, Haber GB. Capsule endoscopy in obscure gastrointestinal bleeding. Gastrointest Endosc Clin N Am 2004;14:87–100.

15. Zuckerman GR, Prakash C, Askin MP, Lewis BS. AGA technical review on the evaluation and management of occult and obscure gastrointestinal bleeding. Gastroenterology 2000;118:201–21.

16. Lo SK, Mehdizadeh S. Therapeutic uses of double-balloon enteroscopy. Gastrointest Endosc Clin N Am 2006; 16:363–76.

17. Kita H, Yamamoto H. Double-balloon endoscopy for the diagnosis and treatment of small intestinal disease. Best Pract Res Clin Gastroenterol 2006;20:179–94.

18. Yamamoto H, Kita H, Sunada K, et al. Clinical outcomes of double-balloon endoscopy for the diagnosis and treatment of small-intestinal diseases. Clin Gastroenterol Hepatol 2004;2:1010–6.

19. Douard R, Wind P, Panis Y, et al. Intraoperative enteroscopy for diagnosis and management of unexplained gastrointestinal bleeding. Am J Surg 2000;180:181–4.

20. Yamamoto H, Kita H. Enteroscopy. J Gastroenterol 2005;40:555–62.

21. Tricarico A, Cione G, Sozio M, et al. Digestive hemorrhages of obscure origin. Surg Endosc 2002;16:711–3.

22. Katz D, Lewis BS, Katz LB. Surgical experience following capsule endoscopy. Gastrointest Endosc 2003;57:AB169.

23. Wolff RS, Cave D, Doherty S, Lopez M, Toth L. Surgical experience after video capsule endoscopy: the fantastic voyage to the operating room. Gastroenterology 2003;124(suppl):A814.

24. Pennazio M, Santucci R, Rondonotti E, Abbiati C, Beccari G, Rossini FP, de Franchis R. Outcome of patients with obscure gastrointestinal bleeding after capsule endoscopy: report of 100 consecutive cases. Gastroenterology 2004;126:643–53.

25. Neu B, Ell C, May A, et al. Capsule endoscopy versus standard tests in influencing management of obscure digestive bleeding: results from a German multicenter trial. Am J Gastroenterol 2005;100:1736–42.

26. Hartmann D, Schmidt H, Bolz G, et al. A prospective two-center study comparing wireless capsule endoscopy with intraoperative enteroscopy in patients with obscure GI bleeding. Gastrointest Endosc 2005;61:826–32.

27. Delvaux M, Fassler I, Gay G. Clinical usefulness of the endoscopic video capsule as the initial intestinal investigation in patients with obscure digestive bleeding: validation of a diagnostic strategy based on the patient outcome after 12 months. Endoscopy 2004;36:1067–73.

28. Mata A, Bordas JM, Feu F, et al. Wireless capsule endoscopy in patients with obscure gastrointestinal bleeding: a comparative study with push enteroscopy. Aliment Pharmacol Ther 2004;20:189–94.

29. Taller J, Lee CM, Feng JJ, Cirangle PT, Jossart GH. Minimally invasive surgery as treatment of obscure GI bleeding and abdominal complaints can be effectively guided by video

capsule endoscopy: a review of 28 patients. J Gastrointest Surg 2005;9:AB191.

30. Kim J, Kim YS, Chun HJ, Hyun JH, Cho MY, Suh SO. Laparoscopy-assisted exploration of obscure gastrointestinal bleeding after capsule endoscopy: the Korean experience. J Laparoendosc Adv Surg Tech A 2005;15:365–73.

31. Rastogi A, Schoen RE, Slivka A. Diagnostic yield and clinical outcomes of capsule endoscopy. Gastrointest Endosc 2004;60:959–64.

32. Hadithi M, Heine GD, Jacobs MA, van Bodegraven AA, Mulder CJ. A prospective study comparing video capsule endoscopy with double-balloon enteroscopy in patients with obscure gastrointestinal bleeding. Am J Gastroenterol 2006;101:52–7.

33. Kita H, Yamamoto H, Nakamura T, Shirakawa K, Terano A, Sugano K. Bleeding polyp in the mid small intestine identified by capsule endoscopy and treated by double-balloon endoscopy. Gastrointest Endosc 2005;61:628–9.

34. Nakamura M, Niwa Y, Ohmiya N, et al. Preliminary comparison of capsule endoscopy and double-balloon enteroscopy in patients with suspected small-bowel bleeding. Endoscopy 2006;38:59–66.

35. De La Mora JG, Rajan E, Knipschield MA. Diagnostic yield of intra-operative endoscopy when guided by capsule endoscopy. Gastrointest Endosc 2005;61:AB105.

36. Hewlett A, Luthra G, Raju GS, Vittal H, Nath SK. Capsule endoscopy findings averted blind surgical intervention. Am J Gastroenterol 2004;99:AB496.

37. Cummings CL. Value of early capsular endoscopy for severe gastrointestinal bleeding. J Natl Med Assoc 2004;96:1653–6.

38. De Leusse A, Landi B, Edery J, et al. Video capsule endoscopy for investigation of obscure gastrointestinal bleeding: feasibility, results, and interobserver agreement. Endoscopy 2005;37:617–21.

39. Lai LH, Wong GL, Chow DK, Lau JY, Sung JJ, Leung WK. Long-term follow-up of patients with obscure gastrointestinal bleeding after negative capsule endoscopy. Am J Gastroenterol 2006;101:1224–8.

40. Lewis BS, Eisen GM, Friedman S. A pooled analysis to evaluate results of capsule endoscopy trials. Endoscopy 2005;37:960–5.

41. de Franchis R, Rondonotti E, Abbiati C, Beccari G, Signorelli C. Small bowel malignancy. Gastrointest Endosc Clin N Am 2004;14:139–48.

42. Cobrin GM, Pittman RH, Lewis BS. Increased diagnostic yield of small bowel tumors with capsule endoscopy. Cancer 2006;107:22–27.

43. Berner JS, Mauer K, Lewis BS. Push and sonde enteroscopy for the diagnosis of obscure gastrointestinal bleeding. Am J Gastroenterol 1994;89:2139–42.

44. Thompson JN, Salem RR, Hemingway AP, et al. Specialist investigation of obscure gastrointestinal bleeding. Gut 1987;28:47–51.

45. Maglinte DT, Reyes BL. Small bowel cancer. Radiologic diagnosis. Radiol Clin North Am 1997;35:361–80.

46. Bessette JR, Maglinte DD, Kelvin FM, Chernish SM. Primary malignant tumors in the small bowel: a comparison of the small-bowel enema and conventional follow-through examination. AJR Am J Roentgenol 1989;153:741–4.

47. Maglinte DD, Lappas JC, Kelvin FM, Rex D, Chernish SM. Small bowel radiography: how, when, and why? Radiology 1987;163:297–305.

48. Boudiaf M, Jaff A, Soyer P, Bouhnik Y, Hamzi L, Rymer R. Small-bowel diseases: prospective evaluation of multi-detector row helical CT enteroclysis in 107 consecutive patients. Radiology 2004;233:338–44.

49. Schwartz GD, Barkin JS. Small bowel tumors. Gastrointest Endosc Clin N Am 2006;16:267–75.

50. Appleyard M, Fireman Z, Glukhovsky A, et al. A randomized trial comparing wireless capsule endoscopy with push enteroscopy for the detection of small-bowel lesions. Gastroenterology 2000;119:1431–8.

51. Schwartz G, Barkin J, and Given imaging tumor study group. Small bowel tumors detected by M2A capsule endoscopy. Am J Gastroenterol 2004;99(suppl):AB190.

52. Mussi C, Caprotti R, Scaini A, et al. Management of small bowel tumors: personal experience and new diagnostic tools. Int Surg 2005;90:209–14.

53. Sunada K, Yamamoto H, Kita H, et al. Clinical outcomes of enteroscopy using the double-balloon method for strictures of the small intestine. World J Gastroenterol 2005;11:1087–9.

54. Ciresi DL, Scholten DJ. The continuing clinical dilemma of primary tumors of the small intestine. Am Surg 1995;61:698–702.

55. Talamonti MS, Goetz LH, Rao S, Joehl RJ. Primary cancers of the small bowel: analysis of prognostic factors and results of surgical management. Arch Surg 2002;137:564–70.

56. Wu TJ, Yeh CN, Chao TC, Jan YY, Chen MF. Prognostic factors of primary small bowel adenocarcinoma: univariate and multivariate analysis. World J Surg 2006;30:391–8.

57. Burke CA, Santisi J, Church J, Levinthal G. The utility of capsule endoscopy small bowel surveillance in patients with polyposis. Am J Gastroenterol 2005;100:1498–502.

58. Schulmann K, Hollerbach S, Kraus K, et al. Feasibility and diagnostic utility of video capsule endoscopy for the detection of small bowel polyps in patients with hereditary polyposis syndromes. Am J Gastroenterol 2005;100:27–37.

59. Hahne M, Adamek HE, Schilling D, Riemann JF. Wireless capsule endoscopy in a patient with obscure occult bleeding. Endoscopy 2002;34:588–90.

60. Voderholzer WA, Beinhoelzl J, Rogalla P, Murrer S, Schachschal G, Lochs H, Ortner MA. Small bowel involvement in Crohn's disease: a prospective comparison of wireless capsule endoscopy and computed tomography enteroclysis. Gut 2005;54:369–73.

61. Basilisco G, Campanini M, Cesana B, Ranzi T, Bianchi P. Risk factors for first operation in Crohn's disease. Am J Gastroenterol 1989;84:749–52.

62. Sands BE, Arsenault JE, Rosen MJ, et al. Risk of early surgery for Crohn's disease: implications for early treatment strategies. Am J Gastroenterol 2003;98:2712–8.

63. Mow WS, Lo SK, Targan SR, et al. Initial experience with wireless capsule enteroscopy in the diagnosis and management of inflammatory bowel disease. Clin Gastroenterol Hepatol 2004;2:31–40.

64. Dubcenco E, Jeejeebhoy KN, Petroniene R, Tang SJ, Zalev AH, Gardiner GW, Baker JP. Capsule endoscopy findings in patients with established and suspected

small-bowel Crohn's disease: correlation with radiologic, endoscopic, and histologic findings. Gastrointest Endosc 2005;62:538–44.

65. Lo SK. Capsule endoscopy in the diagnosis and management of inflammatory bowel disease. Gastrointest Endosc Clin N Am 2004;14:179–93.

66. Chang PK, Holt EG, De Villiers WJ, Boulanger BR. A new complication from a new technology: what a general surgeon should know about wireless capsule endoscopy. Am Surg 2005;71:455–8.

67. Esaki M, Matsumoto T, Hizawa K, Aoyagi K, Mibu R, Iida M, Fujishima M. Intraoperative enteroscopy detects more lesions but is not predictive of postoperative recurrence in Crohn's disease. Surg Endosc 2001;15:455–9.

68. Klein O, Colombel JF, Lescut D, Gambiez L, Desreumaux P, Quandalle P, Cortot A. Remaining small bowel endoscopic lesions at surgery have no influence on early anastomotic recurrences in Crohn's disease. Am J Gastroenterol 1995;90:1949–52.

69. Bourreille A, Jarry M, D'Halluin PN, et al. Wireless capsule endoscopy versus ileocolonoscopy for the diagnosis of postoperative recurrence of Crohn's disease: a prospective study. Gut 2006;55:978–83.

70. Bjarnason I, Price AB, Zanelli G, Smethurst P, Burke M, Gumpel JM, Levi AJ. Clinicopathological features of nonsteroidal antiinflammatory drug-induced small intestinal strictures. Gastroenterology 1988;94:1070–4.

71. Chutkan R, Toubia N. Effect of nonsteroidal anti-inflammatory drugs on the gastrointestinal tract: diagnosis by wireless capsule endoscopy. Gastrointest Endosc Clin N Am 2004;14:67–85.

72. Kelly ME, McMahon LE, Jaroszewski DE, Yousfi MM, De Petris G, Swain JM. Small-bowel diaphragm disease: seven surgical cases. Arch Surg 2005;140:1162–6.

73. Lee DW, Poon AO, Chan AC. Diagnosis of small bowel radiation enteritis by capsule endoscopy. Hong Kong Med J 2004;10:419–21.

74. Romero Vazquez J, Caunedo Alvarez A, Rodriguez-Tellez M, Sanchez Yague A, Pellicer Bautista F, Herrerias Gutierrez JM. Previously unknown stricture due to radiation therapy diagnosed by capsule endoscopy. Rev Esp Enferm Dig 2005;97:449–54.

75. Lewis B. Capsule endoscopy — transit abnormalities. Gastrointest Endosc Clin N Am 2006;16:221–8.

76. Ginsberg GG, Barkun AN, Bosco JJ, et al. Wireless capsule endoscopy: August 2002. Gastrointest Endosc 2002; 56:621–4.

77. Storch I, Barkin JS. Contraindications to capsule endoscopy: do any still exist? Gastrointest Endosc Clin N Am 2006;16:329–36.

78. Mishkin DS, Chuttani R, Croffie J, et al. ASGE Technology Status Evaluation Report: wireless capsule endoscopy. Gastrointest Endosc 2006;63:539–45.

79. Magdeburg R, Riester T, Hummel F, Lohr M, Post S, Sturm J. Ileus secondary to wireless capsule enteroscopy. Int J Colorectal Dis 2006;21:610–3.

80. Gonzalez-Carro P, Picazo Yuste J, Fernandez Diez S, Perez Roldan F, Roncero Garcia-Escribano O. Intestinal perforation due to retained wireless capsule endoscope. Endoscopy 2005;37:684.

81. Mergener K, Schembre DB, Brandabur JJ, Smith MA, Kozarek RA. Clinical utility of capsule endoscopy: a single center experience. Am J Gastroenterol 2002;97:S299.

82. Tang SJ, Zanati S, Dubcenco E, et al. Capsule endoscopy regional transit abnormality revisited. Gastrointest Endosc 2004;60:1029–32.

83. Rondonotti E, Herrerias JM, Pennazio M, Caunedo A, Mascarenhas-Saraiva M, de Franchis R. Complications, limitations, and failures of capsule endoscopy: a review of 733 cases. Gastrointest Endosc 2005;62:712–6.

84. Kastin DA, Buchman AL, Barrett T, Halverson A, Wallin A. Strictures from Crohn's disease diagnosed by video capsule endoscopy. J Clin Gastroenterol 2004;38:346–9.

85. Heine GD, Hadithi M, Groenen MJ, Kuipers EJ, Jacobs MA, Mulder CJ. Double-balloon enteroscopy: indications, diagnostic yield, and complications in a series of 275 patients with suspected small-bowel disease. Endoscopy 2006;38:42–8.

86. De Palma GD, Rega M, Puzziello A, et al. Capsule endoscopy is safe and effective after small-bowel resection. Gastrointest Endosc 2004;60:135–8.

87. Barkin JS, Friedman S. Wireless capsule endoscopy requiring surgical intervention: the world's experience. Am J Gastroenterol 2006;97:S298.

88. Cave DR, Wolff R, Mitty R, Toth L, Lopez M. Indications, contraindications, and an algorithm for the use of the M2A video capsule in obscure gastrointestinal bleeding. Gastrointest Endosc 2002;55:AB136.

89. de Franchis R, Avesani EM, Abbiati C, et al. Unsuspected ileal stenosis causing obscure GI bleeding in patients with previous abdominal surgery — diagnosis by capsule endoscopy: a report of two cases. Dig Liver Dis 2003;35:577–84.

90. Hellmig S, Seeger M, Stuber E, Kiehne K, Schreiber S, Folsch UR. Endoscopic-guided capsule endoscopy in a patient with small-bowel varices after Whipple's operation. Gastrointest Endosc 2005;62:166–9.

91. Beckurts KT, Stippel D, Schleimer K, Schafer H, Benz C, Dienes HP, Holscher AH. First case of isolated small bowel transplantation at the University of Cologne: rejection-free course under quadruple immunosuppression and endoluminal monitoring with video-capsule. Transplant Proc 2004;36:340–2.

92. Chung RS. Laparoscopy-assisted jejunal resection for bleeding leiomyoma. Surg Endosc 1998;12:162–3.

93. Ehrmantraut W, Sardi A. Laparoscopy-assisted small bowel resection. Am Surg 1997;63:996–1001.

94. Felsher J, Brodsky J, Brody F. Laparoscopic small bowel resection of metastatic pulmonary carcinosarcoma. J Laparoendosc Adv Surg Tech A 2003;13:397–400.

95. Kok KY, Mathew VV, Yapp SK. Laparoscopic-assisted small bowel resection for a bleeding leiomyoma. Surg Endosc 1998;12:995–6.

96. Meister TE, Nickl NJ, Park A. Laparoscopic-assisted panenteroscopy. Gastrointest Endosc 2001;53:236–9.

97. Mino A, Ogawa Y, Ishikawa T, et al. Dieulafoy's vascular malformation of the jejunum: first case report of laparoscopic treatment. J Gastroenterol 2004;39:375–8.

98. Teitelbaum DH, Polley TZ Jr, Obeid F. Laparoscopic diagnosis and excision of Meckel's diverticulum. J Pediatr Surg 1994;29:495–7.

99. Canin-Endres J, Salky B, Gattorno F, Edye M. Laparoscopically assisted intestinal resection in 88 patients with Crohn's disease. Surg Endosc 1999;13:595–9.

100. Franklin ME Jr, Gonzalez JJ Jr, Miter DB, Glass JL, Paulson D. Laparoscopic diagnosis and treatment of intestinal obstruction. Surg Endosc 2004;18:26–30.

101. Duepree HJ, Senagore AJ, Delaney CP, Brady KM, Fazio VW. Advantages of laparoscopic resection for ileocecal Crohn's disease. Dis Colon Rectum 2002;45:605–10.

102. Msika S, Iannelli A, Deroide G, et al. Can laparoscopy reduce hospital stay in the treatment of Crohn's disease? Dis Colon Rectum 2001;44:1661–6.

103. Young-Fadok TM, HallLong K, McConnell EJ, Gomez Rey G, Cabanela RL. Advantages of laparoscopic resection for ileocolic Crohn's disease. Improved outcomes and reduced costs. Surg Endosc 2001;15:450–4.

104. Casillas S, Delaney CP. Laparoscopic surgery for inflammatory bowel disease. Dig Surg 2005;22:135–42.

105. Cave DR, Cooley JS. Intraoperative enteroscopy. Indications and techniques. Gastrointest Endosc Clin N Am 1996;6:793–802.

106. Lau WY. Intraoperative enteroscopy — indications and limitations. Gastrointest Endosc 1990;36:268–71.

107. Lewis BS, Wenger JS, Waye JD. Small bowel enteroscopy and intraoperative enteroscopy for obscure gastrointestinal bleeding. Am J Gastroenterol 1991;86:171–4.

108. Agarwal A. Use of the laparoscope to perform intraoperative enteroscopy. Surg Endosc 1999;13:1143–4.

109. Pennazio M. Bleeding update. Gastrointest Endosc Clin N Am 2006;16:251–66.

CHAPTER **6**

Systematization of Terminology for Capsule Endoscopy

Michel Delvaux and Gerard Gay

KEY POINTS

1. Data processing in digestive endoscopy has dramatically changed over the last decade, with the introduction of computers. Capsule endoscopy has been recently introduced to examine the small intestine. Reading of the recordings is computer based and this setting constitutes a unique chance to foster the use of a standardized, structured language to edit the report and improve data exchange.

2. In this perspective, the *Minimal Standardized Terminology* was developed in the 1990s for classical endoscopy. Based on similar principles, the *Capsule Endoscopy Structured Terminology* (CEST) has been developed for the small bowel. It offers a list of terms that are organized in a comprehensive way, linked to attributes allowing further descriptions of the findings and a list of terms for "reasons for" and diagnoses made from the findings.

3. The CEST as been validated in a trial on more than 700 procedures, showing that terms are covering about 93% of findings seen in daily practice.

Introduction

The report is a key feature of any endoscopic procedure, as it contains a description of the observed findings, actions undertaken, and recommendations. It constitutes the link between the endoscopist and the referring physician responsible for the patient. Over the last two decades, computer technology has evolved rapidly and allowed better management of medical data. Advances in imaging techniques and increased data storage capabilities are now routinely used in endoscopy units to provide a better documentation of procedures. This important trend started about 20 years ago with the era of video endoscopes. Since then, several attempts have been made to propose integrated systems for data management in endoscopy.[1,2] Over the same period a substantial effort has been made to standardize endoscopic vocabulary and systematize the terms used to describe endoscopic findings. Text data are key elements of the information to be shared between the physician performing the endoscopic procedure and the referring physician. Two attempts at standardization deserve particular attention, as they were designed to standardize endoscopic reports and facilitate data exchange. The *Minimal Standard Terminology* (MST) was designed as a "minimal" list of terms that could be included within any computer system used to record the results of a gastrointestinal endoscopic examination.[3] It followed the initial attempt by Z Maratka to systematize nomenclature in digestive endoscopy.[4] Despite these efforts, acceptance of standardization of text data has been very slow compared to image formats. Several technical and environmental issues have not been defined, so that the standardization of endoscopic reports is far from being ubiquitous.

In 2001 the development of video capsule endoscopy (VCE) made it possible to noninvasively capture digital images of the entire length of the esophagus, stomach, and small intestine. The automatic storage of these digital images on permanent media allowed reading by one or more eaders at any time. However, the unique capabilities of VCE require specific adaptations of the terminology used to describe both the procedure and the findings that are distinct from conventional endoscopy. The immediate capture of the data on permanent storage media and the unavoidable use of a computer to read the videos constituted a unique opportunity to build, from the bottom up, a standardized layout for the VCE report and a systematic vocabulary. Following the principles of the *Minimal Standard Terminology*, a *Structured Terminology for Capsule Endoscopy* has been designed and proposed by a group of experts which will be available for public use[5] after validation of a large set of existing endoscopic reports.[6]

The aim of this chapter is to describe the environment and the principles of the endoscopic report with special attention paid to the specifics of VCE, including the technical aspects of the procedure and the mucosal patterns observed.

Management of data in an endoscopic unit: General principles

Types of data included in the endoscopic report

The performance of an endoscopic examination requires that data be provided and managed both before and after the procedure. These data will in turn generate other data (Figure 6.1). Before the procedure, the data are mainly of an administrative and historical nature, not specific to VCE, and may include scheduling information and personal data of the patient. Medical data at this step may include the clinical history, the patient's current condition, and results of other tests. These data, when recorded in a computer system, are usually managed in a hospital information system (HIS). The endoscopic procedure itself generates a number of data that are of two types: text and images. The post-procedure data include the description of the findings, i.e. the lesions observed on the capsule recording in the present case, their interpretation, and the clinically relevant conclusions and recommendations.

The American Society for Gastrointestinal Endoscopy (ASGE) has provided guidelines for the content of the endoscopic report listing the items that should be present (Table 6.1).[7] This table shows that most of the items can be translated to VCE.

Organization of the data in an endoscopic database

Several types of endoscopic database have been proposed. However, the most effective one is the "object-oriented" database of the relational type. The database is made up of many separate folders where data are stored according to their specific definition. Thus, one patient whose demographic data are stored in one file may undergo several endoscopic procedures and for each of them a separate file will be created. Each procedure will contain text data and images, the latter being stored in a separate folder, so that a single procedure can include an unlimited number of images

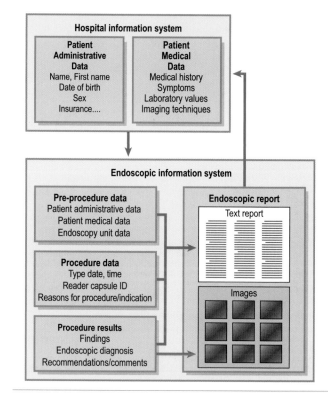

FIGURE 6.1 Organization of the data flow between the Hospital Information System and the Endoscopy Information System or Endoscopic Software. The data are shared in both directions by the two systems. The endoscopic report is built according to the procedure from the data contained in the endoscopic database, and used as a vehicle to transmit information to the Hospital Information System.

(Figure 6.2). When new data are recorded, they are stored in the relevant files. The software of the database is organized in such a way that allows it to retrieve data from the different files to build an "object" made of the dataset relevant for a given procedure and send it back to the screen or the printer as the response to a query. Figure 6.3 shows the structure of an object that would contain all the information needed to describe an endoscopic procedure, which will then be included in the endoscopic report.

This model can be thus be applied almost universally and include all types of endoscopic examinations. It should also allow integration of the results of VCE studies with those of other procedures in one database.

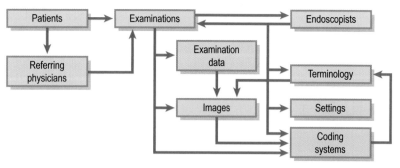

FIGURE 6.2 Organization of a relational database, where data are distributed to different folders linked to each other. The database maintains the links between the folders so that a query about one specific procedure can be answered by a report obtaining information from the different folders. The number of links between the folders is not limited so that one patient may undergo multiple procedures, performed by one or more physicians.

Table 6.1 Structure of an endoscopic record: Comparison of classical endoscopic report and capsule report

ASGE Items[7]	Classical endoscopy	Capsule endoscopy
Patient demographic data Patient Name, First Name Date of Birth Sex Patient ID Patient Insurance Number	Same data format for both types of procedures. May be imported from the Hospital Information System	
Date of procedure	Same format	
Endoscopist	Name of the performing physician	Name of the reader
Type of endoscopic examination performed	EGD, colonoscopy…	Intestinal capsule endoscopy
Instruments used	Instrument type and ID	Capsule ID
Reasons for examination	Include here the medical history of the patient, clinical condition and reasons for performing the study.	
Medication details (Anesthesia, Anaethesiologist, Analgesia, Sedation…)		Not relevant except use of prokinetics
Patient preparation	Bowel cleansing if relevant	Bowel cleansing when used
Anatomical extent of examination	Deepest anatomical landmark reached by the endoscope	Indicate here the transit times of the capsule and the deepest gut segment reached by the capsule
Limitation(s) of examination	Reasons for an incomplete examination	Technical failures limiting the examination
Findings and specimens obtained		No specimen
Endoscopic diagnosis	Diagnosis made from the findings of the procedure	
Therapeutic interventions and results		Not relevant
Notation of images captured	Images are not systematically captured depending on the technical environment	Thumbnails of the relevant images should systematically be included in the report
Complications		Complications
Discharge arrangements		Recommendations
Comments		
Results of biopsies and other late tests		Not relevant
Final diagnosis		Not relevant since no further interpretation of the study results will be possible in the absence of biopsies

Standardization of endoscopic terms

The initial attempt to systematize endoscopic nomenclature was the work done by Maratka and published as the "OMED" Terminology.[4] Following this report, the European Society for Gastrointestinal Endoscopy initiated a project in cooperation with the American and Japanese Societies for Gastrointestinal Endoscopy to devise a "minimal" list of terms that could be included within any computer system used to record the results of a gastrointestinal endoscopic examination. To facilitate implementation and allow a more complete description of observations when necessary, qualifying attributes, which provided additional detail, were added. The attributes are a list of descriptive concepts such as size, number, extent, etc., for which there are a series of values appropriate to that term. Every described lesion is placed in a location by the use of a list of sites relevant to the organ being examined. By this construction, the lists of terms with the specifications given by the attributes translates the concepts evoked by the users into a structured language.

The *Minimal Standard Terminology* is structured in lists of terms that cover the main types of endoscopic examinations, which include upper GI endoscopy, colonoscopy, and ERCP, with an additional complementary list of therapeutic procedures that might be performed (Figure 6.4). These lists contain terms that define concepts describing the medical fields of the endoscopic report (see Table 6.1). The list of terms within the *Reasons for examination* is larger than the one for *Indications* since the former is a broader concept. Some examinations may have been performed for reasons that are not accepted as indications. *Extent of the examination*

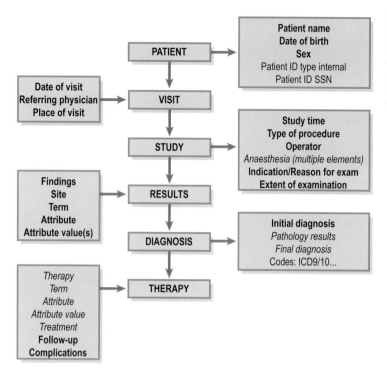

FIGURE 6.3 Model for organizing the data of a procedure in an "object" that can be used by the software to generate a report. The structure follows the logical chain of events that occur before, during, and after the procedure, with the relevant data for each step. Data in bold are those expected to be integrated in the report of a capsule endoscopy. Data in normal fonts are not mandatory, and data fields in italics contain data not relevant for capsule endoscopy.

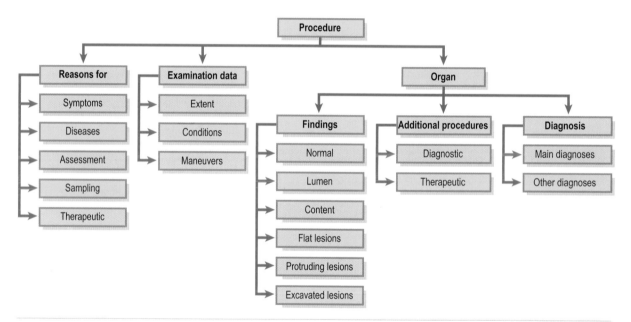

FIGURE 6.4 General structure of the *Minimal Standard Terminology* showing the data fields relevant to each of the steps in creation of an object.

is a section that refers to the characteristics of an examination. *Findings* covers the description of observations made during an endoscopic procedure, without necessarily linking them to a global diagnosis. *Endoscopic diagnosis* lists the diagnosis, single or multiple, that the endoscopist feels is most likely on the basis of macroscopic findings. Lastly, the *Therapeutic and diagnostic procedures* section is intended to describe the additional maneuvers that are undertaken during an endoscopic procedure; this last section is irrelevant to capsule VCE at the present time.

Structured terminology for capsule endoscopy

Principle of a structured language

Human language is based upon the association of concepts that are expressed by words. These words are linked to each other to develop more detailed and precise ideas and are organized in sentences that allow the reader to more easily recognize and understand the concepts. Although this activity is part of the highest level of human intelligence, most of these associations are performed automatically when someone speaks their mother language. The challenge for standardization of terms to be used for endoscopic reports is a difficult process that includes several steps:

- The definition of lists of terms that express, in a common way, concepts that are understood similarly by everyone and encompass the whole activity of the field or at least a significant part of it. As an example, the *Minimal Standard Terminology* was built to cover at least 95% of routine endoscopy.
- The design of lists of attributes that are linked to the main terms and allow a more specific description or a categorization into subclasses of concepts, the level of detail being adapted to each user of the language.
- Linkage between the descriptors that need to meet two requirements that seem opposite in nature: *flexibility* and *stability*. These two conditions are mandatory to make the structured language acceptable by the user on one hand, allowing them to express their ideas with precision and details, and on the other hand manageable in a computerized system with fixed rules and landmarks.

The structured language is thus based on a dual approach, including a first step in which an idea is split into single concepts, and a second where these single concepts are recombined to reconstitute the original idea. The first step is performed by the user who translates their ideas, originally expressed in natural language, into a series of concepts, while the second one is performed by the computer, according to preconfigured rules in the system (Figure 6.5).

Structured Terminology for Capsule Endoscopy

The *Structured Terminology for Capsule Endoscopy* is the proposal of a structured language based on the principles of the Minimal Standard Terminology for Digestive Endoscopy.[3] The terms proposed need to be readily understood, unambiguous, and commonly used. They avoid subjective descriptions and "artistic" comparisons that may not be correctly understood out of their original context. Terms used in less than 0.1% of large series of endoscopic reports, generated in natural language, are rejected. The translation of terms into different languages needs careful consideration to allow exchange of data between systems.

The structured terminology for VCE has been tested against the reports of 766 capsule procedures, created in natural language by non-selected users of capsule endoscopy.[6] After cleaning the database of obvious synonymous expressions, 93.2% of the expressions used to describe the "reasons for performing" a capsule endoscopy and 91.6% of the findings were covered by the proposed lists of terms. Some specific aspects of this terminology are discussed below.

Specific issues in capsule endoscopy

Location of the findings

In general, anatomic location cannot be precisely defined by VCE. Identifiable locations such as esophagus, stomach, pylorus, and the ileocecal valve do enable the observer to provide some accurate anatomic information. In order to approximately define its location, any finding can be characterized by a time point from a known anatomic site. Timer activation begins when the capsule is activated by the data recorder. By definition that time is 0. Total duration of examination is the time when the study ends because the battery runs down, the recording device is disconnected, or the capsule is out of range of the data recorder (naturally excreted). The following locations may be identified by specific time point markers:

- Time of ingestion: first visualization of oral or esophageal mucosa
- Time of gastric entry: first visualization of gastric mucosa
- Time of duodenal entry: first visualization of duodenal mucosa
- Time of colonic entry: first visualization of colonic mucosa.

The anatomic sites are divided into categories that may be visualized by the imaging system. It is understood that, for certain findings, only the time point may be identified. Additionally, the "external mapping locator" system is a component of the reading software used to locate the position of the capsule in the abdomen of the patient.[8] This location is based upon the relative intensity of the signal emitted by the capsule as detected by the eight sensors placed on the abdominal wall. This system gives the reader an indication of the progression of the capsule along the gastrointestinal tract. The correlation between the actual position of the capsule and the position as shown by the software (RAPID, Given Imaging) has not proven clinically useful in localizing small bowel lesions (Figure 6.6).

Characteristics of the procedure

The characteristics of the procedure encompass any technical information that indicates the accuracy of the examination of

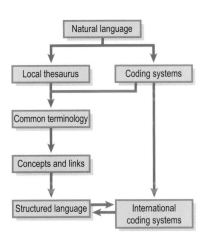

FIGURE 6.5 Diagram of the process for transforming natural language into a structured and standardized language. Concepts expressed in natural language, which have a large cultural and personal diversity, are progressively merged with accepted codes and commonly accepted expressions to be translated into more general and widely accepted terms. In a second step, these terms are linked by hierarchical bonds that create the structured language. At the end of the process, references are created to existing coding systems, mapping the structured language with other standard vocabularies.

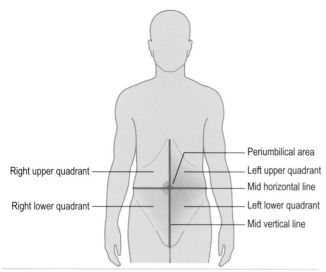

FIGURE 6.6 Sites for external mapping locator of *Findings* using the PillCam SB localization software.

Table 6.2 Example of terms proposed by the *Structured Terminology for Capsule Endoscopy*: Terms in the *Findings* section, describing the changes of the mucosa

Erythematous	Distribution pattern	Localized Patchy Diffuse
	Longitudinal extent	Short segment Long segment Whole organ
Pale	Distribution pattern	Localized Patchy Diffuse
	Longitudinal extent	Short segment Long segment Whole organ
Edematous (congested)	Distribution pattern	Localized Patchy Diffuse
	Longitudinal extent	Short segment Long segment Whole organ
Granular	Distribution pattern	Localized Patchy Diffuse
	Longitudinal extent	Short segment Long segment Whole organ
Nodular	Distribution pattern	Localized Patchy Diffuse
	Longitudinal extent	Short segment Long segment Whole organ
Atrophic	Distribution pattern	Localized Patchy Diffuse
	Longitudinal extent	Short segment Long segment Whole organ
Abnormal villi	Shape	Convoluted Swollen Blunted Absent
	Color	Whitish Yellow
	Distribution pattern	Localized Patchy Diffuse
	Longitudinal extent	Short segment Long segment Whole organ

the mucosa. This section should also describe any restrictions on the examination that may be the result of inadequate preparation, anatomic barriers, or technical failure. Finally, the extent of the examination can defined by the duration of examination and the most distal identifiable anatomic site recognized on the capsule recording, e.g. first view of the colonic mucosa.

Specific terms for findings by capsule endoscopy

The concepts defined by the *Structured Terminology for Capsule Endoscopy* are limited to the small bowel. Any finding or diagnosis represents a biological concept which can then be modified by or related to other concepts. For example, the small bowel mucosa has many characteristics that can be identified (see Table 6.2). Thus, the mucosa can be considered a unique biological concept, and its light absorption or reflectance characteristics a modifying concept. Each is described by a specific term and, when appropriate, a term is attached to it as a modifying concept or attribute that makes the observation more precise. As an example, the small bowel mucosa has the characteristic of color and may appear erythematous, which represents a term describing this specific finding corresponding to an alteration of the color of the mucosa. The extent of this abnormality and the distribution of the pattern on the mucosa may be used as additional information included in the attributes attached to this specific finding. It is recognized that these modifying concepts are subjective, but they represent the consensus of an expert panel. It is anticipated that they will undergo testing and revision as needed.

Color of the mucosa

The descriptors used to define changes in color of the intestinal mucosa were felt to be very subjective but mandatory for a complete description of the mucosal pattern in a segment of the intestine. Changes in color may be influenced by technical factors such as the distance between the capsule and the mucosal surface, which may change according to peristalsis, blood supply, the intensity of lightening of the mucosa, and the presence of food residue or blood in the lumen. These difficulties may explain the low correlation found between the observer and the automatic detector of bleeding areas included in the RAPID software and known as the "suspected blood indicator."[9,10]

Mucosal villi

Due to the magnification of the images taken by the capsule, their resolution, and the presence of a clear fluid/mucosal interface instead of air insufflation, individual villi are often well defined on capsule recordings. In the event of abnormality, a specific term was introduced to characterize them — "abnormal pattern of villi." Additional terms were introduced to further define the abnormality. It should be noted that capsule endoscopy is not intended to replace microscopic examination of biopsies for the diagnosis of celiac disease or other conditions, although a good correlation between capsule and biopsy findings has recently been observed.[11]

Three-dimensional assessment of intestinal lesions

The main list of terms characterizing findings has been divided into subheadings according to the position of the lesion with respect to the linear anatomy of the small intestine. In the absence of air insufflation, the three-dimensional characteristics of lesions may not always be fully appreciated on capsule recordings. However, for clarity and easier implementation of the terminology in a software interface, these subheadings have been maintained. Thus, lesions are classified as changes in the lumen of the organ, content, mucosal pattern, and flat, protruding, and excavated lesions. The principles retained for this classification have been based more on the definition of the lesions than on their actual appearance on the recording.

Endoscopic diagnosis

This part of the *Terminology* provides lists of diseases and conditions that can be used to formulate the conclusion of an endoscopic procedure and the diagnosis supported by the findings. As far as capsule endoscopy is concerned, this endoscopic diagnosis will be regarded as the conclusion and final diagnosis transmitted by the reader to the referring physician. This may be commented upon and accompanied by recommendations for patient management. In the absence of biopsy, there is no element that can later modify this diagnosis.

The list of diagnoses contains a short "top 9" list of the most frequent diagnoses. The others are arranged in alphabetical order in a secondary list. The intent of this classification is mainly to facilitate the implementation of the software interface, by avoiding scrolling long lists of terms.

The attribute proposed as "level of certainty" can be used to indicate to the referring physician how confident the reader can be in the proposed diagnosis. For capsule recordings, the attribute value "suspicion of" might be overused by some users, as they will consider that a firm diagnosis cannot be given in the absence of biopsies. On the other hand, difficulties have been reported in the understanding of the attribute value "exclusion of." The intent of it is to allow the endoscopist to report negative findings. For example, when a procedure is undertaken to confirm or refute the presence of a tumor suspected on other imaging modalities, the attribute "exclusion of an intestinal tumor" may be used to indicate that the gut segment was examined and no tumor was found.

Conclusions and perspectives

Computers are currently widely used in hospitals to manage patient administrative data and distribute information between different physicians caring for a patient. The goal of the standardization process is to provide a lexicon and method for documenting observations in an efficient, unambiguous manner and also to store data in formats that can be exchanged between computer systems operating in different facilities. The architecture of large hospital information systems is based on the use of several standard formats. These formats need to be modified into platforms for smaller facilities as integrated healthcare networks, including small hospitals and other facilities, are increasingly developed on a regional basis in many countries. With this perspective, VCE provides a unique opportunity to promote the use of standardized data in gastrointestinal endoscopy. However there is a reluctance on the part of many endoscopists to use a structured terminology. This can be explained by the difficulty in mastering computer technology and the apparent waste of time encountered during the learning curve when the system is installed. It is also partly related to the relatively poor user interface of software previously dedicated to endoscopy reporting. Endoscopists, who have been trained to dictate their reports, are often reluctant to lose their freedom to use descriptions that they feel are appropriate. VCE requires that the physician uses a computer to access the data, so that a computerized reporting system could be included in the process without an additional time investment for the user and without forcing him or her to use an additional device.

Using a standard format for endoscopic data is also an opportunity to promote research in the field, by allowing the collection of large amounts of data that can be shared by investigators from different centers and countries. Comparative studies of the various modalities used to investigate an organ or a group of diseases could also be more easily designed. This point is particularly important for capsule endoscopy. As an emerging technique, it had to be compared with existing ones, but is now becoming the "gold standard" for the examination of the small bowel, and new techniques will be compared to it, e.g. push-and-pull enteroscopy. The use of terminologies based on the same structure, such as the *Minimal Standard Terminology* and the *Structured Terminology for Capsule Endoscopy*, would make these studies easier and thus help to validate new techniques more quickly.

Finally, standardization of endoscopic data is paramount for their integration in the Hospital Information System. Classical endoscopy and capsule endoscopy, using a similar data format, could then be integrated in the patient's folder, allowing fast access to complete sets of data including the results of radiological investigations and other tests. Technical solutions exist and clinicians must adapt to them and change the way they are used to manage data. This will be a slow but irreversible process. Capsule endoscopy is a real opportunity to accelerate these advances.

References

1. Delvaux M, Escourrou J. Image management: the point of view of the physician. Endoscopy 1992;24:511–5.

2. Kruss DM. The ASGE database: computers in the endoscopy unit. Endosc Rev 1987;4:64–70.

3. Delvaux M, Crespi M and the Computer Committee of ESGE. Minimal Standard Terminology in Digestive Endoscopy. Version 2.0. Endoscopy 2000;32:159–88.

4. Maratka Z. Terminology, definitions and diagnostic criteria in digestive endoscopy, 3rd edn. Normed Verlag, Bad Homburg, 1994.

5. Korman LY, Delvaux M, Gay G, et al. Capsule Endoscopy Structured Terminology (CEST): proposal of a standardaized and structured terminology for reporting capsule endoscopy procedures. Endoscopy 2005; 37: 951–959.

6. Delvaux M, Friedman S, Keuchel M, et al. Structured terminology for capsule endoscopy: results of retrospective testing and validation in 766 small-bowel investigations. Endoscopy 2005; 37: 945–950.

7. Computer Committee. Standard format and content of the endoscopic procedure report. American Society for Gastrointestinal Endoscopy, 1992.

8. Gay G, Delvaux M, Rey JF. The role of video capsule endoscopy in the diagnosis of digestive diseases: a review of current possibilities. Endoscopy 2004;36:913–20.

9. Liangpunsakul S, Mays L, Rex DK. Performance of Given suspected blood indicator. Am J Gastroenterol 2003;98:2676–8.

10. D'Halluin PN, Delvaux M, Lapalus MG, et al. Does the "Suspected Blood Indicator" improve the detection of bleeding lesions by capsule endoscopy? Gastrointest Endosc 2005;61:243–9.

11. Krauss NG, Cellier C, Collin P, et al. Evaluation of capsule endoscopy in coeliac disease patients with ongoing symptoms on a gluten-free diet. Prospective blinded European multicenter trial. Gastroenterology 2005;128:A81 (abstract).

CHAPTER **7**

Normal Small Bowel and Normal Variants of the Small Bowel

Klaus Mergener

"Normal is nothing more than a cycle on a washing machine."
Whoopi Goldberg, b. 1955

Introduction

Defining normality and distinguishing between "normal" and "abnormal" is not always easy. Trainees in conventional gastrointestinal endoscopy spend a considerable amount of time learning to recognize normal anatomy and distinguish it from abnormal, pathologic findings. In situations where this distinction is difficult, the endoscopist has several options: changing the position of the endoscope relative to the area in question; removing intervening fluid, bubbles, and particulate matter by flushing or suctioning; insufflating or removing air, probing a lesion with a catheter to assess its consistency. All of these maneuvers may afford a better look, a different perspective, and clues as to the etiology of a possible abnormality. If this does not solve the problem, sampling by biopsy, brushing, or fluid aspiration may help make a diagnosis through histologic analysis.

Capsule endoscopy represents a fundamental departure from conventional endoscopy in that the current capsule technology does not allow for any of the above interventions. What you see is truly what you get, and a diagnosis, at least a presumed diagnosis, often has to be made on the basis of a few images which cannot be altered or improved. Making such a diagnosis with confidence can initially be challenging even for gastroenterologists with considerable experience in conventional endoscopy. Additionally, capsule endoscopy may produce unfamiliar views or images of commonly seen structures such as the pylorus from unusual angles, e.g. a retrograde view from the duodenal bulb. The interpretation of capsule endoscopy examinations thus requires expertise and specific training which has to be acquired in addition to that obtained in conventional endoscopy. This has recently been recognized by the American Society for Gastrointestinal Endoscopy (ASGE) in their guidelines on credentialing and granting privileges for capsule endoscopy.[1]

This chapter reviews the normal anatomy of the small intestine as seen with capsule endoscopy as well as some artifacts and common normal variants that may be encountered during a capsule examination.

Small bowel segments

The small intestine is approximately 600 cm in length, with its proximal and distal limits defined by the pylorus and the ileocecal valve, respectively.

It is divided into three major segments: the duodenum, the jejunum, and the ileum. Although there are some differences in structure between jejunum and ileum, their precise point of separation cannot be defined. The transition from duodenum to jejunum is accurately indicated by the ligament of Treitz but this landmark cannot be identified from within the lumen of the bowel and is therefore not evident on capsule endoscopy. Unless an abnormality is identified immediately after the capsule passes through the pylorus (and can therefore be presumed to be located in the duodenal bulb), the position of the capsule or any identified abnormality is probably best reported by indicating the time that has elapsed between the passage of the imaging device through the pylorus and its current position, thereby estimating its position in the "proximal" or "distal" portion of the small bowel.

Pylorus

While endoscopists are well familiar with anterograde views of the pylorus, a less familiar retrograde view of the pylorus from the duodenal bulb is sometimes seen during capsule endoscopy if the imaging device is traveling backward (Figure 7.1). The somewhat protuberant appearance of the pylorus in this view should not be mistaken for a polyp or mass lesion. A back and forth movement across the pylorus may also occasionally be observed with retrograde passage of the capsule from the duodenal bulb into the stomach and then again into the bulb (Video 7.1).

Duodenal bulb

Unless transit is delayed, the view of the duodenal bulb is usually brief. Determining whether the capsule has in fact passed the pylorus and entered the duodenal bulb may seem straightforward but can be difficult in individual cases especially if fluid and food particles obscure luminal views. Attention to the surface structure of the mucosa can provide important clues: while the gastric mucosa generally appears smooth and sometimes exhibits a mosaic pattern, the mucosa of the duodenal bulb typically reveals superficial "breaks" and crevices which correspond histologically to the presence of crypts (Figure 7.2).

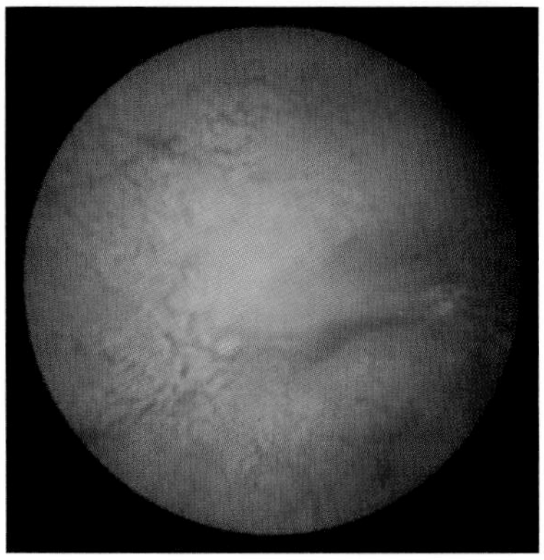

FIGURE 7.2 Normal appearance of mucosa in the duodenal bulb.

Brunner's glands are small lobules of cells that secrete mucin, pepsinogen, and bicarbonate into the crypts. Brunner's glands are mainly located in the duodenal bulb but can also be found in the descending duodenum. They may become hyperplastic and then form either single or multiple nodules (Figure 7.3). The diagnosis is made by histologic evaluation of biopsy specimens. Brunner's gland hyperplasia is typically asymptomatic and discovered incidentally, although individual cases of ulceration, hemorrhage, and obstruction have been described. Foci of heterotopic gastric mucosa may also present as discrete nodules or sessile polyps in the duodenum (Figure 7.4). Microscopically, the mucosa resembles that of the gastric fundus and consists of chief and parietal cells. It may undergo hyperplastic or adenomatous changes but usually remains asymptomatic.

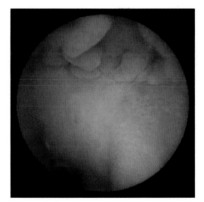

FIGURE 7.3 Nodularity in the duodenal bulb due to Brunner's gland hyperplasia.

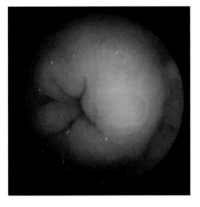

FIGURE 7.1 Pylorus — retrograde view.

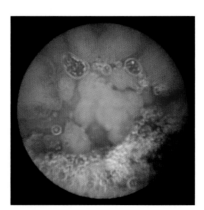

FIGURE 7.4 Gastric metaplasia in the duodenal bulb.

Major and minor papillae

The major papilla, also termed the ampulla of Vater, is located on the posteromedial aspect of the mid part of the descending duodenum. When the duodenum is distended with air during conventional endoscopy, the major papilla protrudes into the lumen and the transmural part of the distal bile duct is often seen as a submucosal bulge. In contrast, the major papilla is difficult to identify in the non-distended duodenum and is, in fact, rarely seen during capsule endoscopy. In a prospective series of 100 capsule examinations reviewed independently by two examiners who specifically focused on the duodenal portion of the exam, the papilla was identified in only 3 of 100 capsule studies (Enns and Mergener, unpublished data). If identified, the major papilla appears as a small nodule with a central pinpoint or slit-like opening which is sometimes marked by the drainage of bile (Figure 7.5). Identification of the minor papilla, which is located 1–2 cm proximal to the major papilla and drains the dorsal pancreatic duct, is even more unusual (Figure 7.6).

Small bowel lumen

The circumferential mucosal folds of the small bowel (plicae circularis of Kerckring or valvulae conniventes) represent invaginations of mucosa and submucosa into the lumen and serve to increase the mucosal surface area. They are more prominent and closely spaced in the duodenum and jejunum, are less well developed and more widely separated in the ileum, and are absent from the terminal ileum. In the non-distended small bowel, the folds are seen in various states of contraction. White lines are sometimes observed at the edges of the folds and probably represent areas of relative hypoperfusion rather than fixed structures such as lymphatic channels as they vary with the state of contraction and disappear with flattening of a fold (Figure 7.7).

The mucosal villi are delicate finger-like structures which extend into the intestinal lumen and are 0.5–1 mm long, tallest in the jejunum and progressively shorter in the ileum. They serve to further increase the luminal surface and absorptive capacity of the small bowel. It is a testament to the extraordinary resolution of capsule images that individual villi can be observed with this examination (Figure 7.8). While mucosal folds and villi are often well visualized, luminal views may be poor during some or all parts of a capsule exam. The lumen may appear collapsed (Figure 7.9) thus limiting the evaluation of the mucosa.

The reviewer should be aware of a number of artifacts that may occur when small intestinal mucosa is viewed through an air bubble: lines may appear which represent the air/water interface at the edge of a large bubble (Figure 7.10). While this may lead to bizarre still images which sometimes resemble worm-like structures or foreign bodies, review of the moving video images should clearly identify this phenomenon. A light reflection next to the air/water interface also provides a clue. Sometimes a frontal reflection of some or all of the capsule light sources may be observed as a ring-like structure

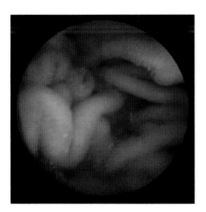

FIGURE 7.5 Major papilla.

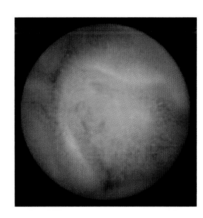

FIGURE 7.7 Normal folds in a non-distended small bowel. The white lines observed at the edges of the folds probably represent areas of relative hypoperfusion.

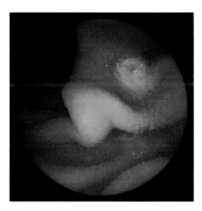

FIGURE 7.6 Minor papilla.

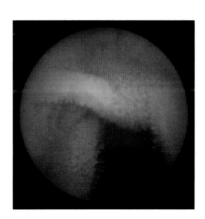

FIGURE 7.8 Normal intestinal villi.

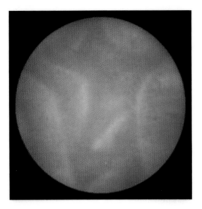

FIGURE 7.9 Collapsed small bowel. No luminal views are obtained.

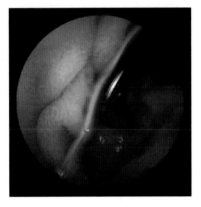

FIGURE 7.10 Artifact lines created at the air/water interface of a large air bubble.

(Figure 7.11). Intestinal villi typically appear blunted or altogether absent when viewed through large air bubbles. Therefore, while the presence of villi in the entire small bowel provides strong evidence against a condition such as celiac disease, the failure to visualize villi may be caused by a variety of exam-related factors and in itself is not sufficient to make a specific diagnosis.

Despite an automatic brightness control mechanism, the clarity of the capsule images varies to some degree dependent on the distance of the imaging device to the small bowel wall and the presence or absence of fluid and/or particulate matter within the lumen of the small intestine. Fluid within the lumen is more concentrated in the ileum and, due to its bile content, the views are often darker in the distal ileum than in the proximal small bowel. Dark brown fluid may

sometimes be difficult to distinguish from dark blood (Figure 7.12). If this is the case, examination of the cecum and the small bowel beyond the stained area can be helpful to determine if melena is accumulating distally. Its absence and the presence of light brown stool in the cecum indicate that the fluid observed was likely not blood-stained.

Terminal ileum

Lymphoid follicles are 2–3 mm nodular elevations which are scattered throughout the small intestine but are found in highest concentrations in the distal ileum (Figure 7.13). They are more prominent during childhood and adolescence but may be seen at all ages and should not be mistaken for polyps.

The small bowel connects to the colon at the ileocecal valve, which is composed of upper and lower lips that protrude into the cecum. The valve is frequently more prominent in children and young adults because of additional lymphoid tissue. Traditional teaching holds that the ileocecal valve opposes reflux of colonic contents into the small bowel and that this appears to be a function of the angulation between the ileum and cecum rather than a true tonic, sphincter-type mechanism. However, reflux of fecal matter can frequently be observed during capsule examinations and may sometimes preclude adequate visualization of the distal aspect of the terminal ileum.

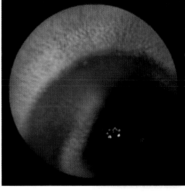

FIGURE 7.12 Dark fluid observed in the distal small bowel (this patient had no history of bleeding and light brown stool was subsequently observed in the cecum).

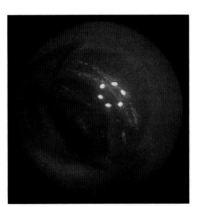

FIGURE 7.11 Reflection of capsule light sources in an air bubble.

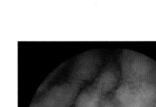

FIGURE 7.13 Nodular lymphoid hyperplasia seen in the terminal ileum.

Diverticula

Small bowel diverticula may occur anywhere along the small intestine but are most commonly found in the second portion of the duodenum adjacent to the major papilla. They are observed in 1–3% of autopsy studies. Duodenal diverticula can attain a large size and are usually asymptomatic. While systematic studies have not been performed, anecdotal evidence suggests that they are rarely visualized during capsule endoscopy.

Meckel's diverticulum represents the most common congenital anomaly of the gastrointestinal tract, occurring in approximately 2% of the population. The omphalo-mesenteric duct, a structure that bridges the yolk sac with the developing gut, is normally obliterated by the 8th week of gestation. Failure to do so may result in either an omphalo-mesenteric fistula, an enterocyst, or, most commonly, a Meckel's diverticulum. A small percentage of Meckel's diverticula may contain ectopic gastric mucosa which may lead to ulceration and painless lower intestinal bleeding. Case reports have described the visualization of a bleeding Meckel's diverticulum during capsule endoscopy.[2]

Bulging lesions

Small bowel tumors are relatively uncommon but can be detected during capsule endoscopy.[3] Distinguishing a submucosal tumor from extrinsic compression of a bowel loop due to an adjacent structure or another loop of bowel can provide a particular challenge especially if luminal views are suboptimal and only a few capsule images show the area in question. Some visual clues may be helpful in making this differentiation: a fixed lesion which does not change its shape or position, and the presence of bridging folds speak for a true tumor (Figure 7.14). Some capsule images may reveal stretching of the mucosa, ulceration, discoloration, or an irregular, lobulated shape of a mass. Conversely, compression of the bowel lumen due to an adjacent loop of bowel is a common phenomenon and can be suspected when a smooth, rounded protrusion is encountered which moves with peristalsis thereby indicating its softness and extrinsic location (Figure 7.15).

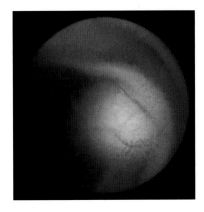

FIGURE 7.15 Extrinsic compression due to an adjacent loop of small bowel creating the impression of a submucosal bulge.

Lymphangiectasias

Lymphatic, vascular, and neural structures within the lamina propria of the small bowel serve as conduits for absorbed material, neural signals, and endocrine mediators. The lymphatic drainage of the small bowel follows its blood supply from lymph channels in individual villi to mesenteric lymph nodes along the superior mesenteric and celiac arteries, and eventually to the cisterna chyli and the thoracic duct.

The term "lymphangiectasia" describes dilation of lymphatic vessels. When involving the small lacteals of individual villi, tiny punctate white flecks may be seen on the mucosal surface (Figure 7.16a). Clustering of such lymphangiectasias may occur and present as bright white nodular protrusions (Figure 7.16b). Cystic dilations of larger lymph vessels in the mucosa and submucosa of the bowel wall are referred to as chylous (lymphangiectatic) cysts or cholesterol cysts. They are cream colored, irregularly shaped, flat or raised into the bowel lumen, and typically up to 1 cm in diameter (Figure 7.16c). Pathologically, they contain amorphous material, foamy macrophages, and scanty lymphocytes. The lymphatics in the overlying mucosa may also be dilated leading to the combination of individual punctate white dots on top of a nodular yellowish base (Figure 7.16d).

Lymphangiectasias may be single or multiple. They represent non-neoplastic lesions which are usually found incidentally and do not produce symptoms or cause protein loss. A more diffuse whitish appearance of the small bowel mucosa can sometimes be observed during capsule endoscopy, sometimes in otherwise asymptomatic individuals (Figure 7.17). Whether this appearance has any clinical significance and correlates with an abnormality of lipid absorption or metabolism is not known.

Phlebectasias

Endoscopists are well familiar with the appearance of the normal vascular pattern of the small bowel. Occasionally, focal dilations of mucosal veins may occur and are referred to as phlebectasias or venous lakes (Figure 7.18). When they are small, they probably represent incidental findings and carry no clinical significance. Rarely, these phlebectasias may increase in size and lead to occult bleeding or overt hemorrhage.

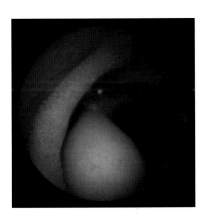

FIGURE 7.14 Submucosal tumor of the small bowel. Note the bridging fold at 12 o'clock.

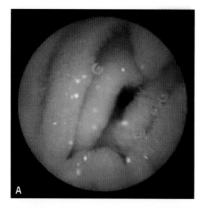

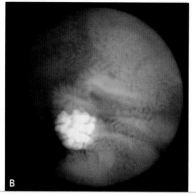

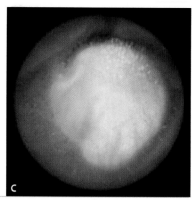

FIGURE 7.16 (a) Punctate lymphangiectasias, (b) cluster of focal lymphangiectasias, (c) chylous cyst, (d) combination of chylous cyst and punctate lymphangiectasias.

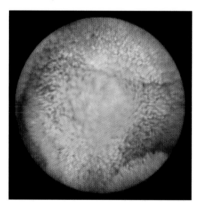

FIGURE 7.17 Whitish appearance of the mucosa in the proximal small bowel presumed to be due to diffuse dilation of lymphatic vessels. The clinical significance of this phenomenon is unknown.

Red spots and angioectasias

Mucosal vascular abnormalities are by far the most common cause of small intestinal bleeding, accounting for at least 50% of cases of obscure gastrointestinal blood loss.[4–6] Several different classifications have been proposed for these vascular anomalies, but none has become universally accepted. An angioectasia is generally defined by the presence of ectasia in normal pre-existing intestinal submucosal veins and overlying mucosal capillaries. Histologically, angioectasias consist of dilated, distorted vessels lined with endothelium, or rarely with a small amount of smooth muscle. Since these lesions appear to represent ectasias of the normal vasculature rather than true malformations, the term "angioectasia" is probably more appropriate than arteriovenous malformation. Endoscopically, angioectasias are flat or slightly raised above the mucosal surface, red in color, and usually 2–10 mm in size. They occur more frequently with increasing age and may be round in contour, stellate, or have sharply circumscribed fern-like margins (Figure 7.19). Angioectasias may be isolated or multiple, as seen in patients with Osler–Weber–Rendu disease.

When red spots are less well defined or very small, it may at times be difficult to determine whether they represent true angioectasias or insignificant findings (Figure 7.20a, b). Given the extraordinary resolution now obtained with capsule endoscopy, some of these lesions are the size of individual villi (1 mm or less). Whether a red spot of such small size can be clinically significant is being debated. If it is seen in a patient who previously presented with severe gastrointestinal

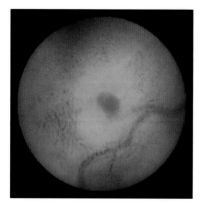

FIGURE 7.18 Small phlebectasia.

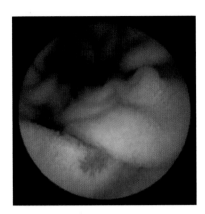

FIGURE 7.19 Typical angioectasia.

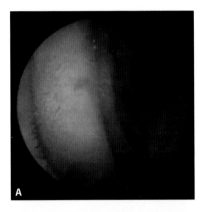

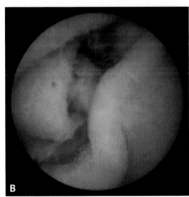

FIGURE 7.20 Small red spots, either poorly defined (a) or very small (b). Do these represent clinically significant lesions?

but may be quite difficult in the middle.[7] Capsule endoscopy presents a particular challenge in this regard as probing and sampling of an indeterminate lesion is not possible. When the technology received its initial approval by the Food and Drug Administration in August of 2001, the initial research projects focused on optimizing the examination, assessing its utility for various clinical indications, describing its limitations, and defining its role within various diagnostic algorithms. At the time this book is being written, more than 5 years later, there is still a striking paucity of literature concerning some of the unique aspects of capsule endoscopy, for example the need to confidently identify clinically relevant abnormalities on the basis of just a few digital images, to report these findings in a standardized fashion, and to develop a system by which different reviewers can use a common frame of reference and arrive at the same presumed diagnosis. The interobserver variability for reviewing capsule studies and identifying abnormalities has been assessed in a pilot trial[8] but needs to be studied systematically on a larger scale. The optimal reading conditions need to be defined: at what speed does the miss rate for small lesions become unacceptably high? Does the multiviewer function affect the accuracy of the reading? Additionally, the reporting of findings needs to be standardized. A workgroup convened by one manufacturer of capsule devices recently proposed a standard format and terminology to be used for reporting capsule examinations.[9] The terminology was modeled after the minimal standard terminology previously developed and published by various professional societies for conventional endoscopy. While this effort provides a useful reporting standard, it falls short of recognizing and addressing some of the challenges that are different from conventional endoscopy and unique to capsule endoscopy. For example, the issue of how best to relay the level of certainty about the significance of a particular finding is not addressed in the current framework. Depending on its exact appearance and the clinical circumstances, a red spot may be considered to be of "probable," "possible," or "indeterminate" significance. While the proposed framework represents a "minimal" terminology and "more detailed descriptors" are specifically encouraged, standardization of the reporting of levels of certainty will be needed to allow for comparisons between different reviewers and different studies. Lastly, additional research is needed to clarify the clinical significance of various small and indeterminate lesions seen at capsule endoscopy. Eventually, it is hoped that this will enable us to know with greater certainty what is "normal" and what is not.

hemorrhage, some might question whether this degree of bleeding can originate from a barely visible lesion. Whether there is a threshold size above which vascular lesions are more likely to bleed is also unknown. Many reviewers tend to err on the side of reporting every questionable and perhaps trivial lesion. In many of the early series investigating the utility of capsule endoscopy in patients with obscure bleeding, punctate red spots were counted towards "positive findings" thereby possibly inflating the true sensitivity of capsule endoscopy.

At the heart of it all — distinguishing between "normal" and "abnormal"

As has been previously recognized, the issue of what is "normal" versus "abnormal" is easy at the poles of the spectrum

References

1. Faigel DO, Baron TH, Adler DG, et al. ASGE guideline: guidelines for credentialing and granting privileges for capsule endoscopy. Gastrointest Endosc 2005;61:503–5.

2. Moon JH, Park CH, Kim JH, et al. Bleeding Meckel's diverticulum detected by capsule endoscopy. Gastrointest Endosc 2006;63:702.

3. Cobrin GM, Pittman RH, Lewis BS. Increased diagnostic yield of small bowel tumors with capsule endoscopy. Cancer 2006;107:22–7.

4. Pennazio M. Bleeding update. Gastrointest Endosc Clin N Am 2006;16:251–66.

5. Dulai GS, Jensen JM. Severe gastrointestinal bleeding of obscure origin. Gastrointest Endosc Clin N Am 2004;14:101–13.

6. Pennazio M, Santucci R, Rondonotti E, et al. Outcome of patients with obscure gastrointestinal bleeding after capsule endoscopy: report of 100 consecutive cases. Gastroenterology 2004;126:643–53.

7. Cave DR. Reading wireless video capsule endoscopy. Gastrointest Endoscopy Clin N Am 2004;14:17–24.

8. Mergener K, Enns R. Interobserver variability for reading capsule endoscopy examinations. Gastrointest Endosc 2003;57:AB85.

9. Korman LY, Delvaux M, Gay G, et al. Capsule Endoscopy Structured Terminology (CEST): Proposal of a standardized and structured terminology for reporting capsule endoscopy procedures. Endoscopy 2005;37:951–9.

Section TWO

Clinical Problems

CHAPTER **8**

Approach to the Patient with Obscure Gastrointestinal Bleeding

Marco Pennazio

KEY POINTS

1. Patients with obscure gastrointestinal bleeding pose difficult diagnostic and management problems.

2. In these patients, although most bleeding sources are in the small bowel, careful repeat studies of upper and lower gastrointestinal tract should be performed before evaluating the small bowel, because of the significant miss rate at initial endoscopy.

3. Capsule endoscopy is currently the preferred test for mucosal imaging of the entire small intestine and should be the next diagnostic step in patients with obscure bleeding for whom there is no suspected obstruction. Its diagnostic yield is high and it can potentially produce earlier diagnosis.

4. When integrated into a global approach to the patient, capsule endoscopy is helpful for effective decision-making concerning subsequent investigations and treatments. This in turn can mean more timely treatment and reduced utilization of resources and costs.

Introduction

The annual incidence of gastrointestinal bleeding in the United States has been conservatively estimated at approximately 100 episodes per 100 000 persons, accounting for approximately 300 000 hospitalizations per year.[1] In most patients, the source of bleeding is readily identified by endoscopy and occasionally by radiological methods. Once identified, the source of bleeding may need endoscopic or surgical treatment but in 80% of patients bleeding stops spontaneously and does not recur. However, approximately 5% of patients continue to bleed from an unidentified source.[2] These patients pose difficult diagnostic and management problems. They may require numerous blood transfusions and repeated hospital admissions, undergo multiple diagnostic procedures, consume increased health-care resources, and have their quality of life significantly affected. Obscure gastrointestinal bleeding (OGIB) is defined as bleeding of unknown origin that persists or recurs, and includes recurrent or persistent iron-deficiency anemia (IDA), fecal occult blood test (FOBT) positivity, or visible bleeding, after negative initial colonoscopy and upper endoscopy. OGIB can be subclassified into two clinical forms: (1) obscure-occult, as manifested by recurrent IDA and/ or recurrent positive FOBT, and (2) obscure-overt, with recurrent passage of visible blood with melena or hematochezia.[3] After bleeding is recognized as recurrent, the focus of care shifts to identifying the site and cause of bleeding; only then can appropriate therapy be instituted. The majority of lesions causing OGIB are located in the small bowel and, rarely, in the stomach, colon, biliary tree or pancreas. Careful utilization of diagnostic tools may lead to early identification of the bleeding source and may help improve diagnostic outcome while decreasing the cost of hospitalization.

Causes of obscure gastrointestinal bleeding

The types of lesion that cause bleeding in the small bowel are similar to those found in other areas of the gastrointestinal tract. They include vascular abnormalities, neoplasms, ulcers, and inflammatory lesions, as well as other less common lesions (Table 8.1). Finding and treating them, however, is much more difficult than with gastroduodenal or colorectal lesions.

Vascular lesions

A variety of vascular lesions affect the small bowel, and are the commonest cause of bleeding in the small intestine, being the underlying cause in

Table 8.1 Causes of small-bowel bleeding

Vascular Lesions	Tumors	Other Causes
Angioectasia	Adenoma[b]	Crohn's disease
Dieulafoy lesion	Hamartoma[c]	Drug-induced small-bowel injury
Telangiectasia[a]	Lipoma	Ulcers in celiac disease
Varices	Adenocarcinoma	Chronic ulcerative jejuno-ileitis
Phlebectasia	Lymphoma	Vasculitis
Aorto-enteric fistula	Gastrointestinal stromal tumors (GISTs)	Radiation enteritis
Aneurysms	Carcinoid tumors	Ischemic injury
	Vascular tumors[d]	Meckel's diverticulum
	Neurofibroma[e]	Diverticulosis
	Metastasis	Zollinger–Ellison syndrome Endometriosis Pancreaticus hemosuccus/hemobilia Infectious causes von Willebrand disease

Associated syndromes: [a]Osler–Weber–Rendu disease, CREST syndrome, Turner's syndrome; [b]familial adenomatous polyposis (FAP); [c]Peutz–Jeghers syndrome; [d]blue rubber bleb nevus syndrome, Klippel–Trenaunay–Weber syndrome; [e]Von Recklinghausen's disease.

70–80% of cases.[4] Angioectasias, often called angiodysplasia, vascular ectasia or arteriovenous malformations, are small superficial red lesions characterized by dilated, distorted blood vessels with thin walls; they can occur anywhere in the gastrointestinal tract and are the commonest cause of small bowel bleeding in elderly patients.

Endoscopically, angioectasias may be flat, excavated, or slightly raised above the mucosal surface, red in color, and usually 2–10 mm in size (Figure 8.1; Video 8.1). They may be rounded, stellate, or have sharply circumscribed fern-like margins. A prominent feeding vessel may be present and in some cases a pale halo may surround the lesions. This halo may represent an area of relative devascularization or blood shunting around the vascular abnormality. Angioectasias have been associated with several clinical disorders, including chronic renal failure, aortic stenosis, and von Willebrand's

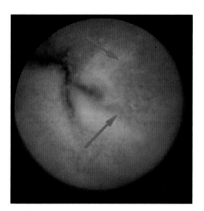

FIGURE 8.1 Large jejunal vascular ectasia (arrows).

disease. They may cause brisk and overt bleeding, melena, or occult bleeding. The reason why mucosal vascular abnormalities bleed remains unclear. Several mechanisms have been postulated including high blood pressure in the mucosal capillaries, abrasion of the mucosa by luminal contents, an ischemic process, or an increased level of vascular endothelial growth factor. The natural history of angioectasia has not been fully clarified because of a lack of long-term prospective trials. It is estimated that less than 10% of all patients with angioectasia will eventually bleed. One study reported a spontaneous cessation of bleeding in 44% of patients with small bowel angioectasia during a mean followup of 13 months.[5]

Telangiectasias differ from angioectasia in their diffuse nature (Figure 8.2; Video 8.2) and tendency to recur. Their macroscopic appearance is virtually identical to that of the angioectasia. Histologically, these lesions consist of dilated blood vessels throughout all layers of the bowel wall, not just in the mucosa or submucosa, as in the case of angioectasia. Thinning of the arterial muscular layer is also considered specific for these lesions. The commonest cause of intestinal telangiectasias is the hereditary hemorrhagic telangiectasia syndrome (HHT or Osler–Weber–Rendu syndrome). HHT is a disorder characterized by vascular lesions involving the skin, mucous membranes, and multiple organ systems outside the gastrointestinal tract. Endoscopically, lesions of HHT are seen more often in the stomach and proximal small bowel. Patients typically present with recurrent episodes of epistaxis by age 10 years. Gastrointestinal bleeding is estimated to occur in 10–40% of affected individuals, usually after age 50, and is generally a chronic low-grade hemorrhage with intermittent melena. Molecular genetic studies have

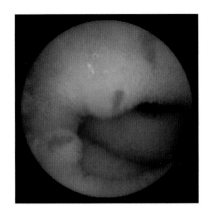

FIGURE 8.2 Multiple small bowel telangiectasias in a patient with Osler–Weber–Rendu syndrome.

shown that HHT is a heterogeneous group of autosomal dominant disorders and that mutations at several different gene sites can produce the clinical syndrome.[6] Telangiectasias may be associated with calcinosis, Raynaud's phenomenon, esophageal motility disorder, sclerodactyly, and telangiectasia, known as the CREST syndrome. Turner's syndrome has also been associated with telangiectasia.

Dieulafoy lesion, also known as caliber-persistent artery, classically occurs in the proximal portion of the stomach but has also been reported throughout the bowel. It tends to affect middle-aged and elderly patients. Its characteristic is that of a larger-than-usual artery found in close proximity to the mucosa surface, and there is often a pinpoint ulcer that causes the bleeding. Establishing the diagnosis of a small bowel Dieulafoy lesion is very difficult; the lesion can easily be missed at endoscopic examination, if it is not bleeding at the time of study. Repeated endoscopies, and some luck, are needed to find this small bleeding site and to treat it.

Small bowel varices are seen in the setting of portal hypertension due to chronic liver disease, portal vein thrombosis, and hepatic vein thrombosis (i.e. the Budd–Chiari syndrome).[7] Varices are usually located within the duodenum and jejunum and may be less likely to rupture because they are deeper within the intestinal wall than esophageal varices. Similar to other types of bleeding due to portal hypertension, such bleeding may be severe. In portal hypertensive enteropathy, small bowel varices may be associated with angioectasias, which are usually minute and petechial in appearance. The latter are usually located in the stomach, but there may also be small bowel involvement. Patients generally present with chronic low-grade bleeding, overt bleeding being less frequent.[8]

Venous ectasia, also called phlebectasia, consists of dilated submucosal veins, usually 3–10 mm in diameter, with thin overlying mucosa. They are a rare cause of obscure bleeding and are not associated with liver disease.

Bleeding from aorto-enteric fistulas often starts with a "herald bleed," an episode of seldom-fatal hemorrhage that ceases spontaneously and is usually followed by massive life-threatening hemorrhage. Over 75% of fistulas communicate with the third or fourth portion of the duodenum. They are most often seen after surgical treatment of aortic aneurysms.[9,10] Mesenteric, gastroduodenal and pancreatic aneurysms may occasionally cause gastrointestinal bleeding. Contrast-enhanced CT usually differentiates pseudocysts and aneurysms; angiography is required to delineate the vascular anatomy.

Neoplasms

Tumors of the small bowel are the second commonest cause of small bowel bleeding and they are the commonest cause in the 30–50 age group.[11] Benign and malignant primary tumors, as well as metastatic tumors, can be found throughout the small intestine. They account for 2–3% of all tumors in the gastrointestinal tract[12] and for 5–10% of cases of small bowel bleeding.[13] Although 75% of tumors found at autopsy are benign, most symptomatic lesions and tumors detected during surgery are malignant. Primary small bowel malignancies may arise from any of the cell types that comprise this organ. The commonest such tumors are adenocarcinomas, accounting for approximately 35–45%. The incidence of other tumors has been reported as follows: carcinoid tumors 20–30%, lymphomas 20%, and sarcomas 10%. Adenocarcinomas are more common in the duodenum and proximal jejunum, whereas lymphomas and carcinoid tumors (Video 8.3) are more frequently found in the distal small bowel. Sarcomas are evenly distributed. Adenocarcinoma may occur sporadically, in association with genetic diseases (e.g. familial adenomatous polyposis coli, Peutz–Jeghers syndrome, and hereditary non-polyposis colorectal cancer (Video 8.4), or in association with chronic intestinal inflammatory disorders such as Crohn's or celiac disease (Figures 8.3, 8.4). Typically, patients

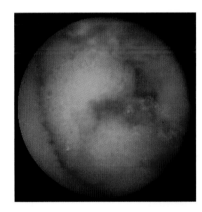

FIGURE 8.3 Infiltrating stenotic mass of the jejunum in a patient with hereditary non-polyposis colorectal cancer syndrome and obscure-occult bleeding.

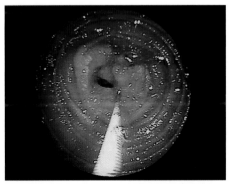

FIGURE 8.4 Same patient as in Figure 8.3. Biopsies performed by double balloon enteroscopy showed an adenocarcinoma.

present with vague, nonspecific abdominal pain, weight loss, and occult or, rarely, overt GI bleeding.[14–17] Benign tumors tend to cause more overt bleeding. Gastrointestinal stromal tumors (GISTs) with smooth muscle differentiation are the commonest tumors associated with episodes of severe bleeding (Video 8.5, 8.6). These tumors are submucosal but often have a mucosal ulcer that causes bleeding. Other lesions, such as adenomatous polyps, adenocarcinoma, lymphoma, polyps associated with syndromes such as the Peutz–Jeghers syndrome (Figures 8.5, 8.6) or familial polyposis, other GISTs, and carcinoid tumors (Figures 8.7–8.9) tend to cause more gradual blood loss. A variety of malignant tumors can metastasize to the small intestine. The commonest are melanoma (Figure 8.10) and breast cancer; others include renal cell cancer, colon cancer, and ovarian cancer. Pancreatic cancer can directly invade the duodenum and present with bleeding.[18]

Vascular tumors

Hemangiomas account for 7–10% of all benign small bowel neoplasms.[19] Although they are formed of proliferating blood vessels, they are rarely malignant. Pathologically they may be divided into capillary, cavernous, and mixed forms. The lesions may be single or, more rarely, multiple. Bleeding from capillary lesions tends to be slow and occult, whereas cavernous lesions cause overt bleeding. The endoscopic presentation of the lesions may be very varied: multiple bluish-colored areas or swollen bluish-colored polypoid formations with a nodular surface and soft elastic consistency.

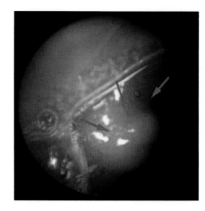

FIGURE 8.7 Small sessile lesion (arrows) in the ileum. Histology revealed a carcinoid tumor.

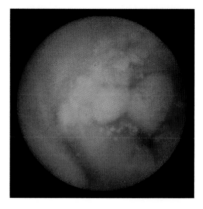

FIGURE 8.8 Vegetation with wide base and nodular surface located in the ileum.

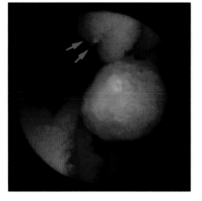

FIGURE 8.5 Pedunculated jejunal polyp (arrows denote stalk) in a patient with Peutz–Jeghers syndrome.

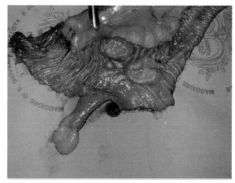

FIGURE 8.9 Same patient as in Figure 8.8. Gross specimen of resected small bowel showing two plaque-like lesions in the ileum. Histology revealed a carcinoid tumor. Note presence of a Meckel's diverticulum.

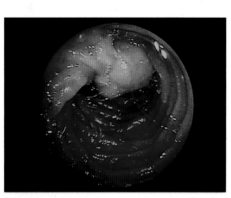

FIGURE 8.6 Same patient as in Figure 8.5 at double balloon enteroscopy.

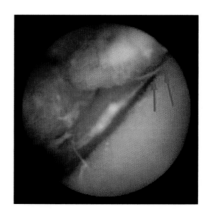

FIGURE 8.10 Infiltrating, stenotic, dark-colored mass (arrows) in the ileum. Histology revealed a metastasis from melanoma.

Hemangiomas of the small bowel may also be associated with cutaneous lesions such as cavernous skin hemangiomas as in the blue rubber bleb nevus syndrome,[20] (Figure 8.11; Video 8.7) or with skin hemangiomas and soft tissue hypertrophy in the Klippel–Trenaunay–Weber syndrome.

Intestinal lymphangiomas are rare neoplasms that account for 3% of benign small bowel tumors. They present with abdominal pain, obstruction or, more rarely, with occult GI bleeding.[21] The lesions appear as circumscribed polypoid masses of soft consistency, with an irregular surface and micronodules.

Kaposi's sarcoma is the most frequent neoplasm in AIDS patients, occurring in about one third of cases. Cutaneous Kaposi's sarcoma generally precedes the intestinal type, which may be found in any part of the gastrointestinal tract. The small bowel is one of the most frequently involved areas. Endoscopically, the lesions appear as macules or nodules of a reddish-purple color that are often ulcerated (Figure 8.12). The diagnostic success of endoscopic biopsy is low, due to the submucosal location of the tumor. In patients with intestinal Kaposi's sarcoma, bleeding is the most frequent sign.[18]

Ulcers, inflammatory lesions, and miscellaneous causes of OGIB

Ulcers and other inflammatory lesions of the small bowel can cause either brisk or slow blood loss in the gastrointestinal tract. Patients with Crohn's disease, the commonest of these conditions, may present with either overt or, more frequently,

chronic blood loss resulting in iron deficiency anemia. Blood loss is rarely the only manifestation of Crohn's disease; in most patients the diagnosis has already been made on the basis of clinical endoscopic and/or radiological findings. However, previously undiagnosed Crohn's disease is incidentally found in 2–6% of patients undergoing capsule endoscopy to evaluate OGIB.[22] Endoscopy may reveal circumscribed alterations such as lymphangiectasia or villous denudation, which may be precursors of the typical aphthous lesions and, in the appropriate clinical context, may be considered as early manifestations of Crohn's disease. Alterations of the mucosa most typical of the advanced stages of the disease are scalloped or shallow aphthae, fissural ulcers, crater-like ulcers that may actively bleed, fistulae, and strictures (Figures 8.13–8.15). These lesions typically show a pattern of discontinuous

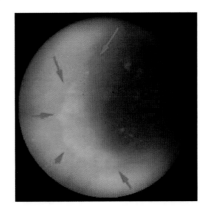

FIGURE 8.13 Ulcer (arrows) in the distal part of the small bowel in a patient with Crohn's disease.

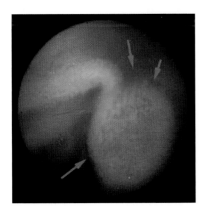

FIGURE 8.11 Swollen bluish-colored polypoid formation in a patient with blue rubber bleb nevus syndrome.

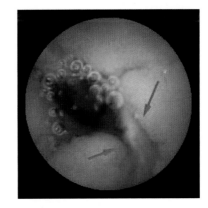

FIGURE 8.14 Fissured ulcer in the ileum (arrows) with slight bleeding in a patient with obscure-occult bleeding. This lesion was proven to be due to Crohn's disease.

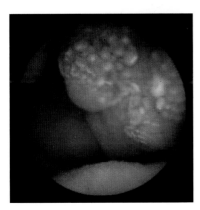

FIGURE 8.12 Nodular reddish-violet small bowel lesion in AIDS patient with biopsy-proven Kaposi's sarcoma.

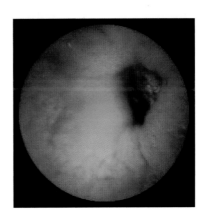

FIGURE 8.15 Ileal stricture in a patient with Crohn's disease in whom the capsule was retained.

involvement, with segments of altered mucosa and intervening segments of normal mucosa ("skip lesions").[23]

A number of different drugs, such as potassium, chemotherapeutic agents, 6-mercaptopurine, and non-steroidal anti-inflammatory drugs (NSAIDs), can cause small bowel ulceration and bleeding. In particular, the intestinal damage due to NSAIDs is probably more common than previously suspected.[24] In NSAID-induced enteropathy, endoscopy shows patchy redness, erosions, ulcers, and strictures that often cause web-like or membrane-like narrowing of the bowel lumen (Figures 8.16, 8.17; Videos 8.8, 8.9).[25–27] All findings are, however, nonspecific (Table 8.2), and may occur with both cyclooxygenase-1 (COX-1) and COX-2 agents. The effects of NSAIDs in the small bowel must be included in differential diagnosis in patients with obscure bleeding.

Patients with chronic mesenteric ischemia may develop small bowel ulcers that are endoscopically indistinguishable from NSAID-induced ulcers (Video 8.10). Small bowel ulcers may also complicate the clinical course of celiac disease, causing occult blood loss and anemia.[28] Ulcers usually occur in the jejunum and ileum and appear endoscopically as aphthous ulcers typical of those seen in Crohn's disease. These ulcers may be difficult to distinguish from lymphoma, which can occur in long-standing celiac disease, and from ulcerative jejuno-ileitis. The latter is a rare condition characterized by the presence of multiple and transverse fissure-type ulcerations located in the jejunum, the ileum, or both, with consequent scarring that can lead to tight intestinal strictures (Figures 8.18, 8.19). Clinically, patients may develop features

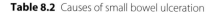

Table 8.2 Causes of small bowel ulceration

Crohn's disease
Drugs (NSAIDs, chemotherapy, enteric coated potassium, 6-mercaptopurine)
Celiac disease
Chronic ulcerative jejuno-ileitis
Vasculitis (systemic lupus erythematosus, Henoch–Schönlein purpura, rheumatoid arthritis, polyarteritis nodosa)
Radiation injury
Mesenteric arterial insufficiency
Infections (cytomegalovirus, tuberculosis, *Yersinia*, typhoid, parasites)
Lymphoma, carcinoma
Hyperacidity syndromes (Zollinger–Ellison syndrome, Meckel's diverticulum)
Toxins (arsenic)
Eosinophilic enteritis
Uremia
Behçet's syndrome
Idiopathic primary ulceration

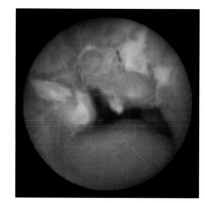

FIGURE 8.18 Multiple jejunal ulcerations with narrowing of lumen in a patient with celiac disease, on a strictly gluten-free diet and with colicky abdominal pain, blood detected in the stool (courtesy of R. de Franchis).

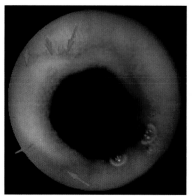

FIGURE 8.16 NSAID-induced jejunal ulcer (arrows) with narrowing of lumen.

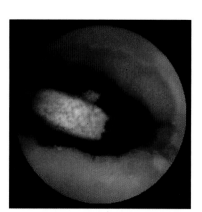

FIGURE 8.17 NSAID-induced membranous stricture; a tablet is visible through the stricture.

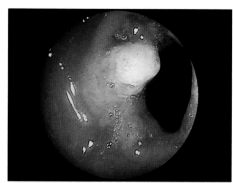

FIGURE 8.19 Same patient as in Figure 8.18 at double balloon enteroscopy. Histology revealed ulcerative jejuno-ileitis.

of malabsorption, colicky central abdominal pain, and occult bleeding with anemia, and do not respond to gluten withdrawal.

Vasculitis is a multisystem disorder characterized by the inflammation and necrosis of blood vessels and is classified by the size of the affected vessels. Organs with the richest vascular supply, such as the gastrointestinal tract, are often affected. Evidence supports the concept that vasculitis, manifesting as a leukocytoclastic process, is linked to immune complex disease with deposition of circulating immune complexes, and abnormal cell-mediated immune response in artery walls, with consequent inflammation and necrosis of the involved tissues. Vasculitis can affect the small bowel in several different ways. Polyarteritis nodosa involves small to medium sized arteries; these may develop aneurysms, which can rupture and bleed massively. Gastrointestinal symptoms are also present in two thirds of cases and include abdominal pain and diarrhea. In Henoch–Schönlein purpura — small vessel vasculitis — the percentage of gastrointestinal symptoms (pain, fever) varies from 29% to 69%. Occult bleeding is common and is related to segmental ischemia and ulceration.

Upper and lower GI bleeding may occur rarely in patients with Wegener's granulomatosis, systemic lupus erythematosus, and rheumatoid arthritis.[29] Infiltrative and infectious processes, usually affecting the mesenteric vessels, may also occur in amyloidosis, sarcoidosis, multiple myeloma, and tuberculosis. Clinically, patients may develop malabsorption, obstruction, and bleeding. Radiation injury to the bowel may initially affect the intestinal mucosa, causing edema, ulceration, and bleeding; progressive occlusive vasculitis with lymphangiectasia, neovascularization, and fibrotic strictures may subsequently develop. Ischemic ulcers can cause acute bleeding, which is typically associated with pain. The endoscopic aspect is characterized by mucosal edema with linear, serpiginous or circumferential ulcers, bleeding, and residual strictures[23] (Figure 8.20).

Small bowel diverticula, like colonic diverticula, occur at the site of perforating blood vessels and may be associated with bleeding. The precise mechanism is not clear. Small bowel diverticulosis, most commonly jejunal, occurs in 0.1–2% of the population. It is estimated that fewer than 5% of all persons with jejunal diverticula actually bleed from them. Evidence of active bleeding is necessary to conclude that a

diverticulum is the site of blood loss. When bleeding does occur from diverticula, it is usually severe and is associated with a high mortality rate. Meckel's diverticulum, a remnant of the vitelline duct, usually located in the distal ileum, is the commonest cause of small bowel bleeding in patients under the age of 25 (Figure 8.9). This anomaly occurs in 2% of the population and is commoner in men than in women. Acid secretion from ectopic gastric tissue in the diverticulum may cause ulceration and acute gastrointestinal bleeding. Occasionally, Meckel's diverticulum can cause intussusception, which is also associated with bleeding. There have also been case reports of inverted Meckel's diverticulum[30] and of angioectasia and submucosal tumors within the diverticulum causing bleeding. In patients with bleeding from a Meckel's diverticulum, surgical resection of the diverticulum is the treatment of choice. In addition to bleeding, pain can be one of the presenting symptoms.[31] Zollinger–Ellison syndrome can also cause small bowel ulceration. Post-bulbar ulceration in the duodenum may occur in 14% of patients with gastrinomas, whereas jejunal ulcers occur in 11%. Small bowel involvement in endometriosis is an uncommon cause of hemorrhage, occurring almost exclusively in the ileum and in approximately 1% of all patients with endometriosis. Small bowel infections, including cytomegalovirus, tuberculosis, *Yersinia* sp., some *Salmonella* species, syphilis, and histoplasmosis, can also cause bleeding.

Hemobilia is caused by communication between the biliary tree and the vascular network of the liver due to neoplasms, vascular aneurysms, liver abscess, or trauma; it can also occur as a result of liver biopsy. Diagnosis of hemobilia may be difficult because of the intermittent nature of the bleeding. Blood may be seen coming from the ampulla of Vater at endoscopy. Hemosuccus pancreaticus can occur in the setting of pancreatic pseudocysts, pancreatitis, or neoplasms with erosion into a major vessel with communication to the pancreatic duct.[9]

It must be pointed out that there are no peculiar endoscopic characteristics for the inflammatory and ulcerative lesions mentioned that are pathognomonic of each specific condition; whenever possible, histological confirmation of such lesions should be obtained.[23]

Diagnostic testing

Diagnosing small bowel bleeding is always challenging. The yield, advantages, and disadvantages of the various diagnostic techniques used for investigating the small bowel in patients with OGIB are presented in Table 8.3.

Radiology

Radiographic contrast studies of the small bowel

The small bowel follow-through (SBFT) has been used to screen the small bowel for a potential bleeding source. SBFT was commonly used because it is simple, readily available, and well tolerated by patients. The problem with SBFT is that it is only possible to visualize gross lesions. Reported diagnostic yields for OGIB range from 0% to 5.6%.[32,33] One study compared the performance of SBFT to that of push enteroscopy

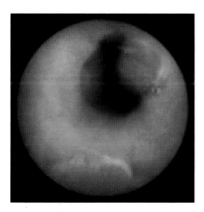

FIGURE 8.20 Ileal stricture in a patient with chronic mesenteric ischemia in whom the capsule was retained.

Table 8.3 Techniques for investigating the small bowel in patients with OGIB: yield, advantages, and disadvantages

Method	Yield	Advantages	Disadvantages
Small bowel follow-through (SBFT)/enteroclysis	0–21%	Minimal side effects or risk	Flat mucosal lesions missed. Enteroclysis requires cooperative patient
CT–MR enteroclysis	—[a]	Reliable methods in the diagnosis of small bowel tumors and extraluminal pathologies. CT enteroclysis may be helpful prior to VCE to detect strictures in high-risk patients	Flat mucosal lesions missed. Increased radiation exposure with CT. Cost and availability of technology
Tagged red blood cell scan	26–78%	Useful for rapid bleeding	Nonspecific, false localizations, and missed bleeding. Cannot determine cause
Meckel's scan	75–100%	Useful in young patients to locate diverticulum	Specific only for Meckel's diverticulum. Usually negative in adults
Angiography	50–86% (massive bleeding); 25–50% (when bleeding has slowed or ceased)	Can intervene in rapid bleeding if source is located	Invasive; risk of i.v. contrast reaction; risk of intestinal infarction with embolization; less likely to determine cause than endoscopy
Helical CT	—[a]	Relatively noninvasive in patients actively bleeding	Radiation exposure
Helical CT angiography	—[a]	Described as useful as a guide for subsequent angiography	Radiation exposure more invasive than helical CT
MR angiography	—[a]	Noninvasive. 3D nature of the examination may help locate the bowel segment that contains the bleeding vessel	Lack of sufficient resolution to visualize hemorrhage from small vessels directly
Capsule endoscopy	40–60%	Allows complete examination of the small bowel. Noninvasive	No intervention capability. Physician interpretation is time-consuming
Push enteroscopy	15–35%	Direct visualization and intervention	Invasive, misses part of jejunum and ileum
Double balloon enteroscopy	50–75%	High success rate of total enteroscopy with therapeutic capabilities	Invasive; time-consuming; requires specialist training
Intraoperative enteroscopy	70–100%	Most complete means of examining the mucosa of the small bowel	Invasive, requires an expert team. Rate of complications

[a] Not known because only a few small series have been published.

(PE) in 40 patients with OGIB. SBFT disclosed a lesion in only one patient (2.5%) while enteroscopy revealed a cause of bleeding in 35% of the patients, although only 15% were located in the small bowel.[34]

Enteroclysis appears to be a more effective tool than SBFT in evaluating patients with OGIB, allowing more detailed visualization of the small bowel. This is accomplished by the passage of a nasoenteric tube into the proximal small bowel, followed by the instillation of barium, methylcellulose, and air. One retrospective study in 128 patients with OGIB found an overall yield of 21% in identifying confirmed or probable lesions.[35] Enteroclysis can be uncomfortable for the patient (e.g. gagging and retching), involves more radiation exposure than SBFT, and is less readily available than SBFT in radiology departments. However, both of these techniques are ineffective in detecting superficial mucosal lesions, particularly angioectasia.[35,36] Because angioectasias are often a major diagnostic concern in patients with small bowel bleeding, radiographic studies have been reserved for those in whom clinical suspicion of a mass lesion is high. Enteroscopy–enteroclysis involves performing a push enteroscopy followed, in the same session, by enteroclysis in cases where the endoscopic examination is negative. Enteroclysis is facilitated by positioning a guidewire in the proximal jejunum during enteroscopy. The guidewire is left in place when the enteroscope is removed; the catheter used to inject contrast medium is pushed along the wire until it reaches the distal limit explored endoscopically. In patients with a negative PE, one study showed that enteroclysis identifies a bleeding source in 8%.[37]

The application of magnetic resonance (MR) imaging technology to enteroclysis is currently being developed; oral magnetic particles provide a negative or black luminal contrast agent, which improves not only visualization of the intestinal lumen but also detection of intestinal wall and extraluminal pathology. Similarly, combining computed tomography (CT) scanning with enteroclysis may improve visualization within the small bowel. Both these methods are described as being reliable for detecting small bowel tumors, Crohn's disease, and small bowel obstruction.[38,39] Overall, the role of radiological evaluation in the elective investigation of patients with OGIB requires re-evaluation in the light of results reported with capsule endoscopy.[40] It is hard to justify the continued use of radiological investigation, with its low sensitivity and poor negative predictive values. Only the use of accurate methods of radiological investigation can justify their continued use and make them complementary to capsule endoscopy in the optimal investigation of small bowel disease.[41]

Nuclear scans

Radioisotope bleeding scans may be helpful when there is evidence of active bleeding. The technetium (^{99m}Tc)-labeled red blood cell (TRBC) scan is most commonly used, although there are limited data on its utility in evaluating OGIB. The overall rate of positivity of TRBC scanning in lower intestinal bleeding is 45% (range, 26–78%). Although relatively sensitive, nuclear medicine scans can only identify a general area of bleeding and are limited in terms of directing treatment. Early scans (e.g. up to 4 hours after injection) may be helpful in gross localization of bleeding when the rate of blood loss exceeds 0.1–0.4 mL/min.[3] Delayed investigation, performed 12–24 hours after injecting the marker, can be deceptive since it does not identify the source of extravasation directly. Because of significant false localization and miss rates, assessment with an alternative test, such as angiography or endoscopy, is usually necessary before an invasive therapeutic intervention can be justified.[42] In one study evaluating technetium-labeled red blood cell scintigraphy, the test failed to localize 85% of bleeding sites[43] and the authors concluded that the scan was of no use either as an investigation preliminary to angiography or as a surgical guide. Overall, bleeding scans are theoretically appealing, but are notoriously disappointing in "real life."

Technetium-99m pertechnetate scintigraphy (Meckel's scan) can be used to show heterotopic gastric mucosa in a Meckel's diverticulum. This test has a sensitivity of 75–100% in children with bleeding.[44] Pentagastrin and cimetidine have been shown to increase the uptake of pertechnetate by parietal cells, and a so-called "enhanced" Meckel's scan with either of these pharmacological agents has been used to increase the sensitivity of this test.[45,46] However, a positive scan only suggests the presence of gastric mucosa and not a definitive bleeding source. Unlike in children, Meckel's scans in adults are usually negative.

Angiography

Visceral angiography may be used to identify the source of major ongoing gastrointestinal bleeding. As with tagged RBC scanning, there are limited data evaluating angiography in the specific clinical setting of OGIB. Angiography may be helpful in evaluating overt OGIB if the bleeding rate is above 0.5 mL/min. Bleeding is manifested as active extravasation of contrast material into the lumen of the bowel. Although less sensitive than nuclear scans, angiography is potentially more effective at localizing the bleeding site and may present a therapeutic opportunity; however, it is more invasive.[47] The yield of angiography ranges from 50% to 86% in patients with massive bleeding, but the percentage drops to 25–50% if bleeding is slower or has ceased.[48] The percentage of cases in which bleeding is active at the time of angiography is below 20%; if the initial angiogram is negative, a repeat study may occasionally be of benefit.[49] Moreover, interventional radiologists can administer embolization therapy, if an appropriate lesion is detected. In patients who are going to surgery, preoperative selective angiographic catheter placement, in conjunction with intraoperative methylene blue dye injection, may be useful to allow more precise localization of bleeding, to minimize the length of small bowel that can be resected.[50] Provocative tests using anticoagulants, vasodilators, or clot-lysing agents to provoke bleeding and increase the likelihood that a bleeding source will be found have been reported.[51] However, since these tests can initiate uncontrolled bleeding, they are rarely used and generally not recommended.

Helical computer aided tomography (CT) has promise as an alternative to more invasive procedures because of its simplicity and its ability to detect a wide variety of causes in intestinal bleeding. However, the specificity and sensitivity of this technique is not yet known.[52]

An innovation in the field of radiology is helical CT angiography.[53,54] This is a technique where the abdominal aorta is catheterized, followed by intra-arterial injections of contrast medium just prior to CT scanning. The site of hemorrhage is identified by extravasation of contrast medium, resulting in a hyperdense area in the intestinal lumen. One study involving 18 patients compared helical CT angiography with conventional angiography.[53] The former technique diagnosed the bleeding site in 13 (72%) patients while standard angiography was diagnostic in only 11 patients. CT angiography was found to be easier and faster than conventional angiography for localizing OGIB and it was useful as a guide for subsequent selective conventional angiography. Preliminary studies on the use of MR angiography to detect GI bleeding have also been reported.[55,56]

Enteroscopy

In evaluating the source of obscure bleeding, it is mandatory that the small bowel be investigated endoscopically. There are four nonsurgical methods available: push enteroscopy, sonde enteroscopy, double balloon enteroscopy, and capsule endoscopy. Intraoperative enteroscopy is considered to be the ultimate endoscopic evaluation of the small bowel. Enteroscopic studies provide an opportunity for both diagnosis and therapy, if a lesion is found.

Push enteroscopy

Push enteroscopy entails peroral insertion of a long endoscope (usually a dedicated enteroscope or a pediatric colonoscope), and allows thorough examination of the distal duodenum and proximal jejunum to approximately 50–100 cm beyond the ligament of Treitz. Use of an overtube backloaded on to the instrument before the examination may help limit looping of the enteroscope within the stomach and facilitate deeper small bowel intubation. The enteroscope is introduced orally into the gastric cavity, taking care not to distend the stomach with excessive insufflation; it is then pushed into the third portion of the duodenum. The enteroscope is retracted to straighten it and the overtube inserted along the enteroscope, which is kept taut to avoid looping, until the distal tip of the overtube reaches the second portion of the duodenum. Further progress of the endoscope within the small bowel is facilitated by changes of position, manual pressure on the abdomen, and hooking and retraction movements. Fluoroscopy is useful, but not indispensable, to position the overtube. Although use of the overtube increases the depth of insertion of a standard enteroscope in the small bowel, its "routine" use is not recommended, since the increased technical complexity of push enteroscopy and the greater risk of complications due to use of the overtube (e.g. perforation and mucosal laceration) do not correspond to a better diagnostic yield.[57] To overcome this problem, new prototype enteroscopes, such as variable stiffness enteroscopes, have been developed.[58]

During both the insertion and retraction phases of push enteroscopy, the entire mucosal surface of the lumen may be accurately evaluated. The use of drugs to reduce gut motility, such as anticholinergic drugs, glucagon, or topical otilonium bromide, may facilitate insertion and optimize visualization. Push enteroscopy is presently considered an effective diagnostic procedure; however, it is time-consuming, technically complex, and carries a moderate risk of complications.[59–64] The main advantages of push enteroscopy are that it is readily available and that biopsy and therapy can be performed through the instrument. The procedure is usually performed under conscious sedation; however, when complex endoscopic treatment is required, monitored or general anesthesia may be appropriate.

Experiences with push enteroscopy have been variable, but the technique has led to identification of a source of bleeding in 38–75% of patients with obscure bleeding.[3] It is striking that most studies report the discovery of lesions using push enteroscopy that should have been within reach of a skillfully employed standard gastroscope; between 28% and 75% of positive findings at push enteroscopy were missed or misinterpreted during previous gastroscopic examinations, often performed several times in many of these patients. Thus, the true diagnostic yield of push enteroscopy for the workup of obscure bleeding in the small bowel may be more realistically in the 15–35% range.[65] Push enteroscopy has been reported to change management in 40–75% of patients[59,66–68] and is especially useful in patients with overt bleeding.[68] Little is known of the long-term outcome in patients with OGIB who undergo investigation by means of push enteroscopy, and published studies are conflicting. One study found that recurrent bleeding occurs in about one third of patients who undergo investigation by push enteroscopy for OGIB, with a trend towards more frequent rebleeding in patients with angioectasia.[69] Push enteroscopy was also found to be effective in improving clinical outcomes by reducing the transfusion requirements and improving quality of life.[67,70–72] However, other investigators came to divergent conclusions.[73–75]

Sonde enteroscopy

Sonde enteroscopy consists of a long, small-caliber endoscope, which is advanced via the nose through the small intestine exploiting normal peristalsis[76] which pulls on a small balloon attached to the tip of the scope. Viewing of the mucosa is only possible on withdrawal of the scope. This technically challenging procedure requires considerable time and does not permit therapy or biopsy. The diagnostic yield of sonde enteroscopy in patients with OGIB has been reported to be between 26% and 54%.[3] With the advent of capsule endoscopy, sonde enteroscopy is now a historical footnote and should not be considered part of the workup of OGIB.

Intraoperative enteroscopy

Intraoperative enteroscopy is the most complete but also the most invasive means of examining the small bowel.[77] It may be carried out with a standard or thin-caliber colonoscope or with a push or sonde enteroscope. The advent of the modern push video-enteroscope has brought a considerable improvement, in terms of reducing trauma to the mucosa, improving endoscopic vision and reaching more distal segments of the small bowel as well as making conventional therapeutic procedures possible. The small bowel should be examined laparoscopically before the scope is introduced into the small bowel at laparotomy, when both direct vision and palpation can be used. Laparoscopy can detect tumors, large vascular lesions, and Meckel's diverticula, obviating the need for intraoperative enteroscopy. The endoscope may be inserted orally, rectally, or via an enterotomy. The risk of infection entailed in the last route can be minimized by using an endoscope covered with sterile cloth or plastic sheathing. If a push enteroscope is available, it may be passed orally and advanced to the ligament of Treitz. An overtube previously backloaded on to the enteroscope is positioned in the second portion of the duodenum. Intubation of the duodenum is usually easier if the enteroscope is inserted before the abdomen is opened. A non-crushing clamp should be placed on the ileocecal junction to prevent colonic distension. If intra-abdominal adhesions are encountered, they should be lysed to facilitate insertion of the enteroscope. The surgeon then grasps the tip of the scope and holds a short segment of small bowel for endoscopic inspection. The mucosa should be examined mainly during anterograde intubation because, on withdrawal, mucosal trauma is difficult to distinguish from vascular lesions. Dimming of the operating room lights facilitates endoscopic visualization. While the endoscopist observes the mucosa, the surgeon examines the serosal surface by transillumination. The mucosa of the small bowel is best visualized by occluding the small bowel distally either with a non-crushing clamp or with an assistant's fingers in 30 cm segments; this latter technique results in less mucosal trauma.

In order to examine the entire small bowel, the surgeon gently telescopes the small bowel on to the enteroscope, and facilitates progress of the instrument with external counterpressure and by reducing loops in the stomach — if an overtube is not used — and in the small bowel. After segmental inspection, the bowel is evacuated of air and the same method is applied for the next 30 cm. Abnormalities are marked serosally or treated endoscopically. Video monitoring allows the endoscopist and the surgeon to work in close cooperation. Each movement requires caution: minimal inflation, progression under visual control, and frequent inspection of the mesentery to avoid excessive stretching and tearing of vessels. The endoscopic procedure usually takes at least one hour.[78]

The diagnostic yield of intraoperative enteroscopy in patients with OGIB has ranged from 70% to 100%.[3] Surgical resection of focal lesions such as neoplasms, ulceration, or strictures may be useful for controlling sources of hemorrhage. It is also possible to endoscopically coagulate isolated vascular lesions; however, finding a lesion does not always equate with cessation of bleeding. In one study, the rebleeding rate after intraoperative enteroscopy was 30% at a mean followup of 19 months.[79]

Intraoperative enteroscopy is a difficult, time-consuming technique, often traumatic to the bowel. Complication rates have ranged from 0% to 52% and include mucosal lacerations and perforations; mortality related to the procedure or to postoperative complications has been as high as 11%.[80,81] Thus, the decision to perform intraoperative enteroscopy requires a careful balance of the risks and benefits of the procedure. It is only considered for patients in whom the source of bleeding is not identified after an in-depth diagnostic evaluation, who have persistent blood transfusion requirement, and in whom the risks of continued bleeding are judged to outweigh the risks of laparotomy. The success of the technique is directly correlated both to a careful preoperative evaluation of the strategy to be adopted and to a close cooperation between surgeon and endoscopist during the examination.[77,78]

The combination of enteroscopy with laparoscopy was recently introduced into clinical practice and appeared to be a promising way of avoiding the laparotomy-related complications of intraoperative enteroscopy. The highest success rate has been found with laparoscopically exteriorizing a loop of mid small bowel and placing the enteroscope through this portal.[82] However, in the approximately 50 cases described in the literature thus far, complete examination of the small bowel was not always possible and almost two thirds of patients required a laparotomy due to the underlying condition.[57] This method is not complication free, and since the advent of VCE and double balloon enteroscopy it has not been further reported.

Double balloon enteroscopy

Double balloon enteroscopy is a new specialized technique. Unlike conventional push enteroscopy, double balloon enteroscopy offers the potential for complete small bowel examination and treatment of previously inaccessible lesions. Compared to intraoperative enteroscopy it has the advantage of enabling biopsies and therapeutic treatments in all parts of the small bowel without laparotomy. Double balloon enteroscopy uses a dedicated video-endoscope with two balloons: one attached to the tip of the endoscope and the other attached at the distal end of a flexible overtube. These may be inflated and deflated with air from a pressure-controlled pump system. The balloons grip the wall of the bowel, thus allowing the endoscope to be advanced without looping. This device can be inserted to the ileocecal valve by timing inflation and deflation of the two balloons so as to alternately push and retract the endoscope and overtube in a coordinated fashion so that the small bowel is telescoped on to the overtube. The procedure can be performed via the oral or anal approach, usually on different days. It is usually performed under fluoroscopic guidance; however, experience in several centers now suggests that fluoroscopy is not always necessary, and that fluoroscopy time can be markedly reduced with increasing experience. Double balloon enteroscopy is a time-consuming technique requiring specialist training and additional staffing. It is safe with a high diagnostic yield in selected patients, and excellent patient tolerability provided that the patient is adequately sedated. Reports on this technique are mainly from Japan and Germany. In one study, a bleeding source in the small intestine was discovered during double balloon enteroscopy in 50 of 66 (76%) patients with OGIB; total enteroscopy was attempted in a subgroup of 28 patients and was successful in 86% of cases, mainly by a combination of both oral and anal approaches.[83] Two recent studies of this technique reported a high frequency of therapeutic intervention. In one study of 137 patients, (66%) with OGIB, a therapeutic procedure was carried out in 104 patients (76%) as a result of double balloon enteroscopy findings.[84] A multicenter trial on 100 patients, of whom 64% had OGIB, came to similar conclusions: the enteroscopic findings played a role in the subsequent treatment in 62% of the patients.[85] Although more studies are required to determine the yield of double balloon enteroscopy versus other currently available imaging modalities, at present it is a complementary procedure to capsule endoscopy for patients with OGIB. In addition, long-term followup data will be necessary to determine whether the interventions performed during double balloon enteroscopy have an impact on patient outcome.

Capsule endoscopy

Video capsule endoscopy (VCE) is a revolutionary procedure that provides direct, noninvasive visualization of the small bowel. The characteristics of this three-part diagnostic system are discussed elsewhere in this book. Since its first clinical use in 2000,[86] VCE has developed from the exotic to a clinical reality. It has greatly extended our diagnostic capabilities in the small intestine, which is of great utility in planning the most appropriate therapeutic strategy. OGIB is now the primary indication for VCE: a potential bleeding source has been identified in 38–93% of patients undergoing VCE,[87] a significant improvement over established methods. The differences in diagnostic yield reported in different studies depend on a combination of factors, among which are varying size of series, use of non-uniform inclusion criteria, variable definitions of obscure bleeding, and quality of pre-VCE endoscopic investigations. In a multi-center trial including

100 patients, the overall diagnostic yield of VCE was 47%.[88] Timing of VCE with respect to the bleeding episode can optimize the diagnostic yield. When stratified by type of bleeding, a positive site of bleeding or active bleeding was seen in 24 of 26 (92%) patients with ongoing obscure-overt bleeding, 4 of 31 (13%) patients with obscure-overt bleeding during the past year, and 19 of 43 (44%) patients with obscure-occult bleeding. These data suggest that patients with ongoing obscure-overt bleeding and with obscure-occult bleeding are most suitable for VCE.[88]

An important issue is the accuracy of diagnostic interpretation in VCE: the clinical significance of some of the lesions observed during capsule recording is not yet fully understood. The assessment of positive and negative predictive values of VCE is hampered by the lack of a gold standard with which to verify diagnoses. However, the few studies that have investigated these parameters to date have been in agreement in reporting a sensitivity of 89%, a specificity of 95%, a positive predictive value between 94% and 97%, and a negative predictive value between 83% and 100%.[88,89] In a recent prospective study comparing VCE with intraoperative enteroscopy, the sensitivity, specificity, and positive and negative predictive values of VCE were 95%, 75%, 95%, and 86%, respectively.[90] In the diagnostic algorithm for OGIB, it is still not entirely clear whether VCE or push enteroscopy should be performed first. Numerous reports have shown VCE to be superior in determining source of bleeding in the small bowel, compared with radiological methods[91–94] (Table 8.4), push enteroscopy[88,95–103] (Table 8.5), and selective mesenteric angiography.[104] Although the currently available capsule technology suffers from some limitations (i.e. it is a purely diagnostic method with no biopsy or therapeutic capability), it has also the undoubted advantage of being a simple, low-risk procedure, and is well tolerated by patients. Based on the results obtained in OGIB patients, it has been suggested that the standard diagnostic protocol for OGIB be modified to start with the least invasive method. Careful repeat studies of the upper and lower GI tract should be performed before evaluation of the small bowel because of the significant miss rate of initial endoscopy; however, VCE should be used immediately if these studies are negative.[88]

This approach is further supported by evidence that the diagnostic yield of push enteroscopy in patients with OGIB is not very high, with the majority of lesions often being identified in the esophagus, stomach, or duodenum.[66,105–107] This suggests indirectly that, before VCE, it would be better to repeat a careful esophagogastroduodenoscopy, rather than performing the more complex push enteroscopy. The results of a recent prospective study conducted on 78 OGIB patients who were randomized to either VCE or push enteroscopy, and in whom the alternative examination was only performed when no lesion was found, or in case of clinical necessity during the one-year followup period, are also in agreement with the strategy of an "early VCE." The percentage of patients having to undergo the alternative examination was 74% for VCE and 77% for push enteroscopy. If the 100% negative predictive value of VCE for small bowel lesions had been taken into account (no push enteroscopy when VCE negative), these percentages would favor VCE (33% vs. 77%). Data from this study show that VCE, as the initial test for OGIB, is the most efficient strategy as regards diagnosis, and that this strategy reduces the number of examinations performed, provided that the negative predictive value of VCE for small bowel lesions is taken into account, and provided also that an upper GI source of bleeding is ruled out before performing VCE.[108]

There are reports on lesions missed by VCE that are subsequently detected by push enteroscopy and the reverse.[88] VCE has also sometimes identified lesions situated in the upper GI tract (Video 8.11) or in the right colon that were missed by previous investigations[88,109,110] (Figures 8.21–8.23). Therefore, although VCE is intended for small bowel examination, the video images from esophagus, stomach, and right colon should be carefully viewed by endoscopists with extensive experience in GI bleeding. In the light of the above, push enteroscopy, double balloon enteroscopy or intraoperative enteroscopy would be relegated to a diagnostic and therapeutic role for lesions previously identified by VCE.[88,89,111–113] In a population at high risk for capsule retention, such as patients with prolonged NSAID use, abdominal radiation injury, known Crohn's disease, or prior major abdominal surgery, screening with a radiological study[114–117] or the patency capsule[118] should precede the capsule examination to minimize the chance of capsule retention caused by a small bowel stricture. Since both small bowel series and enteroclysis often miss strictures, CT enteroclysis with enteral and intravenous contrast enhancement should become the preferred radiological test

Table 8.4 Comparison of capsule endoscopy and small bowel radiology in patients with OGIB

Author	Number of patients	Yield of capsule endoscopy (%)	Yield of small bowel radiology (%)	
Costamagna et al[91]	13	31	5[a]	p < 0.05
Voderholzer et al[92]	8	50	13[b]	p = 0.1
Hara et al[93]	40^	55	3[c]	p < 0.001
Hara et al[93]	19^	63	21[d]	p < 0.02
Golder et al[94]	14	36	0[e]	p < 0.05

[a]SBFT; [b]CT–enteroclysis; [c]SBFT(n = 36)/enteroclysis (n = 4); [d]contrast-enhanced CT; [e]MR enteroclysis; ^majority of patients with OGIB.

Table 8.5 Comparison of capsule endoscopy and push enteroscopy in patients with OGIB

Author	Number of patients	Yield of capsule endoscopy (%)	Yield of push enteroscopy (%)
Lewis & Swain[95]	20	55	30
Ell et al[96]	32	66	28[a]
Hartmann et al[97]	33	76	21[a]
Mylonaki et al[98]	50	76	38[a]
Van Gossum et al[105]	21	52	61
Saurin et al[99]	58	69	38[a]
Adler et al[100]	20	30	10[a]
Mata et al[101]	42	74	19[a]
Pennazio et al[88]	51	59	29[a]

[a]$p < 0.05$.

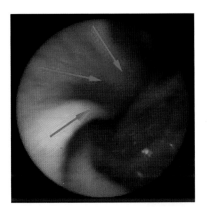

FIGURE 8.21 Prolapsing lesion (arrows) of the second duodenal portion seen at capsule endoscopy in a patient with obscure-overt bleeding.

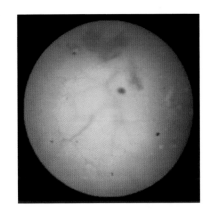

FIGURE 8.23 Angioectasia of the right colon missed at initial endoscopy and subsequently detected at capsule endoscopy.

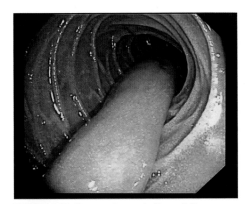

FIGURE 8.22 Same patient as in Figure 8.21. Subsequent push enteroscopy detected a long and narrow polypoid formation with an ulcer on the summit. Histology revealed a lipoma.

prior to VCE when there is a risk of an obstructing small bowel abnormality.[41] Whether the introduction of the patency capsule will impact the use of radiological investigations remains to be seen.

Lastly, it must be stressed that, as for all other diagnostic methods used in OGIB patients, it is unclear how often the results of a capsule examination will alter subsequent treatment of patients. Indeed, much has been reported about the findings at VCE, but considerably less concerning patients' subsequent course. Although most studies appear to indicate a positive influence of VCE diagnosis on clinical outcome,[88,89,119–123] others do not.[124,125] A large prospective multi-center trial with a protocol including a standardized treatment approach after VCE is warranted to answer this question definitively.[126]

Diagnostic and therapeutic approach in patients with OGIB

The patient with chronic unexplained bleeding can be a source of frustration from the standpoints of establishing diagnosis and managing blood loss, especially if exhaustive tests fail to elucidate the cause of bleeding. There are few data on the natural history of OGIB, or its clinical outcome; as a result there is no single cost-effective approach to the management of these patients.[127] Thus the specific approach to diagnostic evaluation of any patient with OGIB will be dictated by the clinical scenario, availability of different technologies, and local expertise. The clinical history and physical examination in a patient with OGIB may suggest a possible cause but is rarely diagnostic. Melena and hematochezia are typically associated with bleeding of the upper and lower GI tracts, respectively, although slow oozing from the distal small bowel or cecum may lead to melena. Heavy bleeding from a site in the upper GI tract can also cause hematochezia. Bloody nasogastric lavage fluid, or a disproportionately high blood urea nitrogen level in relation to the creatinine level, suggests bleeding from the upper rather than the lower GI tract, but these tests are not sensitive for localizing bleeding. A directed history can reveal consumption of medications known to cause mucosal damage or exacerbate bleeding, such as aspirin, anti-platelet agents, or NSAIDs. A coagulation disorder should also be considered in patients with recurrent bleeding (e.g. von Willebrand's disease), whereas a family history of bleeding may indicate the presence of a hereditary syndrome involving the gastrointestinal tract (e.g. Osler–Weber–Rendu syndrome). Endoscopic studies of the upper and lower gastrointestinal tract should be repeated before evaluation of the small bowel, because of the significant miss rate on initial endoscopy. Commonly missed lesions in the upper tract include gastric or duodenal angioectasia, Dieulafoy lesions, Cameron's erosions or ulcers within a hiatal hernia sac, peptic ulcers, neoplasms, esophageal or gastric varices, and gastric antral vascular ectasias. Colonoscopy with ileoscopy should be performed in cases of OGIB, to rule out missed lesions in the colon or an occult ileal process. Lesions most often missed in the colon include angioectasia and neoplasms.[127] The skill and experience of the initial endoscopist, as well as the quality and completeness of the initial evaluation, may be factors that need to be taken into consideration when deciding to repeat upper endoscopy and/or colonoscopy, yet the diagnostic yield of repeat endoscopy may be enough to warrant a second look. Familiarity with bleeding lesions that are rare or subtle is essential when managing patients with OGIB. The gross endoscopic appearance of the proximal small bowel as seen on upper endoscopy can be suggestive of villous atrophy caused by celiac disease leading to iron deficiency anemia, and may identify the need for biopsy. It is equally important to achieve correct visualization of the papilla of Vater, to exclude bleeding from the bilio-pancreatic tract. Once all the standard examinations have been found to be negative, the focus of investigation should be broadened to include the small intestine. The extent of further evaluation will depend on severity of bleeding, patient's age, and also the diagnostic workup that has already been performed. The patient's age is probably the major patient-related factor that could influence strategy in the case of OGIB. Among patients between 30 and 50 years of age, tumors are the most common abnormalities; among patients below 25, a Meckel's diverticulum is the commonest source of bleeding in the small bowel; and among patients above 50, angioectasia and medication-induced ulcers predominate. VCE should be the next diagnostic step in patients with obscure bleeding in whom there is no suspected obstruction. The appropriate subsequent approach should be targeted on the basis of the data acquired by capsule examination. In the patient with overt bleeding, VCE can confirm the small bowel as the site of bleeding, providing a location and guiding further evaluation and therapy.[111] Even if the study is negative for the small bowel in the actively bleeding patient, the study may indicate that the bleeding is actually colonic or even gastric in origin. In a patient with massive hemorrhage, selective mesenteric angiography should also be considered and embolization therapy attempted, if an appropriate lesion is detected. A patient with a small bowel tumor detected by VCE should proceed directly to laparoscopic surgery (Figures 8.24, 8.25). If the site of bleeding is identified in the proximal small bowel and there is no mass, push enteroscopy or double-balloon enteroscopy can be used to re-identify the site and cauterize the lesion (Figures 8.26, 8.27). In cases in which a distal small bowel site is identified, double-balloon enteroscopy or surgical intervention coupled with intraoperative enteroscopy may be necessary. As the entire small bowel has been examined with the capsule examination, surgery can be targeted to examine only the suspected area. If VCE reveals inflammatory disease, histological confirmation should be obtained whenever possible to optimize further management.

If a diffuse small bowel lesion (e.g. angioectasia) is revealed at VCE, surgery can be avoided. Patients with multiple lesions throughout the small bowel are the most difficult to treat,

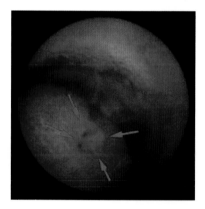

FIGURE 8.24 Ulcerated mass (arrows) in the ileum.

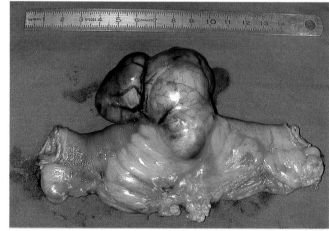

FIGURE 8.25 Same patient as in Figure 8.24. Gross specimen of laparoscopically resected small bowel showing large extraluminal component of the tumor. Histology revealed a GIST.

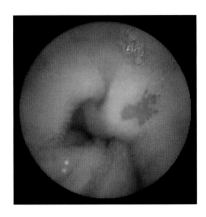

FIGURE 8.26 Jejunal vascular ectasia in a patient with obscure-occult bleeding.

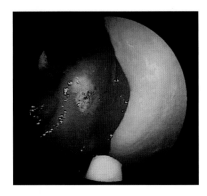

FIGURE 8.27 Same patient as in Figure 8.26. The lesion was cauterized at double balloon enteroscopy.

because of the high rebleeding rate, and they also have the greatest transfusion requirement. Medical therapy including adequate iron supplementation and blood transfusions, together with repeated coagulation sessions of the endo-scopically accessible vascular lesions, should be considered. Although it remains unclear whether medical therapy utilizing hormonal agents (such as compounds of estrogen and progesterone or somatostatin analogues) is effective in stopping or reducing bleeding, this may be an option for these patients.[5,75,128–132]

Repeat VCE has been suggested in patients with recurrent GI bleeding[133] or severe iron deficiency anemia[134] when the initial study is negative or inconclusive. However, if bleeding persists and remains undiagnosed after multiple testing, and blood transfusion requirement persists, the patient should go to surgery with intraoperative enteroscopy. Should the patient be too sick to undergo surgery, sympto-matic treatment must be considered.

In patients with isolated iron deficiency anemia, more occult or intermittent type of bleeding, VCE may be used similarly to identify a bleeding lesion and thus direct subsequent testing or treatment.[111] In this clinical context, VCE may be especially useful in detecting small bowel tumors, which may sometimes also be identified at CT or MR enteroclysis. Although Meckel's diverticulum can occasionally be diagnosed with VCE[135] this lesion should also be excluded via a Meckel's scan. The imminent universal introduction of double balloon

enteroscopy will initially support and strengthen the indication to VCE for patients with OGIB, since after diagnostic clarification with VCE, double balloon enteroscopy allows targeted biopsies and interventional treatment throughout the small bowel, without the need for laparotomy.[113,136] Lastly, it must however be stressed that, despite the use of all available diagnostic methods, in about 15–25% of patients the cause of bleeding is never identified.

References

1. Hussain H, Lapin S, Cappell MS. Clinical scoring systems for determining the prognosis of gastrointestinal bleeding. Gastroenterol Clin North Am 2000;29:445–64.

2. Katz LB. The role of surgery in occult gastrointestinal bleeding. Semin Gastrointest Dis 1999;10:78–81.

3. Anonymous. American Gastroenterological Association medical position statement: evaluation and management of occult and obscure gastrointestinal bleeding. Gastroenterology 2000;18:197–201.

4. Lewis BS. Small intestine bleeding. Gastroenterol Clin North Am 2000;29:67–95.

5. Lewis B, Salomon P, Rivera-MacMurray S, et al. Does hormonal therapy have any benefit for bleeding angiodysplasia? J Clin Gastroenterol 1992;15:99–103.

6. Marchuk D, Guttmacher P, Penner J, et al. Report on the workshop on hereditary hemorrhagic telangiectasia. Am J Med Genet 1998;76:269–73.

7. Tang SJ, Zanati S, Dubcenco E, et al. Diagnosis of small-bowel varices by capsule endoscopy. Gastrointest Endosc 2004;60:129–35.

8. Repici A, Pennazio M, Ottobrelli A, et al. Capsule endoscopy in cirrhotic patients: prevalence and spectrum of small bowel lesions. Gastrointest Endosc 2005;61:158.

9. Bashir RM, Al-Kawas FH. Rare causes of occult small intestinal bleeding, including aortoenteric fistulas, small bowel tumors, and small bowel ulcers. Gastrointest Endosc Clin N Am 1996;9:709–38.

10. Gonzalez-Suarez B, Guarner C, Escudero JR, et al. Wireless capsule video endoscopy: a new diagnostic method for aortoduodenal fissure. Endoscopy 2002;34:938.

11. Lewis BS, Kornbluth A, Waye JD. Small bowel tumours: yield of enteroscopy. Gut 1991;32:763–5.

12. Barelay TH, Schapira DV. Malignant tumors of the small intestine. Cancer 1983;51:878–81.

13. Gill SS, Heuman DM, Mihas AA. Small intestinal neoplasms. J Clin Gastroenterol 2001;33:267–82.

14. Jones DV, Skibber J, Levin B. Adenocarcinoma and other small intestinal neoplasms, including benign tumors. In: Feldman M, Scharschmidt BF, eds. Sleisenger Gastrointestinal and liver disease. WB Saunders, Philadelphia, 1998, pp. 1858–65.

15. Pennazio M, Arrigoni A, Rossini FP. Enteroscopic identification of an adenocarcinoma of the small bowel in a patient with previously unrecognized hereditary nonpolyposis colorectal cancer syndrome. Am J Gastroenterol 1999; 94:1962–6.

16. Wright NH, Howe JR, Rossini FP, et al. Carcinoma of the small intestine. In: Hamilton SR, Aaltonen LA, eds. World Health Organization Classification of tumours. Pathology and genetics of tumours of the digestive system. IARC Press, Lyon, 2000, pp. 71–4.

17. Pennazio M. L'adénocarcinome de l'intestine grêle. Acta Endoscopica 2005;35:179–85.

18. Rossini FP, Risio M, Pennazio M. Small bowel tumors and polyposis syndromes. Gastrointest Endosc Clin N Am 1999;9:93–114.

19. Ramanujam PS, Venkatesh KS, Bettinger L, et al. Hemangioma of the small intestine. Am J Gastroenterol 1995;90:2063–4.

20. Jennings M, Ward P, Madocks JL. Blue rubber bleb naevus disease: an uncommon cause of gastrointestinal tract bleeding. Gut 1988;29:1408–12.

21. Barquist ES, Apple SJ, Jensen DM, et al. Jejunal lymphangioma. An unusual cause of chronic gastrointestinal bleeding. Dig Dis Sci 1997;42:1179–83.

22. Eliakim R, Adler SN. Capsule video endoscopy in Crohn's disease — the European experience. Gastrointest Endosc Clin N Am 2004;14:129–37.

23. Pennazio M. Small-intestinal pathology on capsule endoscopy: inflammatory lesions. Endoscopy 2005;37:769–75.

24. Goldstein JL, Eisen GM, Lewis B, et al. Video capsule endoscopy to prospectively assess small bowel injury with celecoxib, naproxen plus omeprazole, and placebo. Clin Gastroenterol Hepatol 2005;3:133–41.

25. Jonnalagadda S, Prakash C. Intestinal strictures can impede wireless capsule enteroscopy. Gastrointest Endosc 2003;57:418–20.

26. Manetas M, O'Loughlin C, Kelemen K, et al. Multiple small-bowel diaphragms: a cause of obscure GI bleeding diagnosed by capsule endoscopy. Gastrointest Endosc 2004;60:848–51.

27. Yousfi MM, De Petris G, Leighton JA, et al. Diaphragm disease after use of nonsteroidal anti-inflammatory agents: first report of diagnosis with capsule endoscopy. J Clin Gastroenterol 2004;38:686–91.

28. Culliford A, Daly J, Diamond B, et al. The value of wireless capsule endoscopy in patients with complicated celiac disease. Gastrointest Endosc 2005;62:55–61.

29. Sorbi D, Conio M, Gostout CJ. Vascular disorders of the small bowel. Gastrointest Endosc Clin N Am 1999;9:71–92.

30. Hori K, Suzuki Y, Fujimori T. Inverted Meckel's diverticulum. Surgery 2003;133:116–7.

31. Keroack MD, Peralta R, Abramson SD, et al. Case 24-2004. A 48-year-old man with recurrent gastrointestinal bleeding. N Engl J Med 2004;351:488–95.

32. Fried AM, Poulos A, Hatfield DR. The effectiveness of the incidental small-bowel series. Radiology 1981;140:45–6.

33. Rabe FE, Becker GJ, Besozzi MJ, et al. Efficacy study of the small-bowel examination. Radiology 1981;140:47–50.

34. Cellier C, Tkoub M, Gaudric M, et al. Comparison of push-type endoscopy and barium transit study of the small intestine in digestive bleeding and unexplained iron-deficiency anemia. Gastroenterol Clin Biol 1998;22:491–4.

35. Moch A, Herlinger H, Kochman ML, et al. Enteroclysis in the evaluation of obscure gastrointestinal bleeding. Am J Roentgenol 1994;163:1381–4.

36. Rex DK, Lappas JC, Maglinte DD, et al. Enteroclysis in the evaluation of suspected small intestinal bleeding. Gastroenterology 1989;97:58–60.

37. Willis JR, Chokshi HR, Zuckerman GR, et al. Enteroscopy-enteroclysis: experience with a combined endoscopic radiographic technique. Gastrointest Endosc 1997;45:163–7.

38. Schreyer AG, Geissler A, Albrich H, et al. Abdominal MRI after enteroclysis or with oral contrast in patients with suspected or proven Crohn's disease. Clin Gastroenterol Hepatol 2004;2:491–7.

39. Romano S, De Lutio E, Rollandi GA, et al. Multidetector computed tomography enteroclysis (MDCT-E) with neutral enteral and IV contrast enhancement in tumor detection. Eur Radiol 2005;15:1178–83.

40. Liangpunsakul S, Chadalawada V, Rex DK, et al. Wireless capsule endoscopy detects small bowel ulcers in patients with normal results from state of the art enteroclysis. Am J Gastroenterol 2003;98:1295–8.

41. Maglinte DDT. Invited commentary. Radiographics 2005;25:711–8.

42. Zuckerman GR, Prakash C. Acute lower intestinal bleeding. Part I: clinical presentation and diagnosis. Gastrointest Endosc 1998;48:606–16.

43. Voeller G, Bunch G, Britt L. Use of technetium-labeled red blood cell scintigraphy in the detection and management of gastrointestinal hemorrhage. Surgery 1991;110:799–804.

44. Brown CK, Olshaker JS. Meckel's diverticulum. Am J Emerg Med 1988;6:157–64.

45. Baum M. Pertechnetate imaging following cimetidine administration in Meckel's diverticulum of the ileum. Am J Gastroenterol 1981;76:464–5.

46. Yeker D, Buyukunal C, Benli M, et al. Radionuclide imaging of Meckel's diverticulum: cimetidine versus pentagastrin plus glucagon. Eur J Nucl Med 1984;9:316–9.

47. Rollins ES, Picus D, Hicks ME, et al. Angiography is useful in detecting the source of chronic gastrointestinal bleeding of obscure origin. Am J Roentgenol 1991;156:385–8.

48. Browder W, Cerise E, Litwin M. Impact of emergency angiography in massive lower gastrointestinal bleeding. Ann Surg 1986;204:530–6.

49. Lau WY, Ngan H, Chu KW, et al. Repeat selective visceral angiography in patients with gastrointestinal bleeding of obscure origin. Br J Surg 1989;76:226–9.

50. McDonald ML, Farnell MB, Stanson AW, et al. Preoperative highly selective catheter localization of occult small-intestinal hemorrhage with methylene blue dye. Arch Surg 1995;130:106–8.

51. Bloomfeld RS, Smith TP, Schneider AM, et al. Provocative angiography in patients with gastrointestinal hemorrhage of obscure origin. Am J Gastroenterol 2000;95:2807–10.

52. Miller FH, Hwang CM. An initial experience: using helical CT imaging to detect obscure gastrointestinal bleeding. Clin Imaging 2004;28:245–51.

53. Ettorre GC, Francioso G, Garribba AP, et al. Helical CT angiography in gastrointestinal bleeding of obscure origin. Am J Roentgenol 1997;168:727–31.

54. Junquera F, Quiroga S, Saperas E, et al. Accuracy of helical computed tomographic angiography for the diagnosis of colonic angiodysplasia. Gastroenterology 2000;119:293–9.

55. Erden A, Bozkaya H, Turkmen Soygur I, et al. Duodenal angiodysplasia: MR angiographic evaluation. Abdom Imaging 2004;29:12–14.

56. Anderson CM. GI magnetic resonance angiography. Gastrointest Endosc 2002;55:S42–8.

57. Rossini FP, Pennazio M. Small-bowel endoscopy. Endoscopy 2002;34:13–20.

58. Harewood GC, Gostout CJ, Farrell MA, et al. Prospective controlled assessment of variable stiffness enteroscopy. Gastrointest Endosc 2003;58:267–71.

59. Hayat M, Axon TR, O'Mahony S. Diagnostic yield and effect on clinical outcomes of push enteroscopy in suspected small-bowel bleeding. Endoscopy 2000;32:369–72.

60. Foutch G, Sawyer R, Sanowski RA. Push-enteroscopy for diagnosis of patients with gastrointestinal bleeding of obscure origin. Gastrointest Endosc 1990;36:337–41.

61. Barkin JE, Lewis BS, Reiner DK, et al. Diagnostic and therapeutic jejunoscopy with a new, longer enteroscope. Gastrointest Endosc 1992;38:55–8.

62. Pennazio M, Arrigoni A, Risio M, et al. Clinical evaluation of push-type enteroscopy. Endoscopy 1995;27:164–70.

63. Landi B, Tkoub M, Gaudric M, et al. Diagnostic yield of push-type enteroscopy in relation to indication. Gut 1998;42:421–5.

64. Waye JD. Small-intestinal endoscopy. Endoscopy 2001;33:24–30.

65. Goldfarb N, Phillips A, Conn M, et al. Economic and health outcomes of capsule endoscopy: opportunities for improved management of the diagnostic process for obscure gastrointestinal bleeding. Dis Manag 2002;5:249–53.

66. Chak A, Koehler MK, Sundaram SN, et al. Diagnostic and therapeutic impact of push enteroscopy: analysis of factors associated with positive findings. Gastrointest Endosc 1998;47:18–22.

67. Nguyen NQ, Rayner CK, Schoeman MN. Push enteroscopy alters management in a majority of patients with obscure gastrointestinal bleeding. J Gastroenterol Hepatol 2005;20:716–21.

68. Bezet A, Cuillerier E, Landi B, et al. Clinical impact of push enteroscopy in patients with gastrointestinal bleeding of unknown origin. Clin Gastroenterol Hepatol 2004;2:921–7.

69. Landi B, Cellier C, Gaudric M, et al. Long-term outcome of patients with gastrointestinal bleeding of obscure origin explored by push enteroscopy. Endoscopy 2002;34:355–9.

70. Vakil N, Huilgol V, Khan I. Effect of push enteroscopy on transfusion requirements and quality of life in patients with unexplained gastrointestinal bleeding. Am J Gastroenterol 1997;92:425–8.

71. Askin MP, Lewis BS. Push enteroscopic cauterization: long-term follow-up of 83 patients with bleeding small intestinal angiodysplasia. Gastrointest Endosc 1996;43:580–3.

72. Morris AJ, Mokahashi M, Straiton M, et al. Push enteroscopy and heater probe therapy for small bowel bleeding. Gastrointest Endosc 1996;44:394–7.

73. Schmit A, Gay F, Adler M, et al. Diagnostic efficacy of push enteroscopy and long-term follow-up of patients with small-bowel angiodysplasias. Dig Dis Sci 1996;41:2348–52.

74. Romelaer C, Le Rhun M, Beaugerie L, et al. Push enteroscopy for gastrointestinal bleeding: diagnostic yield and long-term follow-up. Gastroenterol Clin Biol 2004;28:1061–6.

75. Barkin JS, Ross BS. Medical therapy for chronic gastrointestinal bleeding of obscure origin. Am J Gastroenterol 1998;93:1250–4.

76. Lewis BS. Enteroscopy. Gastrointest Endosc Clin N Am 2000;10:101–16.

77. Cave LA, Cooley JS. Intraoperative enteroscopy. Indication and techniques. Gastrointest Endosc Clin N Am 1996;6:793–802.

78. Gay G, Pennazio M, Delmotte JS, et al. Intraoperative enteroscopy. In: Rossini FP, Gay G, eds. Atlas of enteroscopy. Springer-Verlag Italia, Milan, 1998, pp. 51–4.

79. Douard R, Wind P, Panis Y, et al. Intraoperative enteroscopy for diagnosis and management of unexplained gastrointestinal bleeding. Am J Surg 2000;180:181–4.

80. Lewis BS, Wenger JS, Waye JD. Small bowel enteroscopy and intraoperative enteroscopy for obscure gastrointestinal bleeding. Am J Gastroenterol 1991;86:171–4.

81. Desa LA, Ohri SK, Hutton KA, et al. Role of intraoperative enteroscopy in obscure gastrointestinal bleeding of small bowel origin. Br J Surg 1991;78:192–5.

82. Matsushita M, Hajiro K, Takakuwa H, et al. Laparoscopically assisted panenteroscopy for gastrointestinal bleeding of obscure origin. Gastrointest Endosc 1997;46:474–5.

83. Yamamoto H, Kita H, Sunada K, et al. Clinical outcomes of double-balloon endoscopy for the diagnosis and treatment of small-intestinal diseases. Clin Gastroenterol Hepatol 2004;2:1010–6.

84. May A, Nachbar L, Ell C. Double-balloon enteroscopy (push-and-pull enteroscopy) of the small bowel: Feasibility and diagnostic and therapeutic yield in patients with suspected small bowel disease. Gastrointest Endosc 2005;62:62–70.

85. Ell C, May A, Nachbar L, et al. Push-and-pull enteroscopy in the small bowel using the double-balloon technique: results of a prospective European multicenter study. Endoscopy 2005;37:613–6.

86. Iddan G, Meron G, Glukhovsky A, et al. Wireless capsule endoscopy. Nature 2000;405:417.

87. Tang SJ, Haber GB. Capsule endoscopy in obscure gastrointestinal bleeding. Gastrointest Endosc Clin N Am 2004;14:87–100.

88. Pennazio M, Santucci R, Rondonotti E, et al. Outcome of patients with obscure gastrointestinal bleeding after capsule endoscopy: report of 100 consecutive cases. Gastroenterology 2004;126:643–53.

89. Delvaux M, Fassler I, Gay G. Clinical usefulness of the endoscopic video capsule as the initial intestinal investigation in patients with obscure digestive bleeding: validation of a diagnostic strategy based on the patient outcome after 12 months. Endoscopy 2004;36:1067–73.

90. Hartmann D, Schmidt H, Bolz G, et al. A prospective two-center study comparing wireless capsule endoscopy with intraoperative enteroscopy in patients with obscure GI bleeding. Gastrointest Endosc 2005;61:826–32.

91. Costamagna G, Shah SK, Riccioni ME, et al. A prospective trial comparing small bowel radiographs and video capsule endoscopy for suspected small bowel disease. Gastroenterology 2002; 123: 999-1005.

92. Voderholzer WA, Ortner M, Rogalla P, et al. Diagnostic yield of wireless capsule enteroscopy in comparison with computed tomography enteroclysis. Endoscopy 2003;35:1009–14.

93. Hara AK, Leighton JA, Sharma VK, et al. Small bowel: preliminary comparison of capsule endoscopy with barium study and CT. Radiology 2004;230:260–5.

94. Golder SK, Schreyer AG, Endlicher E, et al. Comparison of capsule endoscopy and magnetic resonance (MR) enteroclysis in suspected small bowel disease. Int J Colorectal Dis 2006;21:97–104.

95. Lewis BS, Swain P. Capsule endoscopy in the evaluation of patients with suspected small intestinal bleeding: Results of a pilot study. Gastrointest Endosc 2002;56:349–53.

96. Ell C, Remke S, May A, et al. The first prospective controlled trial comparing wireless capsule endoscopy with push enteroscopy in chronic gastrointestinal bleeding. Endoscopy 2002;34:685–9.

97. Hartmann D, Schilling D, Bolz G, et al. Capsule endoscopy versus push enteroscopy in patients with occult gastrointestinal bleeding. Z Gastroenterol 2003;41:377–82.

98. Mylonaki M, Fritscher-Ravens A, Swain P. Wireless capsule endoscopy: a comparison with push enteroscopy in patients with gastroscopy and colonoscopy negative gastrointestinal bleeding. Gut 2003;52:1122–6.

99. Saurin JC, Delvaux M, Gaudin JL, et al. Diagnostic value of endoscopic capsule in patients with obscure digestive bleeding: blinded comparison with video push-enteroscopy. Endoscopy 2003;35:576–84.

100. Adler DG, Knipschield M, Gostout C. A prospective comparison of capsule endoscopy and push enteroscopy in patients with GI bleeding of obscure origin. Gastrointest Endosc 2004;59:492–8.

101. Mata A, Bordas JM, Feu F, et al. Wireless capsule endoscopy in patients with obscure gastrointestinal bleeding: a comparative study with push enteroscopy. Aliment Pharmacol Ther 2004;20:189–94.

102. Appleyard M, Fireman Z, Glukhovsky A, et al. A randomized trial comparing wireless capsule endoscopy with push enteroscopy for the detection of small-bowel lesions. Gastroenterology 2000;119:1431–8.

103. Friedman S. Comparison of capsule endoscopy to other modalities in the small bowel. Gastrointest Endosc Clin N Am 2004;14:51–60.

104. Krauss NG, Hochberger J, Hahn EG. Prospective comparison of wireless capsule endoscopy (CE) with radionuclide dynamic scintiscan (RDS) or selective angiography (SA) in patients with acute gastrointestinal bleeding. Gastroenterology 2005;128:648.

105. Van Gossum A, Hittelet A, Schmit A, et al. A prospective comparative study of push and wireless-capsule enteroscopy in patients with obscure digestive bleeding. Acta Gastroenterol Belg 2003;66:199–205.

106. Descamps C, Schmit A, Van Gossum A. "Missed" upper gastrointestinal tract lesions may explain "occult" bleeding. Endoscopy 1999;31:452–5.

107. Zaman A, Katon RM. Push enteroscopy for obscure gastrointestinal bleeding yields a high incidence of proximal lesions within reach of a standard endoscope. Gastrointest Endosc 1998;47:372–6.

108. de Leusse A, Vahedi K, Edery J, et al. Efficiency of capsule endoscopy and push enteroscopy as the first line exploration of obscure gastrointestinal bleeding. A prospective randomized pragmatic study. Gastroenterology 2007;132:855–862.

109. Gay G, Delvaux M, Fassler I, et al. Localization of colonic origin of obscure bleeding with the capsule endoscope: a case report. Gastrointest Endosc 2002;56:758–762.

110. Tang SJ, Christodoulou D, Zanati S, et al. Wireless capsule endoscopy for obscure gastrointestinal bleeding: a single-centre, one-year experience. Can J Gastroenterol 2004;18:559–65.

111. Lewis BS, Goldfarb N. The advent of capsule endoscopy — a not so futuristic approach to obscure gastrointestinal bleeding. Aliment Pharmacol Ther 2003;17:1085–96.

112. Rey JF, Gay G, Kruse A, et al. ESGE Guidelines Committee. European Society of Gastrointestinal Endoscopy guideline for video capsule endoscopy. Endoscopy 2004;36:656–8.

113. Ell C, May A. Capsule status 2004. Endoscopy 2004;36:1107–8.

114. Ginsberg GG, Barkun AN, Bosco JJ, et al. Wireless capsule endoscopy: August 2002. Gastrointest Endosc 2002;56:621–4.

115. O'Loughlin C, Barkin JS. Wireless capsule endoscopy: summary. Gastrointest Endosc Clin N Am 2004;14:229–37.

116. Pennazio M. Capsule non-passage in clinical practice. In: Jacob H, ed. Proceedings of the Second International Conference on Capsule Endoscopy. Rochash Printing, Haifa, Israel, 2003, pp. 15–17.

117. Jonnalagadda S, Prakash C. Intestinal strictures can impede wireless capsule enteroscopy. Gastrointest Endosc 2003; 57:418–20.

118. Spada C, Spera G, Riccioni M, et al. A novel diagnostic tool for detecting functional patency of the small bowel: the Given patency capsule. Endoscopy 2005;37:793–800.

119. Carey E, Leighton JA, Heigh R, et al. Single center outcomes of 260 consecutive patients undergoing capsule endoscopy. Am J Gastroenterol 2007;102:89–95.

120. Favre O, Jacob P, Daudet J. Impact of videocapsule findings in the management and evolution of unexplained digestive bleeding: 50 patients with 11 months follow-up. Gut 2004;53 (suppl VI):73.

121. Neu B, Ell C, May A, et al. Capsule endoscopy versus standard tests in influencing management of obscure digestive bleeding: results from a German multicenter trial. Am J Gastroenterol 2005;100:1736–42.

122. Schmidt H, Hartmann D, Kinzel F, et al. Long-term outcome in patients with chronic gastrointestinal bleeding: results of a prospective controlled trial comparing capsule endoscopy to intraoperative enteroscopy. Program & Abstracts of the Fourth International Conference on Capsule Endoscopy, Miami, USA, 2005, p. 63.

123. Botelberge T, De Looze D, Beke C, et al. The impact of capsule endoscopy on the outcome of presumed bleeding of small intestinal origin. Program & Abstracts of the Fourth International Conference on Capsule Endoscopy, Miami, USA, 2005, p. 61.

124. Rastogi A, Schoen RE, Slivka A. Diagnostic yield and clinical outcomes of capsule endoscopy. Gastrointest Endosc 2004;60:959–64.

125. Saurin JC, Delvaux M, Vahedi K, et al. Clinical impact of capsule endoscopy compared to push enteroscopy: 1-year follow-up study. Endoscopy 2005;37:318–23.

126. Pennazio M, Eisen G, Goldfarb N. ICCE Consensus for Obscure Gastrointestinal Bleeding. Endoscopy 2005;37:1046–50.

127. Leighton JA, Goldstein J, Hirota W, et al. Obscure gastrointestinal bleeding. Gastrointest Endosc 2003;58:650–5.

128. Van Cutsem E, Rutgeerts P, Vantrappen G. Treatment of bleeding gastrointestinal vascular malformations with oestrogen-progesterone. Lancet 1990;335:953–5.

129. Junquera F, Feu F, Papo M, et al. A multicenter, randomized, clinical trial of hormonal therapy in the prevention of rebleeding from gastrointestinal angiodysplasia. Gastroenterology 2001;121:1073–9.

130. Rossini F, Arrigoni A, Pennazio M. Octreotide in the treatment of bleeding due to angiodysplasia of the small intestine. Am J Gastroenterol 1993;88:1424–7.

131. Orsi P, Guatti-Zuliani C, Okolicsanyi L. Long-acting octreotide is effective in controlling rebleeding angiodysplasia of the gastrointestinal tract. Dig Liver Dis 2001;33:330–4.

132. Bauditz J, Schachschal G, Wedel S, et al. Thalidomide for treatment of severe intestinal bleeding. Gut 2004;53:609–12.

133. Jones BH, Fleischer DE, Sharma VK, et al. Yield of repeat wireless video capsule endoscopy in patients with obscure gastrointestinal bleeding. Am J Gastroenterol 2005;100:1058–64.

134. Bar-Meir S, Eliakim R, Nadler M, et al. Second capsule endoscopy for patients with severe iron deficiency anemia. Gastrointest Endosc 2004;60:711–3.

135. Mylonaki M, MacLean D, Fritscher-Ravens A, et al. Wireless capsule endoscopic detection of Meckel's diverticulum after nondiagnostic surgery. Endoscopy 2002;34:1018–20.

136. Pennazio M. Small-bowel endoscopy. Endoscopy 2004;36:32–41.

CHAPTER **9**

Approach to the Patient with Inflammatory Bowel Disease

Tanja Kühbacher and Stefan Schreiber

KEY POINTS

1. Definition and etiology of inflammatory bowel disease (IBD).

2. Use of capsule endoscopy in diagnosing IBD.

3. Use of capsule endoscopy for treatment decisions in IBD.

4. Advantages and limits of capsule endoscopy in IBD in comparision to conventional techniques.

Definition

Crohn's disease and ulcerative colitis are defined as nonspecific inflammatory bowel diseases (IBD). Both disorders are chronic inflammatory conditions affecting the intestine. A typical course of these conditions is characterized by episodes of active disease interspersed with phases of remission. Maintenance of remission is therefore an important issue, particularly because some patients can develop a chronic state of activity that is characterized by refractoriness to most anti-inflammatory drugs. Since the first description of a Crohn's disease case by Morgagni in 1761, basic and clinical research has led to a great improvement in the understanding of etiology of the diseases, diagnostic techniques, and therapy of IBD. Nevertheless many aspects regarding the molecular pathogenesis still remain unclear and clinical management of both diseases is still imperfect.[1-5]

Etiology and pathophysiology

The lifetime prevalence of inflammatory bowel disease in Europe and the United States is as high as 0.5%. Epidemiological studies have shown an association of a western lifestyle and better hygienic conditions as risk factors for the development of inflammatory bowel diseases. A polygenic predisposition for both diseases has seemed likely, but until recently has been formally established only for Crohn's disease. In 2001 large cohort studies of families and twins identified the first disease gene (*CARD15* encoding for the protein NOD2). In addition to this gene, which carries an odds ratio of up to 40, at least two other disease genes have been identified with smaller associated risks.

Acute disease is characterized by an increase of neutrophil granulocytes and monocytes from the peripheral blood entering the intestinal mucosa. An immunological activation of intestinal granulocytes, macrophages, T- and B-lymphocytes can be seen. Infectious agents such as *Mycobacterium paratuberculosis* have been repeatedly discussed as an etiologic agent, but proof is still lacking. An imbalance of the immune system with an increase of proinflammatory cytokines seems to be an important element in the pathophysiology of inflammatory bowel disease. Recent studies have also demonstrated an interplay between a disturbance of the microbial flora and the loss of the intestinal barrier function, which could promote mucosal invasion of bacterial agents (Figure 9.1; Table 9.1).[6-30]

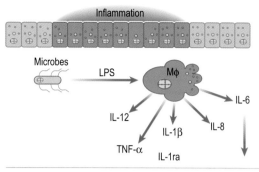

FIGURE 9.1 Immunological activation in IBD. Immunological activation of lymphocytes by monocytes and macrophages is shown by the T-cell antigen-receptor cell–cell contact and the accessory proinflammatory cytokines IL-1β and TNF-α. Macrophages and granulocytes secrete proinflammatory cytokines such as IL-8 and IL-6. The IL-1 receptor-antagonist is able to block the binding of IL-1β to the receptor by competitive binding. Bacterial products, such as lipopolysaccharide (LPS), lead to a nonspecific stimulation in the colonic mucosa.

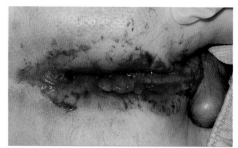

FIGURE 9.2 Severe perianal fistulization in a 20-year-old male patient with Crohn's disease.

Clinical presentation and pathology

Typical clinical symptoms of Crohn's disease and ulcerative colitis include fever, abdominal pain, diarrhea and, especially for ulcerative colitis, bloody stools. Weight loss and malnutrition with the development of anemia and iron deficiency are common. The inflammation in ulcerative colitis is mainly confined to the mucosa and is limited to the large intestine with a continuous inflammation pattern extending distally from the rectum. Depending on the extent of inflammatory lesions, proctitis, proctosigmoiditis, left-sided colitis, and pancolitis are defined as sub-entities. In patients with pancolitis the terminal ileum might be inflamed as a "backwash ileitis." The gastroduodenal tract is never involved. By contrast, Crohn's disease is characterized by transmural inflammation of the mucosa, which can affect the entire gastrointestinal tract from the mouth to the anus. The pattern of inflammation is typically segmental with a tendency to develop fistulae and abscesses (Figure 9.2). Fistulae (e.g. entero-enteral and/or entero-cutaneous) and the development of stenoses may

be associated with active or chronic inflammation but can also occur in the absence of active intestinal inflammation in Crohn's disease. Histologically, crypt abscesses are typical for ulcerative colitis, and epithelioid granulomas are the hallmark of Crohn's disease but are not always present (Figure 9.3). Extra-intestinal complications including liver involvement (both hepatitis and sclerosing cholangitis), various bone and joint disorders, iritis, uveitis, and erythema nodosum are described for both diseases (Figure 9.4). Severe complications such as abscesses, ileus, toxic megacolon, blood loss, perforation and/or the development of colorectal carcinoma can be the sequel of both diseases (Table 9.2).[31–40]

Impact of diagnostic procedures

Disease history, physical examination, and blood test are very important but there are no specific diagnostic criteria for IBD. It is assumed that the rise in disease incidence of the last decades can be partially attributed to the development of modern diagnostic techniques. Most certainly innovations in diagnostic techniques have helped to more precisely distinguish between ulcerative colitis and Crohn's disease. Diagnostic tools include barium contrast studies, endoscopy, CT and MRI scan, capsule endoscopy, and ultrasonography. The general diagnostic workup strategy is quite similar for suspected Crohn's disease and ulcerative colitis. Treatment is influenced by the anatomical site of manifestation, inflam-

Table 9.1 Risk factors for IBD

Risk factors	Crohn's disease	Ulcerative colitis
Genetic predisposition	Association proven	Association suspected, not proven
Smoking	Positive association	Negative association
Medication for contraception	Small studies suggest association, no definite proof	Remains unclear
Bacterial infection in childhood (e.g. measles)	Seems to be associated, not definitely proven	Unclear
Hygienic standards in childhood	Positive association	Association unclear
Environment	Positive association	Positive association

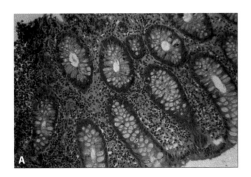

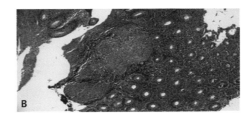

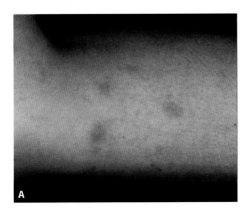

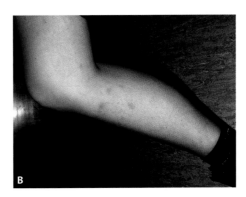

FIGURE 9.3 Histopathological findings of IBD. (a) Typical histopathological picture of ulcerative colitis with granulocyte infiltration and crypt abscesses. (b) Typical histopathological findings in a mucosal biopsy of a Crohn's disease patient with an epithelioid granuloma.

FIGURE 9.4 (a) Extra-intestinal manifestation in IBD. (b) Erythema nodosum in a 33-year-old female patient with Crohn's disease.

Table 9.2 Crohn's disease and ulcerative colitis: disease patterns

Symptoms	Histological findings	Localization	Extra-intestinal manifestation
Crohn's disease			
Abdominal pain: 70–80%	Mucosal ulcers	25–40% small bowel	Anal fistula: 10–40%
Diarrhea: 70–90%	Transmural inflammation	15–35% large bowel	Arthralgia: 10–30%
	Submucosal infiltration	40–55% combined large and small bowel	Erythema nodosum
	Epithelioid granulomas	2–3% complete gastrointestinal tract	Iritis
			Uveitis
			Entero-enteral fistula
			Entero-cutaneous fistula
Ulcerative colitis			
Abdominal pain: 40–80%	Crypt abscesses	50–70% rectum and sigmoid	Anal fistula: 0–5%
Diarrhea: 80–90%	Ulceration of surface epithelium	20–30% pancolitis	Arthralgia: 10–30%
	Purulent exudate	No manifestation in the upper gastrointestinal tract	Erythema nodosum
			Pyoderma gangrenosum
			Uveitis
			Episcleritis
			Primary sclerosing cholangitis (PSC)

Contrast x-ray studies

mation pattern, and course of the disease but also the subtype (Crohn's disease versus ulcerative colitis or indeterminate colitis, respectively). Therapeutic agents include aminosalicylates, oral or topical glucocorticoids, immunosuppressants like azathioprine, methotrexate and cyclosporine, biological therapeutics like various anti-TNF-α antibody drugs, probiotics, and surgical therapies (Figure 9.5).[41–60]

For many years, barium x-ray (enema) studies played a major role in the diagnostic workup of colonic IBD. After the barium contrast agent is administered, air is insufflated in order to achieve a double contrast effect showing the surface contour of the mucosa, including the haustrations. As the lumen is

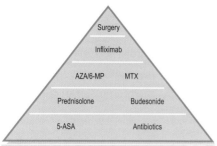

FIGURE 9.5 Therapeutic regimen for Crohn's disease. Treatment is started in mild IBD disease with 5-ASA; in moderate to severe disease, prednisolone is added; and in case of refractoriness to therapy immunosuppressants, e.g. azathioprine and/or biological therapeutics (infliximab or other TNF-α agents), are added. Surgery is in many cases the last resort.

filled with air, the width of large bowel can be assessed and mucosal irregularities defined. With the development of endoscopy and modern imaging techniques without the use of radiation, use of barium techniques has decreased and is now limited to the examination of the small bowel only or is used in case of difficulties, e.g. if endoscopic examination fails as a primary imaging technique.

In contrast to ulcerative colitis, where the inflammation is strictly limited to the colon, the inflammatory pattern in Crohn's disease can involve any part of the gastrointestinal tract. Inflammation of the small bowel can be found in 30–40% of the Crohn's disease patient population. Therefore the examination of the small intestine is important for the diagnosis of Crohn's disease but also in the differentiation between Crohn's disease and ulcerative colitis. Enteroclysis has been used for detection of inflammatory lesions, strictures, stenosis or fistulization in the small bowel. In Crohn's disease,

extra-intestinal inflammatory masses show as a separation of barium-filled bowel loops. Chronic ulceration in the terminal ileum produces a characteristic cobblestone appearance. Fistulae may be found as isolated tracks connecting viscera or leading to the skin, and sinuses may appear as blind-ending tracks with extra-intestinal contrast within inflammatory masses. Chronic or severe inflammation can lead to fibrotic stenosis which may be long (the typical string sign seen on enteroclysis) and, if tight enough, have a prestenotic dilatation (Figure 9.6). A disadvantage of this diagnostic method is the dose of radiation to the patients, who are often of childbearing potential or of young age. In addition, enteroclysis patients are further inconvenienced by the preparation. A nasogastric tube has to be placed in the duodenum and barium contrast is administered via the tube. Placing of the nasogastric tube is unpleasant and sometimes painful for the patient.[61–65]

Magnetic resonance-based small bowel imaging studies

To avoid radiation, magnetic resonance (MR) based imaging is used at many centers instead of enteroclysis. Both techniques, conventional and MR-based enteroclysis, have a similar yield with regards to small bowel lesions. Interestingly, the use of oral gadolinium contrast without a nasogastric feeding tube is equivalent to giving contrast agent via a gastroduodenal tube.

The costs of MR enteroclysis are higher than those of conventional enteroclysis and availability may be a problem. However, in addition to the small bowel itself, MR studies may provide additional information about extraluminal, deep pelvic and perianal anatomy. This is particularly useful when it comes to assessment of perianal and rectal fistulae (Figure 9.7). [66,67]

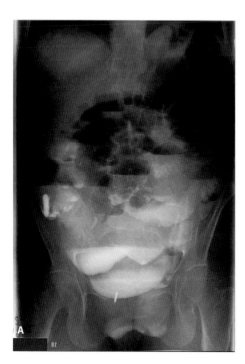

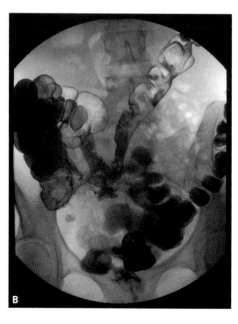

FIGURE 9.6 Contrast x-ray of the small intestine and enteroclysis. (a) Abdominal x-ray after a small bowel follow-through of a 28-year-old female patient with typical signs of obstruction due to stenosis in the small bowel by Crohn's disease. (b) Conventional enteroclysis with fistulization between the transverse and descending colon and a fistula to the sacrum and transverse colon.

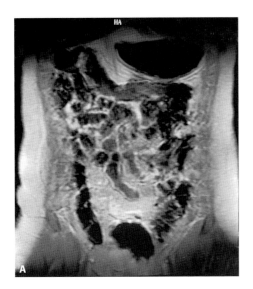
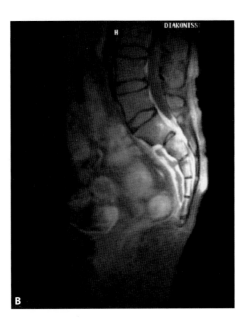

FIGURE 9.7 MR enteroclysis. (a) Stenosis in the small intestine and small fistula in a 42-year-old female with Crohn's disease. (b) Retrosacral abscess in a patient with Crohn's disease.

Computed tomography

The computed tomography (CT) scan is used mostly to detect abscesses, fistulae, or inflammatory masses. The MRI scan is superior to the CT scan in most cases; only abscess detection appears to be better by CT scan. A disadvantage again is the high degree of radiation. An important role for CT scanning is the acute assessment of the critically ill patient as the procedure is fast, readily available, and highly standardized.[68,69]

Endoscopy

Endoscopy has become an important part of the diagnostic investigation of Crohn's disease or ulcerative colitis as lesions can be visualized and tissue obtained using a biopsy forceps for histological or microbiological examinations. The histological pattern of the lesions, together with the anatomical extent of inflammation, have become the major diagnostic criteria that differentiate between the two forms of inflammatory bowel disease and in the differential diagnosis of infectious or ischemic colitis. Endoscopic surveillance for colon cancer has become another important application in patients with long-standing ulcerative or Crohn's colitis.

Typical findings for ulcerative colitis on endoscopy are a friable and erythematous mucosa, with a loss of vascular pattern, a granular mucosal surface, reticular erosive lesions, edema, spontaneous bleeding, deep ulcerations, and pseudopolyps (Figure 9.8). Endoscopic findings in Crohn's disease are much more variable. Inflammatory lesions in the large bowel are usually discontinuous with healthy mucosa between inflammatory lesions. Aphthous ulcers with or without deep, irregular longitudinal ulcerations are often found separated by normal mucosa. Deep longitudinal or serpiginous ulcerations ("snail track ulcers") are typical for Crohn's disease (Figure 9.9). Chronic or recurrent ulceration and inflammation can promote formation of stenoses, which can be caused either by severe edema of the mucosa or by non-inflamed scar tissue. Crohn's disease affects the colon alone in about 30% of cases, while 40% of patients have ileocolonic manifestations of the disease. The rest involve only the small bowel and in a small number of cases also the gastroduodenal and esophageal region. Isolated Crohn's disease in the upper gastrointestinal tract is quite rare (Table 9.3). The form and type of lesions are similar to those seen more distally.

Complications of endoscopy are uncommon and include bleeding after the biopsy procedure, perforation, and anesthesia problems (e.g. overdosage of sedation with midazolam or propofol). Patients complain often about the preparation

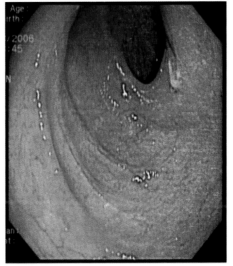

FIGURE 9.8 Endoscopic picture of active ulcerative colitis. Typical signs of inflammation in the sigmoid segment of the colon with redness of the mucosa, friability, and spontaneous bleeding.

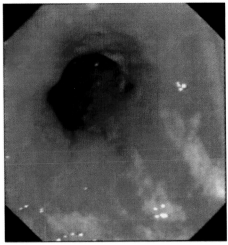

FIGURE 9.9 Endoscopic picture of active Crohn's disease. Typical longitudinal "snail track" ulceration in the ascending colon in a 25-year-old Crohn's disease patient.

the training of physicians. If adequate equipment and a skilled examiner are available, ultrasonography can play a major role in the followup of patients with inflammatory bowel disease. Assessment of blood flow parameters in addition to the diameter of the bowel wall can differentiate between inflammatory and non-inflammatory stenoses (Figure 9.10). Ultrasonography can be used to noninvasively detect and drain abscesses.

While endoscopic ultrasound in the upper GI tract is mainly used for stomach, bile duct and pancreas imaging, this technique plays a major role in the diagnosis of perianal fistulae. Rectal, endoscopic ultrasound (including transperineal examination) is equivalent to magnetic resonance studies in the detection of fistula and abscess formation. Although this technique is much cheaper than MR studies, it requires a skilled examiner and has not been standardized.[77,78]

Open fields — charting lesions in the small bowel

The examination of the mucosa of the large bowel can be easily performed by endoscopy, whereas the complete examination of the small bowel is still a challenge. The small intestine is about 6 meters long and is responsible for the absorption of salts, minerals, nutrients, vitamins, and water. Thirty percent of Crohn's disease patients have inflammatory lesions exclusively in the small intestine. For these patients, safe and exact examination methods that can be repeated at intervals are needed. Enteroclysis with either x-ray or MR contrast agents was for a long time the only choice (with sonography being added in specialized centres). The push-pull/double balloon enteroscope has recently been added as a useful technique but has several disadvantages. Examination times are very long, which in turn requires

procedure that involves an orthograde lavage with either several liters of isotonic saline or the use of a hyperosmolar salt concentrate.[70–76]

Ultrasonography

With the development of new ultrasound machines that feature duplex double flow, contrasting techniques, and real-time 3-dimensional sonography, ultrasound imaging has gained importance. This technique is particularly important in European countries as ultrasound examination is often part of the internal medicine and gastroenterology curriculum for

Table 9.3 Endoscopic findings in IBD

Endoscopic finding	Crohn's disease	Ulcerative colitis
Disease pattern	Discontinuous	Continuous
Strictures	Often	Seldom
Pseudopolyps	Common	Very common
Granularity of the mucosa	Rare	Very common
Cobblestone pattern	Very common	Rare
Longitudinal deep ulcers	Very common	Not seen
Aphthous lesions	Very common	Not seen
Local ulceration	Very common	Common
Purulent secretion	Rare	Very common
Bleeding	Rare	Very common
Friability of the mucosa	Rare	Very common
Erythema and edema	Common	Very common
Inflammation of the rectum	20%	In all cases

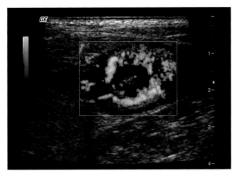

FIGURE 9.10 Sonography of the small intestine in active Crohn's disease. The wall of the small intestine in this 22-year-old female patient is thickened and the double duplex contrast shows enhanced vascularization as a typical sign of inflammation.

prolonged sedation and therefore entails higher risk for the patient. The procedure requires two skilled examiners. Thus the procedure is inconvenient and costly. Additionally, the risk of perforation is three times higher than in conventional endoscopy (Table 9.4).[79,80]

Capsule endoscopy

Capsule endoscopy became widely available with its approval by the Federal Drug Administration (FDA) in 2001. The capsule is about 26 mm in length, disposable, has an optical dome, and transmits images telemetrically. It is able to obtain about 50 000 images during an 8 hour examination. It is noninvasive and the patient needs no special preparation other than fasting for 12 hours. The main contraindication is a suspected stenosis (Figure 9.11) since the capsule may be retained. Other contraindications include an implanted defibrillator or pacemaker.

Before the patient swallows the capsule, sensor leads are attached to the abdomen and a recording belt is placed around the patient. Eight hours after ingestion of the capsule complete transit of the small bowel has occurred in most patients. The patient does not need to stay at the doctor's office or the hospital while the capsule signals are recorded. It takes about 40 minutes with the latest equipment to download the imaging data from the patient recorder to a computer system, and the evaluation of the images takes another 30–120 minutes depending on the length of the examination and observer experience. The capsule will be eliminated naturally via the stool in the next 2–3 days.[81,82] A problem of capsule endoscopy can be the battery lifetime, which in

Table 9.4 Comparison of imaging techniques in Crohn's disease

Imaging technique	Costs	Convenience and availability of the procedure	Risks for the patient	Efficacy
Abdominal x-ray	Low	Broad availability and convenient	Radiation	Very poor except for detection of free air (perforation), large or small bowel obstruction
X-ray enteroclysis	Low	Broad availability; inconvenient for the patient due to nasogastric tube	High radiation	Good in small bowel inflammation: specific inflammatory pattern, strictures, and fistulization
Ultrasonography	Low	Broad availability and convenient	None	Dependent on examiner skills and equipment; large and small bowel can be examined; detection of inflammation, stenosis, fistulization, and abscesses
Endosonography	Medium	Broad availability, but inconvenient for the patient	Rarely perforation or infection	Very useful and efficient in the diagnosis of perianal fistulization
Endoscopy	Medium	Available in all referral centers and hospitals	Perforation, infection, bleeding, risks of sedation	Gold standard for examination of the large bowel and terminal ileum
Capsule endoscopy	Medium	Limited availability; convenient for the patient	Surgery in case of stenosis	Very efficient in the examination of the small bowel
CT/CT-enteroclysis	High	Limited availability (only in hospitals or referral centers); convenient for the patient	High radiation	Very efficient in the detection of abscesses
MRI/MRI-enteroclysis	High	Limited availability (only in large hospitals), convenient for the patient	None	Efficient in the detection of fistulization, abscesses, and extra-intestinal lesions

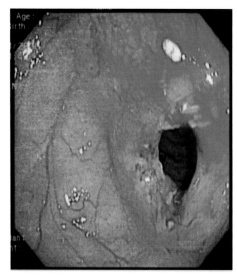

FIGURE 9.11 Endoscopic view of an anastomotic stricture with acute inflammation, 2 years after an ileocecal resection in a 28-year-old female patient with Crohn's disease.

some cases may not be long enough for the capsule to reach the colon.[83,84]

The capsule was initially approved for the detection of bleeding lesions in the small intestine. In 2003 it was approved by the FDA as a first line tool in the evaluation of the small intestine. A meta-analysis of 32 studies demonstrated finding pathology in the small intestine in 71% of patients by capsule endoscopy in contrast to 41% by traditional methods.[85] This included comparative studies against push enteroscopy in which capsule endoscopy was at least equivalent with regards to diagnostic yield in comparison with the much less convenient push enteroscopy.[86,87]

The average time between the onset of symptoms and demonstration of abnormal findings that lead to diagnosis of Crohn's disease is currently more than 36 months. Earlier diagnosis and hence earlier treatment of disease may lead to improved long-term outcomes. As a consequence of the early detection of small bowel lesions by capsule endoscopy, earlier management of the disease could improve quality of life and increase work productivity. Pharmaco-economic studies have modeled the scenario of cost-effectiveness of the additional diagnostic costs of capsule endoscopy and it would offset other health-care expenses.[88,89] A study by Chong et al compared capsule endoscopy with conventional enteroclysis and push enteroscopy in suspected Crohn's disease in 43 patients. Twenty-one patients had suspected Crohn's disease and 22 had known Crohn's disease. The investigators found a greater diagnostic yield in confirming or excluding small bowel Crohn's disease by capsule endoscopy and the management of the patient was changed in 30 patients (70%).[87] Herrerias et al, Eliakim et al, and Fireman et al demonstrated that about 70% of patients without abnormalities on conventional examinations, but with symptoms of chronic diarrhea, weight loss, and abdominal pain had lesions in the small bowel consistent with Crohn's disease.[90-92] Therefore, capsule endoscopy was superior to

conventional techniques for the detection of early lesions in Crohn's disease and this appears to be true in children with suspected Crohn's disease. Argüelles-Arias and Guilhon de Araujo Sant'Anna have demonstrated its applicability for this indication.[93,94]

For patients with ulcerative colitis, capsule endoscopy may be useful only in the initial differential diagnosis against Crohn's disease. Capsule endoscopy may be helpful in the differential diagnosis of indeterminate colitis. In up to 20% the differentiation between Crohn's disease and ulcerative colitis cannot be made based on the known and established diagnostic criteria.[95] Information about even small lesions in the small bowel can be of significant advantage for patients if they develop disease severe enough to require surgical intervention (e.g. colectomy in ulcerative colitis). Mow et al reported typical Crohn's disease ulcerations in a significant fraction of patients previously diagnosed as having ulcerative colitis.[96] In patients planned for colectomy and ileo-anal pouch anastomosis, a capsule endoscopy can therefore provide important additional information.[97,98] If small bowel lesions are found, pouch procedures are better avoided to avoid recurrence at the anastomosis. However the significance of the small lesions described by Mow et al has not been prospectively studied as to whether they truly represent Crohn's disease.

Capsule endoscopy in Crohn's disease has developed a new indication for the followup of Crohn's disease. Capsule endoscopy is able to detect even small lesions.[99] Often such lesions cannot be detected by conventional examinations including ileo-colonoscopy.[100] An example is a series in which enteroclysis detected small bowel lesions in 29% of the study patients, whereas capsule endoscopy found lesions in 61% of the study patients. In the same series, capsule endoscopy detected more ileal lesions than ileo-colonoscopy although mostly in the proximal ileum.[101] A second series confirmed this finding and reported more lesions by capsule endoscopy in both the terminal and the proximal ileum.[102] Capsule endoscopy should be combined with ileo-colonoscopy with biopsies in order to optimize the diagnostic yield, particularly in the more proximal ileum.[103] Capsule endoscopy was superior to other imaging techniques such as CT or MRI enteroclysis in mapping the extent and anatomical localization of small bowel lesions.[104]

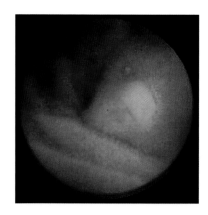

FIGURE 9.12 Capsule endoscopy of active Crohn's disease (with kind permission of the author). Inflammation and ulceration can be seen in the small bowel in a Crohn's disease patient. An aphthous ulcer is seen at 3 o'clock.

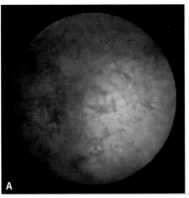
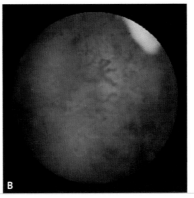
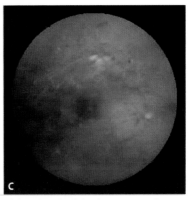

FIGURE 9.13 (a–c) Lesions of the small intestine in three patients with Crohn's disease with endoscopic remission of the colon. (With kind permission of G. Yasih, Venezuela.)

However, the significance of very small lesions in the guidance of therapy is not yet clear. The threshold between normal and pathologic findings needs to be established. Prospective trials will have to be conducted to establish therapeutic goals that include the healing of such lesions. However, capsule endoscopy can also detect large lesions including ulcerated strictures that have a known diagnostic significance (Figures 9.12–9.15).[105]

While a change of therapeutic guidelines based on capsule endoscopy findings requires evidence-based data, clinical practice has anticipated such implications. A study compared capsule endoscopy with small bowel follow-through and reported a change in therapy resulting from the procedure which in turn led to an improvement in quality of life for the study patients.[88] The use of capsule endoscopy together with clinical symptoms and serology led to a change in therapy in 62% of the patients.[102] Chong et al demonstrated that capsule endoscopy is superior to conventional enteroclysis not only in suspected but even in patients with known Crohn's disease and that the detected lesions led to change in disease management.[87] A study by Debinski et al described mucosal healing in the small bowel, seen in the setting of both ulcerated lesions and strictures, after treatment with infliximab.[106]

A problem for capsule endoscopy is the suspected presence of stenoses in the small bowel. Although in most cases the capsule will eventually pass through even tight strictures, in some patients an operation may have to be performed to remove the stricture and recover the capsule.[107] A patency capsule which dissolves after 24–48 hours has been developed. It is filled with an x-ray opaque contrast agent and lactose and also contains a transducer but has no video equipment. The transducer allows anatomic localization with a handheld device. If retained, the device will dissolve and pass the stenosis in most cases of Crohn's disease with suspected or known stenosis.[108] In only one case has there been a failure of dissolution of the capsule, possibly due to a lactase deficiency. Therefore the combined use of the patency and

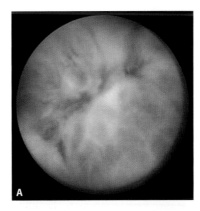

FIGURE 9.15 Capsule endoscopy of (a) a stricture of the small bowel, (b) aphthous ulceration of the small bowel in Crohn's disease. The capsule could pass through. (With kind permission of E. Scapa, Israel.)

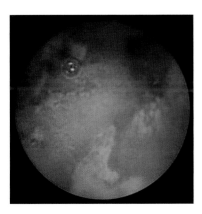

FIGURE 9.14 Capsule endoscopy showing linear ulceration of the small bowel in a Crohn's disease patient. (With kind permission of A.V. Gossum, Belgium.)

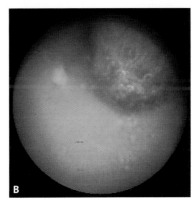

Table 9.5 Advantages and disadvantages of capsule endoscopy in Crohn's disease

Advantages	Disadvantages
Very convenient, no special preparation needed	Limited availability, long evaluation time
Dissolvable patency capsule	Restricted use in patients with lactase deficiency
Detection of early lesions in the small bowel	High rate of false positive findings
Differential diagnosis of indeterminate colitis	Costs often not covered by health insurance
Support for diagnosis in suspected Crohn's disease	Limited number of randomized controlled studies
Detection of additional proximal lesions	
Improved diagnosis leading to improvement in quality of life	

Table 9.6 Consensus Statement from the Fourth International Conference on Capsule Endoscopy

Capsule endoscopy may have a *unique* role in:

- assessment of mucosal healing after medical therapy
- assessment of early postoperative recurrence to guide therapy
- serving as a subclinical marker in asymptomatic family members for exploration of the natural history of IBD

video capsule could evolve as a modality to detect the exact position of a stenosis in the small bowel.[109] Further experience is necessary in patients with long strictures and patients with lactase deficiency in whom disintegration may be prolonged (Table 9.5).

Summary

Diagnostic procedures in suspected or known inflammatory bowel disease are based on endoscopy, MR imaging, CT, and ultrasonography. Conventional x-ray studies have become less frequently used, while capsule endoscopy has evolved as an important novel diagnostic tool to visualize the small bowel (Table 9.6).

References

1. Dalziel TK. Chronic intestinal enteritis. BMJ 1913;1068.

2. Crohn BB, Ginzburg L, Oppenheimer GD. Regional enteritis: A pathological and clinical entity. JAMA 1932;99:1323.

3. Greenstein AJ, Janowitz HD, Sachar DB. The extraintestinal manifestations of Crohn's disease and ulcerative colitis: A study of 700 patients. Medicine 1976;55:401.

4. Adler G. Morbus Crohn-Colitis ulcerosa, 2nd edn. Springer Verlag, Berlin, 1996.

5. Farmer R, Hawk WA, Turnbull RB Jr. Clinical pattern in Crohn's disease: a statistical study of 615 cases. Gastroenterology 1975;68:627–35.

6. Whelan G. Epidemiology of inflammatory bowel disease. Gastroenterol Clin North Am 1990;19:1.

7. Munkholm P, Langholz E, Nielsen OH, Kreiner S, Binder V. Incidence and prevalence of Crohn's disease in the county of Copenhagen, 1962–87: a sixfold increase in incidence. Scand J Gastroenterol 1992;27:609–14.

8. Gent AE, Hellier MD, Grace RH, Swarbrick ET, Coggon D. Inflammatory bowel disease and domestic hygiene in infancy. Lancet 1994;343:766–7.

9. Bjarnason I, MacPherson A, Hollander D. Intestinal permeability: an overview. Gastroenterology 1995;108:1566–81.

10. Blumberg RS, Yockey CE, Gross GG, Ebert EC, Balk SP. Human intestinal intraepithelial lymphocytes are derived from a limited number of T cell clones that utilize multiple V beta T cell receptor genes. J Immunol 1993;150:5144–53.

11. Isaacs KL, Sartor RB, Haskill S. Cytokine messenger RNA profiles in inflammatory bowel disease mucosa detected by polymerase chain reaction amplification. Gastroenterology 1992;103:1587–95.

12. Taylor C, Jobin C. Ubiquitin protein modification and signal transduction: implications for inflammatory bowel diseases. Inflamm Bowel Dis 2005;11:1097–107.

13. Schreiber S, Nikolaus S, Hampe J, et al. Tumour necrosis factor alpha and interleukin 1 beta in relapse of Crohn's disease. Lancet 1999;353:459–61.

14. Danese S, Gasbarrini A. Chemokines in inflammatory bowel disease. J Clin Pathol 2005;58:1025–7.

15. Targan SR, Karp LC. Defects in mucosal immunity leading to ulcerative colitis. Immunol Rev 2005;206:296–305.

16. Cobrin GM, Abreu MT. Defects in mucosal immunity leading to Crohn's disease. Immunol Rev 2005;206:277–95.

17. Macdonald TT, Monteleone G. Immunity, inflammation, and allergy in the gut. Science 2005;307:1920–5.

18. Schreiber S. Of mice and men: what to learn about human inflammatory bowel disease from genetic analysis of murine inflammation. Gastroenterology 2005;129:1782–4.

19. Rosenstiel P, Fantini M, Brautigam K, Kuhbacher T, Waetzig GH, Seegert D, Schreiber S. TNF-alpha and IFN-gamma regulate the expression of the NOD2 (CARD15) gene in human intestinal epithelial cells. Gastroenterology 2003;124:1001–9.

20. Hampe J, Grebe J, Nikolaus S, et al. Association of NOD2 (CARD 15) genotype with clinical course of Crohn's disease: a cohort study. Lancet 2002;359:1661–5.

21. Hampe J, Cuthbert A, Croucher PJ, et al. Association between insertion mutation in NOD2 gene and Crohn's disease in German and British populations. Lancet 2001;357:1925–8.

22. Hugot JP, Chamaillard M, Zouali H, et al. Association of NOD2 leucine-rich repeat variants with susceptibility to Crohn's disease. Nature 2001;411:599–603.

23. Cho JH. Update on the genetics of inflammatory bowel disease. Curr Gastroenterol Rep 2001;3:458–63.

24. Ogura Y, Bonen DK, Inohara N, et al. A frameshift mutation in NOD2 associated with susceptibility to Crohn's disease. Nature 2001;411:603–6.

25. Liu Y, van Kruiningen HJ, West AB, Cartun RW, Cortot A, Colombel JF. Immunocytochemical evidence of Listeria, Escherichia coli, and Streptococcus antigens in Crohn's disease. Gastroenterology 1995;108:1396–404.

26. Lisby G, Andersen J, Engbaek K, Binder V. Mycobacterium paratuberculosis in intestinal tissue from patients with Crohn's disease demonstrated by a nested primer polymerase chain reaction. Scand J Gastroenterol 1994;29:923–9.

27. MacDonald TT, Gordon JN. Bacterial regulation of intestinal immune responses. Gastroenterol Clin North Am 2005;34:401–12.

28. Cario E. Bacterial interactions with cells of the intestinal mucosa: Toll-like receptors and NOD2. Gut 2005;54:1182–93.

29. Ott SJ, Musfeldt M, Wenderoth DF, et al. Reduction in diversity of the colonic mucosa associated bacterial microflora in patients with active inflammatory bowel disease. Gut 2004;53:685–93.

30. Ott SJ, Musfeldt M, Ullmann U, Hampe J, Schreiber S. Quantification of intestinal bacterial populations by real-time PCR with a universal primer set and minor groove binder probes: a global approach to the enteric flora. J Clin Microbiol 2004;42:2566–72.

31. Brignola C, Campieri M, Bazzocchi G, Farruggia P, Tragnone A, Lanfranchi GA. A laboratory index for predicting relapse in asymptomatic patients with Crohn's disease. Gastroenterology 1986;91:1490–4.

32. Farmer RG, Easley KA, Rankin GB. Clinical patterns, natural history, and progression of ulcerative colitis. A long-term follow-up of 1116 patients. Dig Dis Sci 1993;38:1137–46.

33. Farmer RG, Hawk WA, Turnbull RB Jr. Clinical patterns in Crohn's disease: a statistical study of 615 cases. Gastroenterology 1975;68:627–35.

34. Rao SS, Holdsworth CD, Read NW. Symptoms and stool patterns in patients with ulcerative colitis. Gut 1988;29:342–5.

35. Baron JH, Conell AM, Lennard-Jones JE. Variation between observers in describing mucosal appearance in proctocolitis. Br Med J 1964;5375:89–92.

36. Trulove SC, Richards WC. Biopsy studies in ulcerative colitis. Br Med J 1956;(4979):1315–8.

37. Rankin GB, Watts HD, Melnyk CS, Kelley ML Jr. National Cooperative Crohn's Disease Study: extraintestinal manifestations and perianal complications. Gastroenterology 1979;77:914–20.

38. Mekhjian HS, Switz DM, Melnyk CS, Rankin GB, Brooks RK. Clinical features and natural history of Crohn's disease. Gastroenterology 1979;77:898–906.

39. Parks AG, Gordon PH, Hardcastle JD. A classification of fistula-in-ano. Br J Surg 1976;63:1–12.

40. Ekbom A, Helmick CG, Zack M, Holmberg L, Adami HO. Survival and causes of death in patients with inflammatory bowel disease: a population-based study. Gastroenterology 1992;103:954–60.

41. Beck IT. Laboratory assessment of inflammatory bowel disease. Dig Dis Sci 1987;32:26S–41S.

42. Landi B, Anh TN, Cortot A, et al. Endoscopic monitoring of Crohn's disease treatment: a prospective, randomized clinical trial. The Groupe d'Etudes Therapeutiques des Affections Inflammatoires Digestives. Gastroenterology 1992;102:1647–53.

43. Maglinte DD, Chernish SM, Kelvin FM, O'Connor KW, Hage JP. Crohn disease of the small intestine: accuracy and relevance of enteroclysis. Radiology 1992;184:541–5.

44. Wijers OB, Tio TL, Tytgat GN. Ultrasonography and endosonography in the diagnosis and management of inflammatory bowel disease. Endoscopy 1992;24:559–64.

45. Pera A, Bellando P, Caldera D, et al. Colonoscopy in inflammatory bowel disease. Diagnostic accuracy and proposal of an endoscopic score. Gastroenterology 1987;92:181–5.

46. Potzi R, Walgram M, Lochs H, Holzner H, Gangl A. Diagnostic significance of endoscopic biopsy in Crohn's disease. Endoscopy 1989;21:60–2.

47. Summers RW, Switz DM, Sessions JT Jr, Becktel JM, Best WR, Kern F Jr, Singleton JW. National Cooperative Crohn's Disease Study: results of drug treatment. Gastroenterology 1979;77:847–69.

48. Rutgeerts P, Lofberg R, Malchow H, et al. A comparison of budesonide with prednisolone for active Crohn's disease. N Engl J Med 1994;331:842–5.

49. Singleton JW, Hanauer SB, Gitnick GL, Peppercorn MA, Robinson MG, Wruble LD, Krawitt EL. Mesalamine capsules for the treatment of active Crohn's disease: results of a 16-week trial. Pentasa Crohn's Disease Study Group. Gastroenterology 1993;104:1293–301.

50. Candy S, Wright J, Gerber M, Adams G, Gerig M, Goodman R. A controlled double blind study of azathioprine in the management of Crohn's disease. Gut 1995;37:674–8.

51. Pearson DC, May GR, Fick GH, Sutherland LR. Azathioprine and 6-mercaptopurine in Crohn disease. A meta-analysis. Ann Intern Med 1995;123:132–42.

52. Campieri M, Gionchetti P, Belluzzi A, et al. Optimum dosage of 5-aminosalicylic acid as rectal enemas in patients with active ulcerative colitis. Gut 1991;32:929–31.

53. Bullen TF, Hershman MJ. Surgery for inflammatory bowel disease. Hosp Med 2003;64:719–23.

54. Cummings JH, Kong SC. Probiotics, prebiotics and antibiotics in inflammatory bowel disease. Novartis Found Symp 2004;263:99–111; discussion 111–4, 211–8.

55. Isaacs KL, Lewis JD, Sandborn WJ, Sands BE, Targan SR. State of the art: IBD therapy and clinical trials in IBD. Inflamm Bowel Dis 2005;11:S3–12.

56. Sandborn WJ. New concepts in anti-tumor necrosis factor therapy for inflammatory bowel disease. Rev Gastroenterol Disord 2005;5:10–8.

57. Loftus CG, Egan LJ, Sandborn WJ. Cyclosporine, tacrolimus, and mycophenolate mofetil in the treatment of inflammatory bowel disease. Gastroenterol Clin North Am 2004;33:141–69.

58. Shanahan F. Probiotics in inflammatory bowel disease — therapeutic rationale and role. Adv Drug Deliv Rev 2004;56:809–18.

59. Ardizzone S, Bianchi Porro G. Biologic therapy for inflammatory bowel disease. Drugs 2005;65:2253–86.

60. Kusugami K, Ina K, Ando T, Hibi K, Nishio Y, Goto H. Immunomodulatory therapy for inflammatory bowel disease. J Gastroenterol 2004;39:1129–37.

61. Rubesin SE, Laufer I, Dinsmore B. Radiologic investigation of inflammatory bowel disease. Inflammatory Bowel Disease. Elsevier, New York, 1992, p. 458.

62. Bernstein CN, Boult IF, Greenberg HM, van der Putten W, Duffy G, Grahame GR. A prospective randomized comparison between small bowel enteroclysis and small bowel follow-through in Crohn's disease. Gastroenterology 1997;113:390–8.

63. Dixon PM, Roulston ME, Nolan DJ. The small bowel enema: a ten year review. Clin Radiol 1993;47:46–8.

64. Furukawa A, Saotome T, Yamasaki M, et al. Cross-sectional imaging in Crohn disease. Radiographics 2004;24:689–702.

65. Lipson A, Bartram CI, Williams CB, Slavin G, Walker-Smith J. Barium studies and ileoscopy compared in children with suspected Crohn's disease. Clin Radiol 1990;41:5–8.

66. Rohr A, Rohr D, Kuhbacher T, Schreiber S, Heller M, Reuter M. Radiological assessment of small bowel obstructions: Value of conventional enteroclysis and dynamic MR-enteroclysis. Rofo 2002;174:1158–64.

67. Broglia L, Gigante P, Papi C, Ferrari R, Gili L, Capurso L, Castrucci M. Magnetic resonance enteroclysis imaging in Crohn's disease. Radiol Med (Torino) 2003;106:28–35.

68. Hyer W, Beattie RM, Walker-Smith JA, McLean A. Computed tomography in chronic inflammatory bowel disease. Arch Dis Child 1997;76:428–31.

69. Rollandi GA, Curone PF, Biscaldi E, Nardi F, Bonifacino E, Conzi R, Derchi LE. Spiral CT of the abdomen after distention of small bowel loops with transparent enema in patients with Crohn's disease. Abdom Imaging 1999;24:544–9.

70. Quinn PG, Binion DG, Connors PJ. The role of endoscopy in inflammatory bowel disease. Med Clin North Am 1994;78:1331–52.

71. Carbonnel F, Lavergne A, Lemann M, et al. Colonoscopy of acute colitis. A safe and reliable tool for assessment of severity. Dig Dis Sci 1994;39:1550–7.

72. Itzkowitz SH, Present DH. Crohn's and Colitis Foundation of America Colon Cancer in IBD Study Group. Consensus conference: Colorectal cancer screening and surveillance in inflammatory bowel disease. Inflamm Bowel Dis 2005;11:314–21.

73. Theodossi A, Spiegelhalter DJ, Jass J, et al. Observer variation and discriminatory value of biopsy features in inflammatory bowel disease. Gut 1994;35:961–8.

74. Arrowsmith JB, Gerstman BB, Fleischer DE, Benjamin SB. Results from the American Society for Gastrointestinal Endoscopy/U.S. Food and Drug Administration collaborative study on complication rates and drug use during gastrointestinal endoscopy. Gastrointest Endosc 1991;37:421–7.

75. Lee EY, Stenson WF, DeSchryver-Kecskemeti K. Thickening of muscularis mucosae in Crohn's disease. Mod Pathol 1991;4:87–90.

76. Fefferman DS, Farrell RJ. Endoscopy in inflammatory bowel disease: indications, surveillance, and use in clinical practice. Clin Gastroenterol Hepatol 2005;3:11–24.

77. Parente F, Greco S, Molteni M, Anderloni A, Porro GB. Imaging inflammatory bowel disease using bowel ultrasound. Eur J Gastroenterol Hepatol 2005;17:283–91.

78. Di Sabatino A, Armellini E, Corazza GR. Doppler sonography in the diagnosis of inflammatory bowel disease. Dig Dis 2004;22:63–6.

79. Ell C, May A, Nachbar L, Cellier C, Landi B, di Caro S, Gasbarrini A. Push-and-pull enteroscopy in the small bowel using the double-balloon technique: results of a prospective European multicenter study. Endoscopy 2005;37:613–6.

80. May A, Nachbar L, Ell C. Double-balloon enteroscopy (push-and-pull enteroscopy) of the small bowel: feasibility and diagnostic and therapeutic yield in patients with suspected small bowel disease. Gastrointest Endosc 2005;62:62–70.

81. Lewis B. Enteroscopy. Gastrointest Endosc Clin N Am 2000;1:101–16.

82. Meron GD. The development of the swallowable video capsule (M2A). Gastrointest Endosc 2000;52:817–9.

83. Iddan G, Meron G, Glukhovsky A, Swain P. Wireless capsule endoscopy. Nature 2000;405:417.

84. Appleyard M, Glukhovsky A, Jacob H. Transit times for the capsule endoscope. Gastrointest Endosc 2001;53:122.

85. Given Imaging, 2 Hacarmel Street, Yoqneam 20692, Israel. Data supporting FDA non-adjunctive use labelling for capsule endoscopy, March 2003: Metaanalysis of 691 patients. Performance evaluation of Given diagnostic system in the diagnosis of small bowel diseases and disorders.

86. Lewis B. Metaanalysis of capsule endoscopy versus alternative modalities in the diagnosis of small bowel pathologies. Gastrointest Endosc 2004;54AB:105.

87. Chong AK, Taylor A, Miller A, Hennessy O, Connell W, Desmond P. Capsule endoscopy vs. push enteroscopy and enteroclysis in suspected small-bowel Crohn's disease. Gastrointest Endosc 2005;61:255–61.

88. Goldfarb NI, Pizzi LT, Fuhr JP Jr, Salvador C, Sikirica V, Kornbluth A, Lewis B. Diagnosing Crohn's disease: an economic analysis comparing wireless capsule endoscopy with traditional diagnostic procedures. Dis Manag 2004;7:292–304.

89. Carey E J. Single center outcomes of 260 consecutive patients undergoing capsule endoscopy for obscure GI bleeding. Gastroenterology 2004;126 AB 96.

90. Herrerias JM, Caunedo A, Rodriguez-Tellez M, Pellicer F, Herrerias JM Jr. Capsule endoscopy in patients with suspected Crohn's disease and negative endoscopy. Endoscopy 2003;35:564–8.

91. Eliakim R, Fischer D, Suissa A, Yassin K, Katz D, Guttman N, Migdal M. Wireless capsule video endoscopy is a superior diagnostic tool in comparison to barium follow-through and computerized tomography in patients with suspected Crohn's disease. Eur J Gastroenterol Hepatol 2003;15:363–7.

92. Fireman Z, Mahajna E, Broide E, et al. Diagnosing small bowel Crohn's disease with wireless capsule endoscopy. Gut 2003;52:390–2.

93. Arguelles-Arias F, Caunedo A, Romero J, et al. The value of capsule endoscopy in pediatric patients with a suspicion of Crohn's disease. Endoscopy 2004;36:869–73.

94. Guilhon de Araujo Sant'Anna AM, Dubois J, Miron MC, Seidman EG. Wireless capsule endoscopy for obscure small-bowel disorders: final results of the first pediatric controlled trial. Clin Gastroenterol Hepatol 2005;3:264–70.

95. Whitaker DA. Can capsule endoscopy help to differentiate the etiology of indeterminate colitis? Gastrointest Endosc 2004;59 AB177.

96. Mow WS, Lo SK, Targan SR, et al. Initial experience with wireless capsule enteroscopy in the diagnosis and management of inflammatory bowel disease. Clin Gastroenterol Hepatol 2004;2:31–40.

97. Swain P. Wireless capsule endoscopy and Crohn's disease. Gut 2005;54:323–6.

98. Lo SK. Capsule endoscopy in the diagnosis and management of inflammatory bowel disease. Gastrointest Endosc Clin N Am 2004;14:179–93.

99. Ge ZZ, Hu YB, Xiao SD. Capsule endoscopy in diagnosis of small bowel Crohn's disease. World J Gastroenterol 2004;10:1349–52.

100. Bourreille A, Jarry M, D'Halluin PN, et al. Wireless capsule endoscopy versus ileocolonoscopy for the diagnosis of post-operative recurrence of Crohn's disease: a prospective study. Gut 2006;55:978–83.

101. Voderholzer WA, Beinhoelzl J, Rogalla P, Murrer S, Schachschal G, Lochs H, Ortner MA. Small bowel involvement in Crohn's disease: a prospective comparison of wireless capsule endoscopy and computed tomography enteroclysis. Gut 2005;54:369–73.

102. Tabibzadeh S. Utility of wireless capsule endoscopy versus serology in the evaluation of small bowel Crohn's disease. Gastrointest Endosc 2003;57:AB174.

103. Bloom PD. Wireless capsule endoscopy is more informative than ileoscopy and SBFT for the evaluation of the small intestine in patients with known or suspected Crohn's disease. Gastroenterology 2004;124:A203.

104. Albert JG, Martiny F, Krummenerl A, et al. Diagnosis of small bowel Crohn's disease: a prospective comparison of capsule endoscopy with magnetic resonance imaging and fluoroscopic enteroclysis. Gut 2005;54:1721–7.

105. Cheifetz A, Sachar D, Lewis B. Small bowel obstruction — indication or contraindication for capsule endoscopy. Gastrointest Endosc 2004;59:AB102.

106. Debinski HS, Hooper J, Farmer C. Mucosal healing in small bowel Crohn's disease following therapy with infliximab. Assessment using Crohn's disease capsule endoscopic index. Fourth International Conference on Capsule Endoscopy March 5–8, 2005.

107. Chang PK, Holt EG, De Villiers WJ, Boulanger BR. A new complication from a new technology: what a general surgeon should know about wireless capsule endoscopy. Am Surg 2005;71:455–8.

108. Spada C, Spera G, Riccioni M, et al. A novel diagnostic tool for detecting functional patency of the small bowel: the Given patency capsule. Endoscopy 2005;37:793–800.

109. Gay G, Delvaux M, Laurent V, Reibel N, Regent D, Grosdidier G, Roche JF. Temporary intestinal occlusion induced by a "patency capsule" in a patient with Crohn's disease. Endoscopy 2005;37:174–7.

CHAPTER **10**

Approach to the Patient with Abdominal Pain

Martin Keuchel

KEY POINTS

1. Chronic abdominal pain is a frequent complaint in gastroenterology. Video capsule endoscopy (VCE) is sometimes requested as part of the workup. Nevertheless, data on diagnostic yield, therapeutic impact, and clinical outcome in patients with abdominal pain, with or without additional conditions, are still sparse.

2. Video capsule endoscopy is of limited value in the workup of abdominal pain.

3. Abdominal pain with additional fever, inflammatory signs, weight loss, anemia or bleeding, should raise the suspicion of Crohn's disease. After negative conventional endoscopy, VCE is the most sensitive noninvasive diagnostic test for the detection of small intestinal mucosal abnormalities. Care should be taken to avoid possible capsule retention by unexpected strictures.

4. In patients with celiac sprue and recurring symptoms such as abdominal pain in spite of diet, VCE seems to be a valuable tool in the search for complications.

5. VCE facilitates diagnosis of small intestinal tumors. However, the diagnosis of tumor is usually made by VCE looking for the cause of obscure digestive bleeding rather than of abdominal pain.

6. Enteropathy in asymptomatic NSAID users has been observed with VCE in clinical trials. Single cases of NSAID-induced strictures causing obstruction have been diagnosed by VCE.

7. Abdominal pain together with diarrhea is a common constellation in IBS, which does not require VCE for workup.

8. Suspected intestinal obstruction is a relative contraindication to VCE. In symptomatic patients with unclear diagnosis, VCE can help to make a diagnosis and to prove a suspected stenosis prior to surgery.

9. Data on the use of VCE in patients with chronic abdominal pain and suspected adhesions, chronic intestinal ischemia or malabsorption are presently too sparse for recommendations.

Introduction

The appropriate application of video capsule endoscopy (VCE) in patients with chronic abdominal pain is a difficult task. This is quite different from gastrointestinal (GI) bleeding. In patients with established bleeding and normal findings at upper and lower GI endoscopy, it is most likely that the bleeding source is within the small intestine. This scenario is not very frequent but is clearly defined, has been investigated in several prospective studies, and is generally accepted as an indication for VCE. A positive effect of therapy guided by VCE findings on the outcome in patients with obscure bleeding has been documented (Chapter 9).

In contrast, chronic abdominal pain is a frequent problem in clinical practice with a wide range of possible causes, including functional, organic, metabolic, toxicological or psychiatric disorders.[1-5] As most patients with abdominal pain have functional complaints, organic disease of extraintestinal origin or intestinal diseases that can be diagnosed by conventional methods, there is only a limited range of indications for VCE in these patients. On the other hand, some patients with abdominal pain request a variety of investigations, including VCE, rather than accepting a functional origin of their complaints as in irritable bowel disease (IBS). Nevertheless, abdominal pain, together with headache and lower back pain, is likely to remain medically unexplained in frequent users of secondary health care.[6] In contrast, organic small bowel diseases such as Crohn's disease or tumors are often diagnosed with significant delay. Here, VCE with its high sensitivity might help to provide earlier diagnosis and therapy. Some aspects of the potential application of VCE and preceding testing in patients with chronic abdominal pain are discussed in this chapter.

Diagnostic tests in chronic abdominal pain

A thorough history and careful physical examination are necessary to set up an adequate diagnostic and therapeutic strategy. If this basic evaluation and laboratory tests prove insufficient, a "second level" evaluation with imaging techniques such as abdominal ultrasound or computed tomography (CT) is often considered.[7]

Transabdominal ultrasound is a noninvasive, generally available technology which is able to diagnose multiple organic causes of chronic abdominal pain such as cholelithiasis, pancreatitis, nephrolithiasis, aortic aneurysm, lymphomas, mass lesions, and others, including inflammatory bowel disease, especially Crohn's disease of the ileum and right cecum.

Thus, ultrasound can also be used as a first-line investigation of the intestine[8]; however, its sensitivity is too low to categorically exclude small bowel disease.[9]

Formerly, radiographic techniques using distension of the small lumen with contrast medium such as the small bowel follow-through (SBFT) and enteroclysis with methylcellulose were the mainstay of small bowel diagnostics.[10] However, diagnostic yield in patients with abdominal pain is low. Enteroclysis documented significant findings in 8 of 84 patients (10%) with chronic abdominal pain, including adhesions, Crohn's disease, diverticulitis, jejunal carcinoma, stenosis due to adnexitis or relapse of sigmoid carcinoma; 5 of these 8 patients had a stenosis.[11] CT enterography and MRI enterography use similar techniques to distend the small bowel lumen with different contrast media, while cross-sectional imaging enables additional visualization of extra-intestinal pathology. These latter techniques are probably the most valuable if any radiologic tests are to be considered prior to VCE to exclude complications of intestinal disease such as stenosis, fistula or abscesses as well as other extra-intestinal causes of pain.

Endoscopy is not necessary for the diagnosis of irritable bowel syndrome[12] but is used in the presence of alarm symptoms (weight loss, iron deficiency anemia, positive fecal occult blood test, dysphagia), higher age, and positive family history of gastrointestinal carcinoma. Frequent and serious gastrointestinal diseases such as peptic ulcer disease and colorectal cancer[13] can be ruled out by upper and lower intestinal endoscopy. Ileo-colonoscopy is the gold standard for diagnosis of inflammatory bowel disease (IBD).[14]

In a retrospective study, 6 of 8 patients with a diagnostic VCE performed for abdominal pain had also undergone endoscopic procedures, which were sufficient to make a diagnosis in all cases. Additionally, the rate of impacted capsules was 3.8%, being twice as high as in patients with obscure GI bleeding.[15] This confirms the current practice of performing VCE only after inconclusive esophagogastro-duodenoscopy (EGD) and colonoscopy.

'Push' enteroscopy allows endoscopic investigation of the proximal small intestine including the possibility of biopsy. However, diagnostic yield in patients with chronic abdominal pain is low, between 0% and 10%.[16,17] Consequently this investigation has been considered as not helpful in the investigation of chronic abdominal pain.[18]

The further development of double balloon enteroscopy (DBE) permits investigation of the entire small bowel in up to 80% of patients.[19] It has also been applied in patients with chronic abdominal pain, especially in suspected Crohn's disease. DBE requires sedation, fluoroscopy, a skilled endoscopy team, and often the need to use both oral and anal approaches. Hence, it does not seem to replace VCE in the primary diagnosis of small intestinal diseases, perhaps with the exception of patients with a strong suspicion of Crohn's stenosis, where DBE can provide biopsy and balloon dilation[20] and avoid the risk of capsule retention.

Laparoscopy has been advocated as a helpful diagnostic and therapeutic procedure in patients with chronic abdominal pain, especially after prior abdominal surgery.[21,22] Diagnoses are predominantly adhesions, appendiceal pathology, and gynecological diseases. The performance of a definite therapy during laparoscopy is reported in nearly half of the patients undergoing this procedure for diagnostic reasons.[21]

VCE in patients with chronic abdominal pain

In many series on VCE, one or few patients with chronic abdominal pain are included, whereas few studies have focussed on this indication. In a prospective study by Bardan et al[23] on 20 patients with chronic abdominal pain who had a negative workup including upper and lower gastrointestinal endoscopy, barium follow-through, and abdominal CT scan, 17 patients had normal findings on VCE. In 2 cases, very few erosions in the distal small bowel were found, and 2 small sessile polyps in 1 patient. All findings were found not to be related to the abdominal pain. In a multi-center series by Fireman et al[24] with various indications, only 1 out of 24 patients with abdominal pain/IBS had a positive finding at VCE, compatible with Crohn's disease. Romero-Vázquez et al[25] reported normal findings in 27 of 60 patients with abdominal pain but without alarm symptoms: 20% had unrelated findings, 33% had signs of minimal unspecific enteropathy, and only in one patient (1.7%) were multiple jejunal erosions and ulcers detected. Spada et al[26] investigated 15 patients with abdominal pain. Twelve of these 15 patients (80%) had a normal investigation. Only one patient had ileal erosions and a stricture, which was diagnosed at surgery as stenosing carcinoid. The authors of this abstract commented that VCE does not play an important role in the evaluation of patients with chronic abdominal pain, due to its low diagnostic yield.

In a series on 15 children (age 5–16 years) with recurrent abdominal pain, Argüelles-Arias et al[27] obtained VCE findings described as lymphoid hyperplasia in the terminal ileum in 7 (47%), invagination, considered as irrelevant, and bleeding in the cecum without source in one child each.

VCE has made it possible to investigate the entire small bowel noninvasively. Nevertheless, only structural changes of the small bowel such as vascular abnormalities, inflammation, tumor or obstruction are accessible with VCE. In detecting such lesions, VCE has been shown to be more sensitive than competitive methods in many indications. Costs, time-consuming review of the video, and low incidence of intestinal diseases jeopardize the use of VCE as a screening tool.

In patients with abdominal pain alone, diagnostic yield of VCE is low, in accordance with results from enteroclysis and push enteroscopy. Hence, it seems important to predict the likelihood of detecting alterations of the small bowel mucosa from additional clinical symptoms and findings in order to provide early diagnosis to patients with organic disease of the small bowel and to avoid VCE in those with functional complaints or extra-intestinal disease. Data on this complex issue, especially data systematically addressing the impact of certain clinical features on the diagnostic yield of VCE, are still sparse. Table 10.1 gives a suggestion for possible applications of VCE in patients with chronic

Table 10. 1 Possible fields of application of VCE in patients with chronic abdominal pain

Signs and symptoms accompanying abdominal pain	Suspected diagnosis	VCE indicated after inconclusive diagnostic tests	Evidence based on
Diarrhea, fever, elevation of leukocytes, CRP, anemia	Crohn's disease	Yes	Prospective studies, retrospective series
Recurrent complaints in celiac sprue under diet	Refractory sprue, neoplasia	Yes	Prospective studies
Intestinal bleeding	Tumor	Yes	Retrospective series Case reports
Long-term NSAID intake	NSAID-induced stricture	Only if surgery is indicated	Small series Case reports
Localized pain, previous surgery, intermittent obstruction	Adhesions	?	Single cases
Postprandial pain, weight loss, diarrhea, generalized atherosclerosis	Ischemic enteritis	Only in unclear cases	Case reports
Diarrhea, Rome II criteria	Irritable bowel syndrome	No	Prospective studies without Rome II criteria
Malabsorption, hypoproteinemic edema, exudative enteropathy	Primary lymphangiectasia Various other entities.	In rare cases	Case reports
Crampy post-prandial pain, progressive, vomiting, weight loss recurrent ileus	Obstruction	Only in unclear cases if surgery is indicated	Small retrospective series Case reports

CRP, C-reactive protein; NSAID, non-steroidal anti-inflammatory drug.

abdominal pain according to accompanying clinical features and suspected underlying diseases as discussed below.

Abdominal pain in Crohn's disease

In the first prospective trial from Israel on diagnosis of suspected Crohn's disease by Fireman et al,[28] 12 of 17 patients had a positive finding on capsule endoscopy. Clinical suspicion was based on abdominal pain (71%), anemia (59%), diarrhea (35%), and weight loss (18%). However, among those patients with VCE findings compatible with Crohn's disease, anemia was more frequent than pain (75% vs. 67%).

Similar observations were made in a prospective Chinese study by Ge et al.[29] Clinical suspicion of Crohn's disease was based on a variety of symptoms and findings. Initially, the most frequent symptom was abdominal pain (14 of 20 patients, 70%). However, when only those 13 patients with a VCE study compatible with Crohn's disease were considered, 85% had a positive fecal occult blood test, 77% were anemic, and only 54% had abdominal pain. Herrerias et al reported on VCE images compatible with Crohn's disease in 9 of 21 patients studied prospectively for suspicion of Crohn's disease based on abdominal pain and diarrhea, accompanied in different percentages by weight loss, fever, anemia, leukocytosis, and elevated C-reactive protein (CRP). Prior endoscopy and small bowel follow-through had been normal.[30]

In a prospective Australian study by Chong et al, 21 patients had a suspicion of Crohn's disease.[31] In 3 of these 21 patients, VCE was diagnostic. In 2 cases, Crohn's disease was suspected by VCE, but only one of the patients had abdominal pain, together with diarrhea and weight loss. In a third patient with abdominal pain, diarrhea, mouth ulcers, and iron deficiency anemia, VCE showed a circumferential jejunal ulcer, which was resected and attributed to ischemia.

In 7 of 12 children (58%) aged between 12 and 16 years,[32] small intestinal lesions suggestive of Crohn's disease were observed with VCE in spite of normal ultrasonography, small bowel follow-through, and upper and lower GI endoscopy. Fifty per cent additionally had normal ileoscopy preceding VCE. Clinical suspicion of Crohn's disease was based on abdominal pain together with weight loss and fever in all, laboratory changes (anemia, leukocytosis, elevated CRP) in 58%, and diarrhea in 50%.

In a series reported by Mow et al,[33] a subgroup of patients with suspected Crohn's disease consisted of 8 patients. Two had a history of small bowel obstruction and VCE findings suggestive of Crohn's disease, while 2 patients with chronic abdominal pain alone had a normal VCE. Abdominal pain together with diarrhea in patients with inconclusive endoscopy does not seem to predict findings typical for Crohn's disease at VCE, which were normal in 9 patients, whereas in 5 patients with chronic abdominal pain, diarrhea, and additionally inflammatory signs such as fever or leukocytosis VCE findings were compatible with Crohn's disease.[34]

In a prospective study from Israel by Eliakim et al on 35 patients with suspected Crohn's disease (based on abdominal pain in 88%, diarrhea in 83%, and weight loss in 69%), diagnostic yield of capsule endoscopy was 77%, three times as high as for CT or SBFT.[35] Ileo-colonoscopy was only performed in 17 cases with discrepancy between the other tests. As ileo-colonoscopy confirmed findings of VCE in all cases, it should have been possible to make a diagnosis in these patients without VCE. These results further justify the current practice of using VCE only after complete and thorough endoscopy, which additionally provides histology, differentiation from ulcerative colitis, and colon cancer screening.

These studies, although quite heterogeneous, show that VCE is superior to radiologic imaging studies in the detection of mucosal Crohn's lesions of the small bowel. Abdominal pain alone does not seem to be a good predictor of Crohn's disease, whereas additional fever, inflammatory signs, weight loss, anemia, and bleeding may raise suspicion. In rare cases where small intestinal Crohn's disease spares the terminal ileum, VCE can provide a diagnosis in spite of negative endoscopy.

It should be noted that a fibrotic stenosis may be the reason for obstructive-type pain in patients with Crohn's disease, even with low activity. These strictures can be detected by VCE in rare cases, and surgery may be indicated rather than escalation of medical therapy.

VCE findings in Crohn's disease Fissuring (Figure 10.1a), aphthous or serpiginous ulcers, focal loss of villi (villous denudation), edema, reddening, and cobblestone appearance (Figure 10.1b) of the mucosa are typical but not specific findings in Crohn's disease. Occasionally, complications such as ulceration (Figure 10.2) or fibrosis (Figure 10.3) stenosis, bleeding or fistula may be visualized.

Value of VCE in suspected Crohn's disease Abdominal pain with or without diarrhea which is accompanied by signs of bleeding, inflammation or malabsorption is suggestive of Crohn's disease. After negative endoscopy, VCE is the most effective noninvasive diagnostic tool in suspected Crohn's disease. Although radiologic imaging tests are less sensitive than VCE in detecting mucosal lesions of the small intestine, their initial application may be prudent to exclude severe stenosis before VCE. In doubtful cases, a test with the biodegradable patency capsule (Given Imaging, Yoqneam, Israel) may be helpful. In patients with stenosis, double balloon enteroscopy can be a diagnostic alternative.

Abdominal pain in celiac disease

Besides diarrhea with malabsorption, celiac disease may present with various gastrointestinal symptoms, including abdominal pain.[36] However, in Canadian and Turkish children with recurrent abdominal pain, prevalence of anti-endomysial antibodies as a serologic marker for celiac disease was too low (1.2% and 2.7%) to recommend screening for celiac disease in recurrent abdominal pain.[37,38]

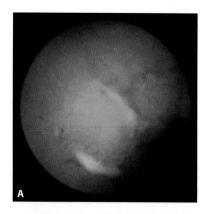

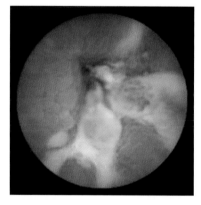

FIGURE 10.1 Crohn's disease. (a) Fissured ulcers and (b) cobblestone relief and swelling of the mucosa in the ileum of a 70-year-old woman with abdominal pain, short episode of fever, anemia, and elevated CRP.

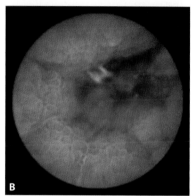

FIGURE 10.2 Ulcerated Crohn's stenosis of the terminal ileum, uneventful passage of the capsule into the cecum.

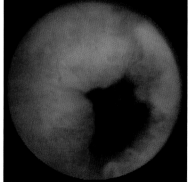

FIGURE 10.3 Fibrotic Crohn's stenosis of the mid jejunum, delayed excretion of the capsule after 14 days. This patient with mild activity of known Crohn's disease complained of postprandial pain and intermittent vomiting. Previous upper and lower endoscopy, and enteroclysis had been inconclusive. Laparoscopic lysis of adhesion was ineffective. Stenosis could be confirmed during open surgery. The patient was without complaints after segmental resection.

In adults, it has been reported that up to 5% of patients with irritable bowel syndrome (IBS) had celiac disease; most of them had positive anti-endomysial antibodies.[39]

Endoscopic findings such as villous atrophy are typically seen in the duodenum and jejunum, but may involve the entire small intestine. Underwater high-resolution endoscopy provides an optimized view of the villi.[40] This underwater view is present most of the time during VCE, making it possible to diagnose villous atrophy. A good correlation of VCE findings with histology has been reported in a small series.[41] Thus, a presumptive diagnosis of extensive celiac disease by VCE should be possible in patients with chronic abdominal pain. Mucosal changes in less extensive celiac disease may be limited to the duodenum. These changes might easily be missed by VCE. In a study by Culliford et al,[42] discussed below, all patients with proven celiac disease and normal findings at VCE had endoscopic signs of celiac disease diagnosed at conventional endoscopy. Due to the risk of missing mucosal changes limited to the duodenum, the inability to obtain histology, costs, and time-consuming evaluation, VCE is presently not a first-line test for suspected celiac disease. Tests for anti-endomysial or the recombinant antigen tissue-transglutaminase (t-TG) antibodies provide a highly sensitive and specific, noninvasive diagnostic tool at reasonable cost. The anti-gliadin antibody tests should be avoided due to low sensitivity and specificity. It seems unlikely that VCE will provide a diagnosis of celiac disease in patients with normal conventional workup including negative t-TG/endomysial antibodies, or even after normal duodenoscopy and normal duodenal biopsy, although there are no data available yet.

However, there is emerging evidence for a potential role of VCE in the diagnosis of complications during the course of celiac sprue. Initial reports demonstrated the feasibility of VCE in detecting ulcerative jejunoileitis[43] and enteropathy-associated T-cell lymphoma.[44] In the first single-center prospective study on 47 patients with complicated celiac sprue, VCE revealed pathologic findings in a high percentage.[42] This group from New York found in 87% of the patients signs of celiac sprue, such as villous atrophy, fissuring, and mosaic pattern. These alterations extended to the ileum in 34%. Additionally, 52% of the subgroup of patients with abdominal pain in spite of using a gluten-free diet (n = 27) had unexpected findings, predominantly ulcerations. Also stricture and intussusception was found in one case each with recurrent episodes of abdominal pain. Nodularity in the small intestine was seen in 6 patients. Two of these 6 patients had abdominal pain. Both had ulcerated nodularity as well as an aberrant T-cell clone in duodenal biopsies, suspicious for lymphoma. However, the only adenocarcinoma detected in this study was found in a patient with occult bleeding. It should be noted that most patients in this study, including the patient with carcinoma, had undergone repeated inconclusive radiologic studies such as CT, small bowel follow-through or enteroclysis.

Preliminary results of an European multi-center study are similar, demonstrating mucosal alterations in 32 of 43 patients (74%) with ongoing symptoms while on gluten-free diets; 2 strictures and tumors each were found (4.6%).[45]

There are no recommendations for the application of VCE in the followup of asymptomatic patients with celiac sprue yet. However, it seems appropriate to investigate patients with recurrent symptoms in spite of good dietary compliance. By analogy to comparative studies in obscure gastrointestinal bleeding and in Crohn's disease, VCE could provide a diagnosis in spite of inconclusive radiological examinations in patients with complicated celiac sprue. VCE might be able to replace SBFT and enteroclysis in the search for neoplasia in these patients.

VCE findings in celiac disease Signs of celiac sprue are total or partial villous atrophy, mosaic pattern of the mucosa, reduction and scalloping of folds (Figure 10.4a). These findings are potentially reversible on a gluten-free diet, but persist in a high percentage of patients with ongoing or recurring symptoms. Small erosions are seen in a significant proportion of these patients. Ulcerations, thickened folds (Figure 10.4b), masses or stenosis are signs of complication and may be indicative of refractory sprue, ulcerative jejuno-ileitis, enteropathy-associated T-cell lymphoma or adenocarcinoma.

Value of VCE in celiac disease Anti-endomysial/t-TG antibody tests and upper GI endoscopy with duodenal biopsy are still the mainstay in the search of suspected celiac disease. In surveillance of patients with complicated sprue, however, VCE seems to be the most sensitive noninvasive test.

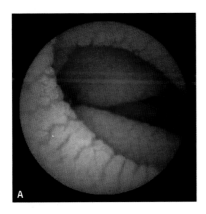
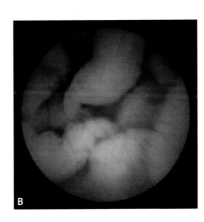

FIGURE 10.4 Celiac sprue with recurrent abdominal complaints. (a) Villous atrophy, mosaic pattern of the mucosa, and scalloped folds affecting the entire jejunum. (b) Additionally, a thickened fold is visible. Enteroscopy with biopsy of suspicious lesions was performed to rule out lymphoma. A 66-year-old patient with celiac sprue and abdominal pain after years of consequent gluten-free diet.

Abdominal pain and small bowel tumors

Small bowel tumors are rare and are often diagnosed late. Since early diagnosis is an important prognostic factor, concerns may arise in missing such a tumor in patients with chronic abdominal pain. However, pain and intermittent obstruction are considered signs of advanced tumor, whereas occult bleeding and iron deficiency anemia should raise early suspicion of small bowel tumor.[46]

Adenocarcinoma is the most frequent primary malignant small bowel tumor. As these tumors are often located in the upper small bowel, especially in the duodenum, diagnosis can be made already by upper endoscopy in about 1 in 3 patients.[47] Several other benign and malignant tumor entities can be found in the small intestine such as benign mesenchymal tumor, carcinoids, gastrointestinal stromal tumors, lymphomas, and others (Table 10.2).

Tumors of the small intestine found on VCE were reported from patients with obscure bleeding. In a first retrospective series by Mascarenhas-Saraiva et al on 5 small bowel tumors seen by VCE, one of the patients with a small ileal carcinoid had chronic abdominal pain.[48] However, some carcinoids have been suggested to be indolent tumors, detected incidentally.[49] Table 10.3 shows the data from Hamburg Altona. The majority of tumors were detected because of obscure bleeding. Three patients with intestinal carcinoid and abdominal complaints without bleeding already had hepatic metastasis; another one had obstructive symptoms. In an Australian multi-center analysis, Bailey et al identified 26 patients with small bowel tumor by VCE out of 416 investigations.[50] The indication for VCE was obscure GI bleeding in 21 patients and abdominal pain in only one. In a French series by Delvaux et al on 275 patients with obscure GI bleeding, 22 proved to have a small bowel tumor at VCE.[51] Between 56% and 69% of these tumors were malignant.[50-52] The vast majority of small bowel tumors detected by VCE were associated with intestinal bleeding. Only rare cases of tumors were diagnosed with VCE as a result of abdominal pain, mainly in an advanced stage or causing obstruction. There is no evidence to support the application of VCE in the workup of abdominal pain without bleeding and without obstruction to exclude intestinal tumor. Although prognosis of small bowel tumors depends on early diagnosis, abdominal pain does not seem to be a typical symptom of early tumor. On one hand, IBS is a frequent cause of abdominal pain with a presumed prevalence of 15 million in the United States.[13] On the other hand, an incidence of 5300 small bowel carcinomas per year has been reported.[53] Furthermore, small bowel tumors have predominantly been detected by VCE associated with obscure bleeding. Thus, it seems unlikely that VCE is able to detect a significant number of small bowel tumors at an early stage in patients with abdominal pain but without warning signs.

VCE findings in small bowel tumor Benign small bowel tumors are mostly diagnosed as submucosal masses with

Table 10. 2 Small bowel tumors

Benign small bowel tumors
Hyperplasias
Hyperplastic polyps
Brunner's gland hyperplasia
Hamartomas
Peutz–Jeghers polyps
Juvenile polyps
Ectopic tissues
Ectopic pancreatic tissue
Ectopic gastric mucosa
Epithelial tumors
Adenoma
Mesenchymal tumors
Hemangioma
Lymphangioma
Leiomyoma
Lipoma
Neurofibroma
Malignant small bowel tumors
Primary small bowel malignancies
Epithelial tumors
Adenocarcinoma
Neuroendocrine tumors
Mesenchymal tumors
Gastrointestinal stromal tumors
Sarcomas
Lymphomas
Metastasis

Table 10. 3 Indications for VCE in patients with intestinal tumor — bleeding versus pain

Indication for VCE	Tumors seen at VCE	Tumors seen by radiology
Obscure bleeding	9 malignant[a] 4 benign[b] 4 no histology[c]	3/5 3/4
Pain and hepatic metastasis	3 carcinoids	2/3
Pain and obstruction	1 carcinoid	1/1
Pain and neurofibromatosis	1 neurofibroma	1/1
Pain and weight loss and history of carcinoid	1 leiomyoma	0/1

[a] Adenocarcinoma, GIST, melanoma, metastasis of bronchial carcinoma.
[b] Pancreatic ectopia, adenoma, lipoma, fibrolipoma.
[c] Clinical and endoscopic suspicion: large hyperplastic polyp, lipoma, Kaposi sarcoma.

intact overlying mucosa or with superficial ulceration. However, malignant tumors, especially carcinoids and gastrointestinal stromal tumors, can also present as submucosal tumors. Malignant tumors may show ulceration, diffuse infiltration, polypoid growth pattern, and obstruction (Figure 10.5).

Value of VCE in the search of small bowel tumor Small bowel tumors have been detected by VCE on occasion of intestinal bleeding rather than of abdominal pain. Many tumors causing abdominal pain are in an advanced stage or cause obstruction. VCE may be helpful in patients with intermittent obstruction if radiological methods are inconclusive, provided surgery is indicated and possible.

Abdominal pain in NSAID enteropathy

Enteropathy caused by non-steroidal anti-inflammatory drugs (NSAIDs) is an underestimated entity. Weight loss, abdominal pain, and diarrhea have been attributed to NSAID enteropathy. The most frequent complication is iron deficiency anemia, whereas massive small bowel bleeding, perforation or obstruction is rare.[54] NSAID-associated lesions

were described in patients undergoing VCE for obscure bleeding.[55] The majority of data on VCE findings in NSAID users have been obtained from volunteers. Maiden et al found new lesions after 2 weeks of diclofenac intake in 27 of 40 volunteers (68%). In 13%, these lesions were bleeding or blood without visible source was observed by VCE.[56] In another controlled trial by Graham et al., injuries of the small intestine such as red spots, erosions, and ulcers were detected in 15 of 21 (71%) NSAID users, compared to 10% in controls.[57] In the largest trial by Goldstein et al,[58] mucosal changes were observed by VCE in 57 of 413 (14%) of healthy controls. In patients without initial lesions, new lesions were seen after 2 weeks of placebo in 7%, in 16% in the celecoxib group, and in 55% after naproxen with omeprazole. This phenomenon of unexplained mucosal damage in healthy volunteers should be kept in mind when diagnosing NSAID enteropathy or Crohn's disease by VCE.

VCE has proven to be a very sensitive tool for the detection of mucosal lesions in NSAID-induced enteropathy, possibly overestimating the true incidence. This high sensitivity is of relevance in the search for bleeding lesions in the small intestine. However, possibly due to the primary

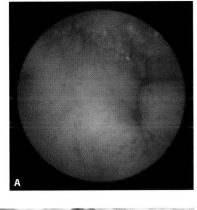
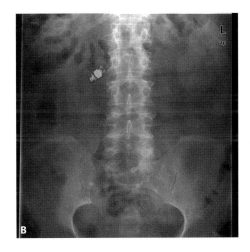
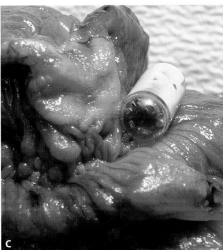
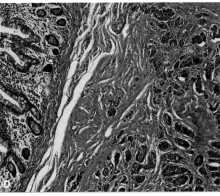

FIGURE 10.5 Stenosing carcinoid tumor. Infiltrating tumor of the proximal ileum with petechiae and stenosis at VCE (a), not traversed by the capsule, as demonstrated by plain abdominal x-ray (b). Note that the position of the capsule might easily be interpreted erroneously as being in the transverse colon. (c) The surgical specimen shows infiltrating tumor and retained capsule (courtesy of Christopher Pohland, MD). (d) Histology reveals carcinoid (courtesy of Renate Höhne, MD). This 49-year old-patient had suffered from post-prandial pain for several months. Enteroclysis gave suspicion of stenosis of an ileal segment.

analgesic action of NSAIDs, these often small mucosal lesions are unlikely to cause significant pain. The above-mentioned studies have shown a high rate of mucosal lesions in NSAID consumers, but do not report on complaints of these patients or volunteers, although this topic was not specifically addressed by these trials. Thus, the present data do not suggest that VCE will play a major role in the search for NSAID-induced mucosal lesions as cause of abdominal pain.

The situation is different in patients with NSAID-induced diaphragms of the small intestine causing obstructive pain. A case of VCE diagnosis of multiple small intestinal diaphragms caused by NSAIDs has been reported. This patient had no abdominal pain besides recurrent episodes of obstruction.[59] In another patient with diaphragm disease, diagnosed by double balloon endoscopy, the clinical presentation was gastrointestinal bleeding requiring transfusion, and, later on, ileus.[60] NSAID-related strictures were detected by Cave and co-workers with VCE in 11 patients, but only 2 of them were studied because of abdominal pain; the other 9 patients suffered from obscure bleeding.[61] VCE can be helpful in detecting significant strictures, which may be overlooked even at surgery. As detection of strictures in these patients is associated with a significant risk of capsule retention, the patient should be fit for surgery and the severity of the complaints should justify an operation. In doubtful cases, prior application of the patency capsule might be considered.

VCE findings in NSAID-induced enteropathy Erosions, ulcers, red spots, focal destruction of villi (villous denudation), and bleeding are seen in NSAID enteropathy (Figure 10.6). They cannot reliably be distinguished from Crohn's disease. Complicating strictures typically have a diaphragm-like appearance.

Value of VCE in the search for NSAID-induced enteropathy in patients with abdominal pain Enteropathy is a frequent complication in NSAID users. However, this enteropathy rarely seems to cause abdominal pain unless complicating strictures occur.

Abdominal pain and adhesions

Adhesions are a frequent finding at laparoscopy in patients with chronic abdominal pain.[21,22] Laparoscopic lysis of adhesions is controversial. Most of the patients benefit from lysis.[22,62] The number of previous operations had a significant influence on the completeness of lysis, but not on the short-term benefit.[63] On the other hand, improvement of complaints after laparoscopy without any therapeutic procedure in some patients suggests a possible placebo

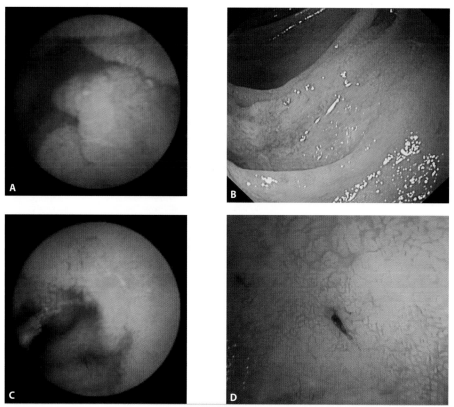

FIGURE 10.6 NSAID enteropathy. (a) An area in the jejunum with superficial inflammation showing reddening of mucosa, loss of villi, and discrete swelling at VCE. (b) Corresponding push enteroscopy. (c) VCE further shows small aphthous ulcers in the ileum. (d) Corresponding ileoscopy reveals small ulcers with hematin and diffuse bleeding (not shown). Biopsy diagnosed nonspecific ulcers, no suspicion of Crohn's disease. This 80-year-old woman, taking aspirin for coronary heart disease and diclofenac for joint pain, presented with severe intestinal bleeding. Bleeding stopped after cessation of NSAIDs. She did not complain of any abdominal pain or diarrhea.

effect in some cases[22] and long-term benefit was only noted in 45% in a small series.[64] Hence, a noninvasive test able to predict a benefit from laparoscopic treatment in patients with suspected adhesions could significantly improve management of these patients. From a theoretical point of view, it might be interesting to observe the effect of adhesions on the wall and lumen of the small intestine by video capsule. However, up to now, there are no clear criteria to establish the diagnosis of small intestinal adhesions by VCE or to predict a possible effect of lysis. On one hand, minor changes at VCE can be observed in patients with severe adhesions at laparoscopy; on the other, impaction of a capsule can occur due to adhesions (with no stenosis seen at enteroclysis), requiring surgical removal.[65]

Suspicion of adhesion may arise if a "string" impressing the lumen is seen at VCE. Sharply bent intestinal loops may be found in adhesions, but are also a frequent finding in normal studies. Delayed progression of the capsule or dilation of the lumen, causing dark images, might support the diagnosis. However, dark images due to dilated small intestinal loops can also be caused by lavage, used for bowel cleansing prior to VCE. There are no studies on the application of VCE in the diagnosis of adhesions. Hence, VCE cannot presently be recommended for this indication.

The use of the patency capsule, if available, prior to VCE may be prudent in patients with abdominal pain and other conditions, such as iron deficiency anemia, if adhesions are likely. Whereas in Crohn's disease a patency capsule might get impacted in a long stricture and not fully dissolve, long stenoses are unlikely to occur as a result of adhesions. Presently, there are no data on a potential role of the patency capsule in the search for adhesions in patients with abdominal pain.

VCE findings in patients with small intestinal adhesions "Strings" may be seen traversing the intestinal lumen (Figure 10.7). Obstruction can cause dilation of the intestinal lumen, resulting in dark images and delayed capsule progression.

Value of VCE in patients with small intestinal adhesions

There are no data on diagnosing small intestinal adhesions by VCE. If diagnostic tests are required for the decision to perform laparoscopy for suspected adhesions or not, radiological imaging techniques are presently applied. Whether VCE has a place in the search for adhesions in the future remains to be seen. In patients with suspected adhesions undergoing VCE for another indication, prior use of a patency capsule might be prudent.

Abdominal pain in chronic mesenteric ischemia

Suspicion of chronic ischemia of the small bowel is usually based on a patient's history, including atherosclerosis, typical post-prandial abdominal angina, weight loss, and sometimes chronic diarrhea. The diagnostic gold standard is angiography, which also allows for intervention with infusion of vasodilator agents as well as dilatation of circumferential stenosis and stent implantation.[66] However, the quality of CT angiography for noninvasive diagnosis is approximating that of standard angiography.[67]

Endoscopy may augment the diagnosis. Findings include ulcers, often circular on the edges of folds, edema, lymphangiectasia, and strictures. Some unclear, benign strictures might be of ischemic origin. The risk of development of strictures during the course of ischemic enteropathy limits the application of VCE. High-resolution spiral CT prior to VCE allows exclusion of severe long stenosis and provides valuable information on the vascular state. Three-dimensional reconstruction of the mesenteric arteries and the celiac trunk may provide more detailed information. VCE has only been applied in a few patients with suspected ischemic enteritis. One patient with ischemia and diffuse mucosal changes including villous atrophy at VCE has been reported,[68] while another one with severe stenosis of the superior mesenteric artery seen on CT had a normal capsule endoscopy.[69] At present, VCE should not be considered a useful tool in the diagnosis of chronic mesenteric ischemia.

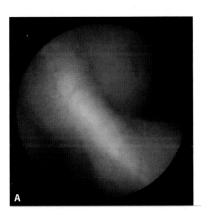
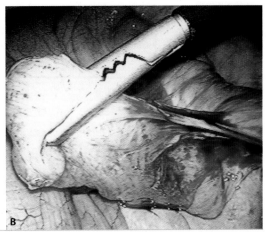

FIGURE 10.7 Adhesions. (a) A "string" crosses the lumen of a small bowel loop. (b) Adhesions seen at laparoscopy. A 24-year-old woman with localized abdominal pain after resection of a Meckel's diverticulum. Laparoscopic lysis of adhesions had no major benefit after 6 months. From Keuchel et al (2006): Postoperative Changes. In Keuchel M, Hagenmüller F, Fleischer D (eds). Atlas of Video Capsule Endoscopy with permission from Springer Verlag.

However, ischemia should be included in the differential diagnosis of intestinal ulcers, especially if they are circular, on the edge of folds, segmental, and accompanied by a circumferential stenosis.

VCE findings in ischemic enteropathy Endoscopic findings in ischemic enteropathy can be ulcers, often semicircular or circular, on the edge of a Kerckring's fold (Figure 10.8a). In severe cases, these ulcers may comprise an entire segment of the small intestine and cause strictures. Nonspecific findings accompanying ulcers include erythema, edema, and lymphangiectasia (Figure 10.8b).

Value of VCE in chronic ischemic enteropathy The low incidence, necessity of vascular imaging for correct diagnosis and for planning of therapy, and lack of experience with VCE in this disease limit the application of this method in ischemic enteropathy. VCE should be reserved for unclear cases. A high risk of stenosis has to be considered, including the possible need for surgery with small bowel resection.

Abdominal pain in irritable bowel syndrome

Irritable bowel syndrome (IBS) is a functional disorder with different qualities of chronic abdominal discomfort, arbitrarily defined, for instance by the Rome II criteria.[70] These complaints may be predominantly pain and/or diarrhea or constipation. Patients with IBS have an increased incidence of multiple somatic complaints and obtain frequent consultations for minor illness. Those patients with IBS who consult a doctor have an increased level of psychological disturbance.[71] The guidelines of the British Society of Gastroenterology[71] recommend no further diagnostic tests in patients under 45 years with typical complaints, a normal physical examination, and no warning signs such as weight loss, anemia, rectal bleeding or symptoms responsible for night wakening. This should also apply for VCE, which was shown to have a low diagnostic yield in patients with abdominal pain. Although not addressed specifically in these studies,[23–27] it is probable that most of the patients suffered from functional complaints/IBS.

As implied by the functional character of the condition, visible alterations of the small bowel mucosa are not to be expected at VCE. Abnormal motility has been proposed as one of the pathophysiological factors.[12] Future academic research on motility patterns observed during VCE may contribute to this field, but at the moment VCE plays no role in the diagnosis of IBS. IBS is a "safe" diagnosis,[12] but some patients fulfilling the criteria of IBS have been shown to have celiac disease.[39] However, diagnosis of celiac sprue can be made serologically and in these patients is much more cost-effective than VCE. Further concerns may arise as to other organic diseases, mainly Crohn's disease or intestinal tumors. The present, although limited, experience from VCE in patients with abdominal pain with or without diarrhea does not justify the implementation of VCE in the workup of patients with suspected IBS. This initial recommendation

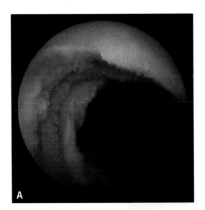
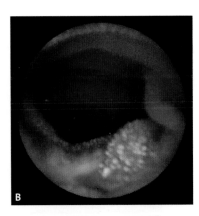
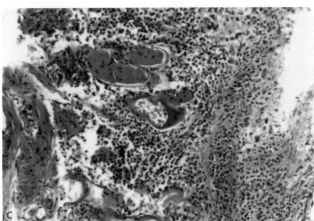

FIGURE 10.8 Ischemic enteropathy. (a,b) VCE demonstrates linear, semicircular ulcers, predominantly on the edges of folds. Additionally, edema and lymphangiectasia (white villi) are present. Ischemic enteritis was confirmed by biopsies obtained during push enteroscopy, showing transmural inflammation and hyaline thrombi (c, H&E stain, courtesy of Volker Hartmann, MD). The 63-year-old patient with a history of "spontaneous" duodenal perforation, microangiopathy, diabetes, and stenosis of the celiac trunk presented with abdominal pain, fever, and elevated CRP and leukocyte count.

should be confirmed by future prospective studies in larger groups of IBS patients.

VCE findings in IBS Findings in patients with IBS are generally normal. As in some healthy volunteers, nonspecific findings such as red spots, lymphangiectasia, and single mucosal breaks may be seen.

Value of VCE in IBS There is no evidence to support the use of VCE in the management of patients with IBS. Discrete nonspecific findings bear the risk of false stigmatization of patients, for instance as suffering from Crohn's disease, or of escalation of diagnostic tests such as push enteroscopy, double balloon enteroscopy or radiological imaging techniques, or of leading to surgery (Figure 10.9).

Abdominal pain in patients with obscure GI bleeding

Obscure GI bleeding is the most common indication for VCE. Hence, the additional symptom of abdominal pain does not add a further indication to the decision whether or not to perform VCE. As many patients suffer from abdominal pain, it seems likely that a significant proportion of patients with obscure bleeding will also have IBS independently. However, abdominal pain in bleeding patients should raise the possibility of obstruction. A detailed history and informed consent focusing on the possible need for surgery in case of capsule retention are necessary. The patency capsule may be used in doubtful cases. Ultrasound and/or CT scan can be used to exclude severe stenosis, tumor infiltration or aortic aneurysm. Repeated upper GI endoscopy might be considered in the search for overlooked bleeding peptic lesions.

VCE findings in patients with abdominal pain and obscure bleeding VCE findings depend on the individual diagnosis, e.g. angioectasia, Crohn's disease or tumor, whether or not related to abdominal pain. When reading VCE studies of patients with bleeding and abdominal pain,

special care should be taken to look for possible strictures or intussusception, but also for peptic gastroduodenal lesions possibly missed at upper GI endoscopy.

Value of VCE in patients with abdominal pain and bleeding The indication for VCE in these patients is based on obscure bleeding, with or without pain. However, abdominal pain should raise the possibility of obstruction (Figure 10.10).

Abdominal pain associated with malabsorption

Malabsorption may be associated with abdominal pain and may be caused by a variety of diseases including chronic pancreatitis, defects of mucosal enzymes, bacterial overgrowth, inflammation related to celiac sprue or Crohn's disease, infections, and other conditions.

Lactose intolerance is a common inherited disorder causing diarrhea and abdominal pain. Diagnosis is provided by a positive hydrogen breath test after ingestion of lactose and cessation of symptoms with a lactose-free diet. Symptomatic celiac sprue can be excluded with serological tests. In unclear cases, biopsies from the duodenum, optimally also from the proximal jejunum, can be helpful in the search for infections such as giardiasis or Whipple's disease. In rare situations VCE may give further information on mucosal changes not accessible to routine endoscopy.[72]

A rare cause of malabsorption is intestinal lymphangiectasia[73] (Waldmann's disease) presenting with typical although not specific findings at VCE. In this condition an exudative enteropathy leads to hypoalbuminemia and edema. The diagnosis can be proven by finding an elevated α_1-antitrypsin clearance in association with lymphopenia and hypoglyceridemia.

VCE findings in primary lymphangiectasia Diffusely distributed whitish, swollen villi affecting a long intestinal segment are the typical finding (Figure 10.11). These

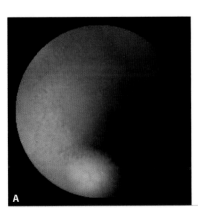
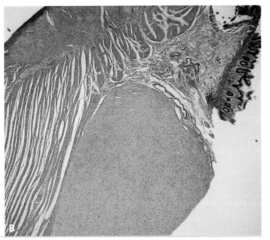

FIGURE 10.9 Leiomyoma. (a) A small submucosal tumor. VCE cannot differentiate between carcinoid and benign mesenchymal tumor. (b) Histology of the resected tumor showed a leiomyoma (H&E, courtesy of Renate Höhne, MD). Immunostain for gastrointestinal stromal tumor, using CD117, was negative. A 41-year-old female patient with abdominal pain, weight loss, and a history of bronchial carcinoid. CT scan of thorax and abdomen, enteroclysis, octreotide scintigraphy, bronchoscopy, EGD, and ileo-colonoscopy were all normal. Abdominal pain recurred shortly after surgery. Laparoscopic fundoplication for hiatal hernia with reflux esophagitis was performed later, but also had no long-standing beneficial effect. The abdominal pain appeared to be of functional origin.

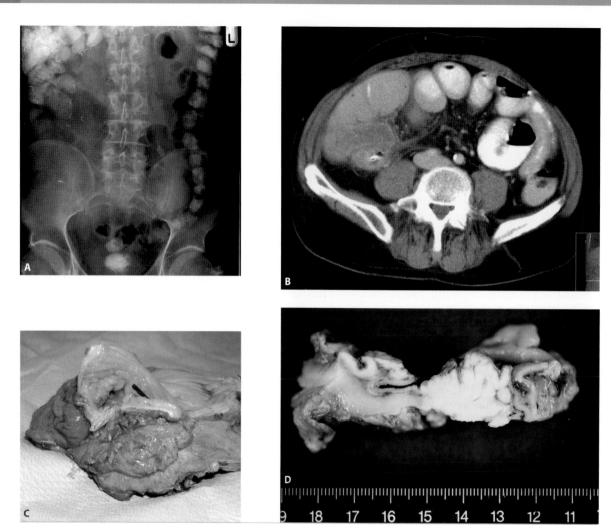

FIGURE 10.10 Metastasis of colon carcinoma to the small bowel. (a) The coil of a dissolved patency capsule is visible on plain abdominal x-ray. Clips are also seen after right-sided hemicolectomy, as is contrast medium after inconclusive enteroclysis. (b) CT scan shows the coil of the patency capsule in a short thickened small bowel segment (courtesy of Ernst Malzfeldt, MD). Surgical specimen with neoplastic stenosis, retained coil, and coating of the dissolved patency capsule (c, courtesy of Christopher Pohland, MD). Pathology revealed infiltrating adenocarcinoma (d, courtesy of Renate Höhne, MD). The 72-year-old patient with iron deficiency anemia, positive FOBT, and intermittent colicky pain had a history of hemicolectomy for colon cancer. Retention of the patency capsule augmented CT diagnosis of suspected relapse of colon carcinoma. Due to stenosis and strong suspicion of tumor relapse, surgery was performed without VCE. Tumor was confirmed and resected. From Costamagna G, Keuchel M, Riccioni M (2006): Patency Capsule. In Keuchel M, Hagenmüller F, Fleischer D (eds). Atlas of Video Capsule Endoscopy with permission from Springer Verlag.

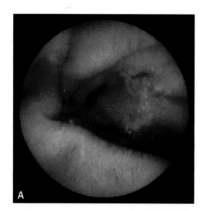

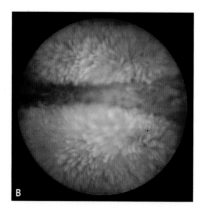

FIGURE 10.11 Diffuse primary lymphangiectasia. Villi in the duodenum are almost normal (a), whereas in the jejunum diffusely distributed whitish villi are visible (b). Lymphangiectasia was proven histologically in jejunal biopsies taken at push enteroscopy. This 26-year-old male patient suffered from abdominal pain, exudative enteropathy, and weight loss of 30 kg. He improved on a low-fat diet with medium chain triglycerides (MCT) and temporary treatment with somatostatin.

alterations may begin in the jejunum, whereas functional lymphangiectasia is usually present already in the duodenum. Causes of secondary lymphangiectasia such as tumor, infection, and inflammation should be excluded.

Value of VCE in malabsorption Workup of malabsorption requires functional and serological tests, as well as duodenal biopsies. In rare cases, VCE can demonstrate mucosal changes of the jejunum or ileum. However, enteroscopy with biopsy is still required to confirm and differentiate positive VCE findings by histology.

Abdominal pain in intestinal obstruction

Intestinal obstruction can cause crampy abdominal pain. Ultrasonography or plain abdominal x-ray film may be used as first-line tests, optimally during an attack. The next step is enteroclysis or small bowel series to further define whether there is a stenosis. CT or MRI enterography may be used alternatively. However, the initial world experience with retained video capsules in patients with negative small bowel series as communicated by Barkin and Friedman[74] suggests that VCE is more sensitive. Patients at risk for retention of the capsule are those with Crohn's disease,[75,76] prior partial resection of the small bowel,[72] abdomino-pelvic radiation,[77] tumor[78] (Figures 10.5, 10.10), and long-term intake of NSAIDs.[79]

Suspected obstruction is generally considered as a contraindication to VCE. In spite of negative x-ray, VCE should not be performed in patients with suspected obstruction unless they are potential candidates for surgery. Informed consent should be obtained, making it clear that surgery may be required if the capsule is retained for a prolonged period. Patients with inflammatory Crohn's stenosis or with radiation enteritis should not be forced into unnecessary surgery because of a retained capsule. However, in certain cases of fibrotic (Figure 10.3), ulcerated (Figure 10.12) or tumorous stenosis (Figure 10.5), capsule impaction may lead to adequate therapy, either surgical with stricturoplasty or segmental resection, or endoscopic balloon dilatation.

Prior to VCE, a trial with a new biodegradable "patency capsule," visible by fluoroscopy, could be helpful in patients at risk for intestinal strictures. In a multi-center study, excretion of the intact patency capsule was found to predict an uneventful VCE.[80–82] However, it should be noted that even the biodegradable patency capsule itself may cause intestinal obstruction. This has been reported in 2 cases of long tight strictures in Crohn's disease.[82,83] Especially in patients with established or strongly suspected Crohn's disease, it is prudent to perform imaging tests such as CT or MRI first to exclude long strictures. Voderholzer et al[84] excluded 27% of their patients with Crohn's disease from VCE because of stenosis < 10 mm seen at CT enteroclysis. In one series of suspected Crohn's disease, as many as 15% of the capsules were retained.[29] All 3 patients with capsule retention were asymptomatic.

In cases with enough evidence from history and prior tests, the retention of a patency capsule might lead to the decision to proceed directly to surgery without performing VCE (Figure 10.10).

The possibility of extracting a retained video capsule from the small bowel with a push enteroscope[78] or a double balloon enteroscope has been reported.[85] This might reduce concern about capsule retention but should not lead to the thoughtless application of VCE in high-risk patients.

VCE findings in intestinal obstruction Stenosis can be visualized by a narrowed lumen due to fibrotic, ulcerated or irregularly infiltrated mucosa. Intermittent pressing of the capsule against the stenosis may be suggested by a white, bloodless ring in the mucosa.

Value of VCE in intestinal obstruction VCE is contraindicated in suspected obstruction. Severe stenosis can be excluded by radiologic tests. In doubtful cases, a test with the patency capsule can be helpful. In symptomatic patients with inconclusive diagnostic tests VCE can be used to document strictures in rare cases where surgery may be indicated.

Future needs

Although abdominal pain is a frequent complaint in gastroenterologic practice, evidence for widespread use of VCE is still insufficient. Future studies should focus on the predictive value of certain symptoms and findings for a positive VCE, for instance in suspected Crohn's disease. With larger numbers of patients studied in a systematic manner, a scoring system might be developed.

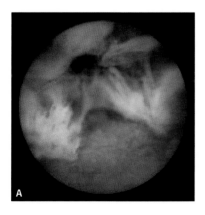

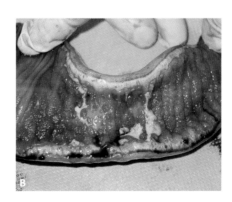

FIGURE 10.12 Stenosis of the jejunum. (a) Circular ulcerated stenosis with edema and nodularity of the visible mucosa. The capsule did not pass the stenosis during recording time. At surgery, a mid-jejunal segment was resected; the capsule had traversed the stenosis in the meantime (b, courtesy of Thomas Fox, MD). Histology revealed a nonspecific benign stenosis with transmural ulceration without granulomas. The 74-year-old lady suffered from progressive crampy abdominal pain for several weeks. CT demonstrated thickening of a jejunal loop and severe stenosis of the celiac trunk. An ischemic origin of the stenosis seems likely.

The investigation of suspected adhesions is a relevant task in the management of patients with chronic abdominal pain. Prospective studies should elucidate whether there is any role for VCE in the workup of suspected adhesions or even in predicting long-term benefit of laparoscopic lysis of adhesions.

References

1. DeBanto JR, Varilek GW, Haas L. What could be causing chronic abdominal pain? Anything from common peptic ulcers to uncommon pancreatic trauma. Postgrad Med 1999;106:141–6.

2. Kalloo AN. Overview of differential diagnoses of abdominal pain. Gastrointest Endosc 2002;56(Suppl 2): S255–7.

3. Guthrie E, Thompson D. Abdominal pain and functional gastrointestinal disorders. BMJ 2002;325:701–703.

4. Zackowski SW. Chronic recurrent abdominal pain. Emerg Med Clin North Am 1998;16:877–94, vii.

5. Srinivasan R, Greenbaum DS. Chronic abdominal wall pain: a frequently overlooked problem. Practical approach to diagnosis and management. Am J Gastroenterol 2002;97:824–30.

6. Reid S, Wessely S, Crayford T, Hotopf M. Medically unexplained symptoms in frequent attenders of secondary health care: retrospective cohort study. BMJ 2001;322:767.

7. Olden KW. Rational management of chronic abdominal pain. Compr Ther 1998;24:180–6.

8. Astegiano M, Bresso F, Cammarota T, et al. Abdominal pain and bowel dysfunction: diagnostic role of intestinal ultrasound. Eur J Gastroenterol Hepatol 2001;13:927–31.

9. Hollerbach S, Geissler A, Schiegl H, et al. The accuracy of abdominal ultrasound in the assessment of bowel disorders. Scand J Gastroenterol 1998;33:1201–8.

10. Maglinte DD, Kelvin FM, O'Connor K, Lappas JC, Chernish SM. Current status of small bowel radiography. Abdom Imaging 1996;21:247–57.

11. Lankisch PG, Gaetke T, Gerzmann J, Becher R. The role of enteroclysis in the diagnosis of unexplained gastrointestinal symptoms: a prospective assessment. Z Gastroenterol 1998;36:281–6.

12. Camilleri M, Heading RC, Thompson WG. Clinical perspectives, mechanisms, diagnosis and management of irritable bowel syndrome. Aliment Pharmacol Ther 2002;16:1407–30.

13. Sandler RS, Everhart JE, Donowitz M, et al. The burden of selected digestive diseases in the United States. Gastroenterology 2002;122:1500–11.

14. Hommes DW, van Deventer SJ. Endoscopy in inflammatory bowel diseases. Gastroenterology 2004;126:1561–73.

15. Carey E, Leighton J, Shiff A, High R, Sharma V, Fleischer D. The value of capsule endoscopy for evaluation of abdominal pain and/or diarrhea. Gastroenterology 2004;126(Suppl 2): A-460.

16. Landi B, Tkoub M, Gaudric M, et al. Diagnostic yield of push-type enteroscopy in relation to indication. Gut 1998;42:421–5.

17. Sharma BC, Bhasin DK, Makharia G, et al. Diagnostic value of push-type enteroscopy: a report from India. Am J Gastroenterol 2000;95:137–40.

18. Swain CP. The role of enteroscopy in clinical practice. Gastrointest Endosc Clin N Am 1999;9:135–44.

19. Yamamoto H. Double-balloon endoscopy. Clin Gastroenterol Hepatol 2005;3(Suppl 1):S27–S29.

20. Sunada K, Yamamoto H, Kita H, et al. Clinical outcomes of enteroscopy using the double-balloon method for strictures of the small intestine. World J Gastroenterol 2005;11:1087–9.

21. Salky BA, Edye MB. The role of laparoscopy in the diagnosis and treatment of abdominal pain syndromes. Surg Endosc 1998;12:911–4.

22. Lavonius M, Gullichsen R, Laine S, Ovaska J. Laparoscopy for chronic abdominal pain. Surg Laparosc Endosc 1999;9:42–4.

23. Bardan E, Nadler M, Chowers Y, Fidder H, Bar-Meir S. Capsule endoscopy for the evaluation of patients with chronic abdominal pain. Endoscopy 2003;35:688–9.

24. Fireman Z, Eliakim R, Adler S, Scapa E. Capsule endoscopy in real life: a four-centre experience of 160 consecutive patients in Israel. Eur J Gastroenterol Hepatol 2004;16:927–31.

25. Romero-Vázquez J, Caunedo AA, Argüelles-Arias F, Pellicer-Bautista F, Herrerías-Gutiérrez JM. Capsule endoscopy in patients with abdominal pain and negative alarm symtoms. 4th Int Conf Capsule Endosc, Miami Beach, FL, March 2005.

26. Spada C, Pirozzi G, Iacopini F, et al. Diagnostic yield of capsule endoscopy in patients with chronic abdominal pain. Gastroenterology 2005;28(Suppl 2):A-649.

27. Argüelles-Arias F, Caunedo AA, Romero-Vázquez J, Pellicer-Bautista F, Argüelles -Martin F, Herrerías-Gutiérrez JM. Use of the capsule endoscopy in children with recurrent abdominal pain. 4th Intern Conf Capsule Endoscopy, Miami Beach, FL, March 2005.

28. Fireman Z, Mahajna E, Broide E, et al. Diagnosing small bowel Crohn's disease with wireless capsule endoscopy. Gut 2003;52:390–2.

29. Ge ZZ, Hu YB, Xiao SD. Capsule endoscopy in diagnosis of small bowel Crohn's disease. World J Gastroenterol 2004;10:1349–52.

30. Herrerias JM, Caunedo A, Rodriguez-Tellez M, Pellicer F, Herrerias JM Jr. Capsule endoscopy in patients with suspected Crohn's disease and negative endoscopy. Endoscopy 2003;35:564–8.

31. Chong AK, Taylor A, Miller A, Hennessy O, Connell W, Desmond P. Capsule endoscopy vs. push enteroscopy and enteroclysis in suspected small-bowel Crohn's disease. Gastrointest Endosc 2005;61:255–61.

32. Arguelles-Arias F, Caunedo A, Romero J, et al. The value of capsule endoscopy in pediatric patients with a suspicion of Crohn's disease. Endoscopy 2004;36:869–73.

33. Mow WS, Lo SK, Targan SR, et al. Initial experience with wireless capsule enteroscopy in the diagnosis and management of inflammatory bowel disease. Clin Gastroenterol Hepatol 2004;2:31–40.

34. Keuchel M, Hagenmuller F. Video capsule endoscopy in the work-up of abdominal pain. Gastrointest Endosc Clin N Am 2004;14:195–205.

35. Eliakim R, Suissa A, Yassin K, Katz D, Fischer D. Wireless capsule video endoscopy compared to barium follow-through and computerised tomography in patients with suspected Crohn's disease — final report. Dig Liver Dis 2004;36:519–22.

36. Sanders DS, Hurlstone DP, Stokes RO, et al. Changing face of adult coeliac disease: experience of a single university hospital in South Yorkshire. Postgrad Med J 2002;78:31–3.

37. Fitzpatrick KP, Sherman PM, Ipp M, Saunders N, Macarthur C. Screening for celiac disease in children with recurrent abdominal pain. J Pediatr Gastroenterol Nutr 2001;33:250–2.

38. Saltik IN, Kocak N, Yuce A, Gurakan F. Celiac disease screening of Turkish children with recurrent abdominal pain. J Pediatr Gastroenterol Nutr 2002;34:424.

39. Sanders DS, Carter MJ, Hurlstone DP, et al. Association of adult coeliac disease with irritable bowel syndrome: a case-control study in patients fulfilling ROME II criteria referred to secondary care. Lancet 2001;358:1504–8.

40. Cammarota G, Martino A, Pirozzi GA, et al. Direct visualization of intestinal villi by high-resolution magnifying upper endoscopy: a validation study. Gastrointest Endosc 2004;60:732–8.

41. Petroniene R, Dubcenco E, Baker JP, et al. Given capsule endoscopy in celiac disease: evaluation of diagnostic accuracy and interobserver agreement. Am J Gastroenterol 2005;100:685–94.

42. Culliford A, Daly J, Diamond B, Rubin M, Green PH. The value of wireless capsule endoscopy in patients with complicated celiac disease. Gastrointest Endosc 2005;62:55–61.

43. Apostolopoulos P, Alexandrakis G, Giannakoulopoulou E, et al. M2A wireless capsule endoscopy for diagnosing ulcerative jejunoileitis complicating celiac disease. Endoscopy 2004;36:247.

44. Joyce AM, Burns DL, Marcello PW, Tronic B, Scholz FJ. Capsule endoscopy findings in celiac disease associated enteropathy-type intestinal T-cell lymphoma. Endoscopy 2005;37:594–6.

45. Krauss N, Cellier C, Collin P, et al. Evaluation of capsule endoscopy in celiac disease patients with ongoing symptoms on a gluten-free diet — a prospective, blinded European multicenter trial. Gastroenterology 2005;128(Suppl 2):A-81.

46. Rossini FP, Risio M, Pennazio M. Small bowel tumors and polyposis syndromes. Gastrointest Endosc Clin N Am 1999;9:93–114.

47. Abrahams NA, Halverson A, Fazio VW, Rybicki LA, Goldblum JR. Adenocarcinoma of the small bowel: a study of 37 cases with emphasis on histologic prognostic factors. Dis Colon Rectum 2002;45:1496–502.

48. Mascarenhas-Saraiva MN, da Silva Araujo Lopes LM. Small-bowel tumors diagnosed by wireless capsule endoscopy: report of five cases. Endoscopy 2003;35:865–8.

49. Hemminki K, Li X. Incidence trends and risk factors of carcinoid tumors: a nationwide epidemiologic study from Sweden. Cancer 2001;92:2204–10.

50. Bailey A, Debinski H, Appleyard M, Remedios M, Hooper J, Selby W. Diagnosis and outcome of small bowel tumours found by capsule endoscopy: a three centre Australian experience. Gastrointest Endosc 2005;61:AB159.

51. Delvaux M, Laurent V, Klopp I, Regent D, Gay G. Intestinal tumors: frequently revealed by an obscure digestive bleeding (ODB) and more easily diagnosed by capsule endoscopy (VCE). Gastrointest Endosc 2005;61:AB162.

52. Keuchel M, Thaler C, Caselitz J, Hagenmüller F. Diagnosis of small bowel tumors with video capsule endoscopy: report of 16 cases. Gastroenterology 2004;126(Suppl 2):A347.

53. Kummar S, Ciesielski TE, Fogarasi MC. Management of small bowel adenocarcinoma. Oncology (Huntingt) 2002;16:1364–9.

54. Morris AJ. Nonsteroidal anti-inflammatory drug enteropathy. Gastrointest Endosc Clin N Am 1999;9:125–33.

55. Chutkan R, Toubia N. Effect of nonsteroidal anti-inflammatory drugs on the gastrointestinal tract: diagnosis by wireless capsule endoscopy. Gastrointest Endosc Clin N Am 2004;14:67–85.

56. Maiden L, Thjodleifsson B, Theodors A, Gonzalez J, Bjarnason I. A quantitative analysis of NSAID-induced small bowel pathology by capsule enteroscopy. Gastroenterology 2005;128:1172–8.

57. Graham DY, Opekun AR, Willingham FF, Qureshi WA. Visible small-intestinal mucosal injury in chronic NSAID users. Clin Gastroenterol Hepatol 2005;3:55–9.

58. Goldstein JL, Eisen GM, Lewis B, Gralnek IM, Zlotnick S, Fort JG. Video capsule endoscopy to prospectively assess small bowel injury with celecoxib, naproxen plus omeprazole, and placebo. Clin Gastroenterol Hepatol 2005;3:133–41.

59. Yousfi MM, De Petris G, Leighton JA, et al. Diaphragm disease after use of nonsteroidal anti-inflammatory agents: first report of diagnosis with capsule endoscopy. J Clin Gastroenterol 2004;38:686–91.

60. Nosho K, Endo T, Yoda Y, et al. Diaphragm disease of small intestine diagnosed by double-balloon enteroscopy. Gastrointest Endosc 2005;62:187–9.

61. Cave D, Bhinder F, Schneider D, Wolff R, Toth L, Ferris K. Small intestinal NSAID injury: An expanding spectrum. Abstracts of the 2nd Conference on capsule endoscopy, Berlin, March 23–25, 2003, p. 19.

62. Schietroma M, Carlei F, Altilia F, et al. The role of laparoscopic adhesiolysis in chronic abdominal pain. Minerva Chir 2001;56:461–5.

63. Swank DJ, van Erp WF, Repelaer van Driel OJ, Hop WC, Bonjer HJ, Jeekel J. Complications and feasibility of laparoscopic adhesiolysis in patients with chronic abdominal pain. A retrospective study. Surg Endosc 2002;16:1468–73.

64. Dunker MS, Bemelman WA, Vijn A, et al. Long-term outcomes and quality of life after laparoscopic adhesiolysis for chronic abdominal pain. J Am Assoc Gynecol Laparosc 2004;11:36–41.

65. Keuchel M, Thaler C, Csomós G, Klick M, Neumann-Grutzeck C, Hagenmüller F. Video capsule endoscopy: technical and medical failures. Endoscopy 2003;35(Suppl):A6.

66. Brandt LJ, Boley SJ. AGA technical review on intestinal ischemia. American Gastrointestinal Association. Gastroenterology 2000;118:954–68.

67. Kozuch PL, Brandt LJ. Review article: diagnosis and management of mesenteric ischaemia with an emphasis on pharmacotherapy. Aliment Pharmacol Ther 2005;21:201–15.

68. Fork F, Toth E. Given capsule enteroscopy in ischemic enteropathy. Abstract of the 2nd Conference on capsule endoscopy, Berlin, March 23–25, 2003. p. 115.

69. Leighton J, Sharma V, Hara A, Fleischer D. Video Capsule endosopy (CE) compared to small bowel follow through (SBFT) and abdominopelvic CT scan (CT) for detecting lesions in the small intestine (SI). Am J Gastroenterol 2002;97(Suppl):S80–81.

70. Thompson WG, Longstreth GF, Drossman DA, Heaton KW, Irvine EJ, Muller-Lissner SA. Functional bowel disorders and functional abdominal pain. Gut 1999;45 Suppl 2:II43–II47.

71. Jones J, Boorman J, Cann P, et al. British Society of Gastroenterology guidelines for the management of the irritable bowel syndrome. Gut 2000;47 Suppl 2:ii1–19.

72. Keuchel M, Thaler Ch, Csomós G, Klick M, Hagenmüller F. Video capsule endoscopy for the diagnosis of small bowel disease. Endo heute 2002;15:153–6.

73. Bliss CM, Schroy III PC. Primary intestinal lymphangiectasia. Curr Treat Options Gastroenterol 2004;7:3–6.

74. Barkin J, Friedman S. Wireless capsule endoscopy requiring surgical intervention: the world's experience. Am J Gastroenterol (Suppl) 2002;97:S298.

75. Keuchel M, Hagenmüller F. [Small bowel endoscopy with the wireless video capsule]. Dtsch Ärzteblatt 2002;99:A2702–10.

76. Kastin DA, Buchman AL, Barrett T, Halverson A, Wallin A. Strictures from Crohn's disease diagnosed by video capsule endoscopy. J Clin Gastroenterol 2004;38:346–9.

77. Lee DW, Poon AO, Chan AC. Diagnosis of small bowel radiation enteritis by capsule endoscopy. Hong Kong Med J 2004;10:419–21.

78. Madisch A, Schimming W, Kinzel F, et al. Locally advanced small-bowel adenocarcinoma missed primarily by capsule endoscopy but diagnosed by push enteroscopy. Endoscopy 2003;35:861–4.

79. Bhinder F, Schneider D, Farris K, et al. NSAID associated small intestinal ulcers and strictures: diagnosis by video capsule endoscopy. Gastroenterology (Suppl) 2002;122:A345.

80. Spada C, Spera G, Riccioni M, et al. A novel diagnostic tool for detecting functional patency of the small bowel: the Given patency capsule. Endoscopy 2005;37:793–800.

81. Delvaux M, Ben Soussan E, Laurent V, Lerebours E, Gay G. Clinical evaluation of the use of the M2A patency capsule system before a capsule endoscopy procedure, in patients with known or suspected intestinal stenosis. Endoscopy 2005;37:801–7.

82. Boivin ML, Lochs H, Voderholzer WA. Does passage of a patency capsule indicate small-bowel patency? A prospective clinical trial. Endoscopy 2005;37:808–15.

83. Gay G, Delvaux M, Laurent V, et al. Temporary intestinal occlusion induced by a «patency capsule» in a patient with Crohn's disease. Endoscopy 2005;37:174–7.

84. Voderholzer WA, Beinhoelzl J, Rogalla P, et al. Small bowel involvement in Crohn's disease: a prospective comparison of wireless capsule endoscopy and computed tomography enteroclysis. Gut 2005;54:369–73.

85. May A, Nachbar L, Ell C. Extraction of entrapped capsules from the small bowel by means of push-and-pull enteroscopy with the double-balloon technique. Endoscopy 2005;37:591–3.

CHAPTER **11**

Approach to the Patient with Obstruction

Maria Elena Riccioni • Syed Shah • Cristiano Spada, and Guido Costamagna

KEY POINTS

1. Adhesions, Crohn's disease and chronic radiation-induced strictures are common causes of chronic, recurrent (partial) small bowel obstruction (SBO).

2. In patients with suspected SBO but equivocal plain abdominal films, small bowel series, either small bowel follow-through (SBFT) or enteroclysis (SBE), may help in confirming the diagnosis and degree of small bowel obstruction.

3. Video capsule endoscopy (VCE) has been shown to detect small intestinal lesions consistent with Crohn's disease in 43–71% of patients, when conventional tests, including flexible endoscopy and SBFT, have been negative.

4. However, with the advent of the Given Patency Capsule®, a self-dissolvable "dummy" capsule, the need for SBFT or SBE may become relatively obsolete in the investigation of patients with suspected partial small bowel obstruction, prior to VCE.

5. The newly developed Given Patency Capsule has been shown to be a promising tool for assessing the degree of small intestinal luminal narrowing prior to performing VCE.

Diagnosis and clinical evaluation of patients with suspected small bowel obstruction

Small bowel obstruction (SBO) occurs when the normal luminal flow of intestinal contents is interrupted resulting in abdominal pain and distension, nausea, and vomiting. The cause of SBO may be due to either intrinsic or extrinsic compression of the small intestine. Post-surgical adhesions, hernias, and metastatic cancer are the commonest causes of SBO (approximately 85% of cases), resulting in extrinsic compression of the small bowel, whereas intrinsic causes, such as tumors (either primary or secondary), strictures of the small bowel, congenital malformations, intussusception, Meckel's diverticulum, foreign body and gallstones (gallstone ileus) are less frequent. Strictures may be inflammatory due to Crohn's disease, ischemic, or secondary to radiation enteritis. More recently, long-term use of non-steroidal anti-inflammatory drugs (NSAIDs) has been shown to be associated with both small and large bowel strictures.[1] SBO may be classified as acute or chronic, partial versus complete, or simple versus closed-loop. In partial obstruction, small intestinal contents (chyme) and gas are able to pass across the site of obstruction whereas this is not the case in complete obstruction. In simple obstruction, there is occlusion of the bowel at a single point along the intestinal tract leading to small bowel dilatation and bacterial overgrowth proximal to the obstruction and decompression distally, whereas in closed obstruction there is occlusion of both proximal and distal ends of a segment of bowel and attached mesentery, with the risk of vascular compromise, ischemia, necrosis, and perforation (strangulation). The most common causes of simple obstruction are intra-abdominal adhesions, tumors, and strictures whereas closed-loop obstruction is usually secondary to hernias, adhesions, and volvulus. Rarely, patients with eosinophilic gastroenteritis or angioneurotic edema may present with transient partial small bowel obstruction.

In a recent population study of hospital discharges, adhesiolysis for SBO accounted for more than 300 000 hospitalizations and over 800 000 days of inpatient care.[2] The incidence of SBO is reported to be up to 11–15% within 1–2 years following abdominal surgery,[3] the risk being dependent on the type of operation performed.[4,5] Adhesions,[6–8] Crohn's disease, and chronic radiation-induced strictures are common causes of chronic, recurrent (partial) small bowel obstruction.

The initial diagnosis of small bowel obstruction is based on history, physical examination, and plain abdominal x-ray. Abdominal pain is often described as peri-umbilical and crampy with paroxysms of pain occurring every 4–5 minutes in proximal obstruction and less frequently (15–20 minute intervals) in distal SBO. A combination of gradual change in bowel habit, progressive abdominal distension, early satiety, mild crampy pain after meals, and weight loss is also suggestive of chronic partial SBO. Patients may or may not complain of absolute constipation or inability to pass flatus. A history of previous episodes of SBO, previous upper or lower abdominal surgery, previous surgery for SBO, intra-abdominal malignancy, previous radiotherapy, and possible Crohn's disease should be sought. Patients should also be questioned about the use of NSAIDs. Physical examination may reveal abdominal distension (distal > proximal SBO), any surgical scars, hernias, an abdominal mass, or signs of peritonitis (in case of strangulation). Laboratory tests are largely unhelpful in diagnosing SBO, although serum lactate may indicate impending gut ischemia.[9,10]

Plain abdominal x-ray

Basic radiologic examination should include an upright chest film to rule out the presence of free air as well as supine and erect abdominal films. Ideally, this should be performed during the acute episode. Multiple distended loops of small bowel with air–fluid levels within the distended loops are typical of SBO. A dilated loop of small bowel appearing in the same location on supine and upright films is suggestive of mechanical obstruction by an adhesion or an internal hernia. If the patient cannot be placed into an upright position then a left lateral decubitus film may reveal the presence of free air and/or air–fluid levels. Although a diagnosis of SBO can usually be made on history, physical examination, and plain abdominal x-rays, in 20–30% plain films may be equivocal or "normal."[11,12]

Small bowel series

In patients with suspected SBO but equivocal plain abdominal films, small bowel series, either small bowel follow-through (SBFT) or enteroclysis (SBE), may help in confirming the diagnosis and degree of small bowel obstruction. Enteroclysis is generally considered the most sensitive method of distinguishing between ileus and partial mechanical small bowel obstruction.[13–19] These studies are highly sensitive and traditionally have been considered to be the gold standard for determining whether an obstruction is partial or complete. In partial obstruction, SBE is superior to SBFT, because the technique of enteroclysis exaggerates the pre-stenotic dilatation that is typical of small bowel obstruction. SBE is reported to have a diagnostic sensitivity of 87% for adhesive obstruction.[20] The presence of water-soluble contrast in the cecum within 24 hours predicts resolution of adhesive small bowel obstruction and may also have a therapeutic role.[21,22] SBE has also been shown to be useful in differentiating between obstruction secondary to metastatic disease and adhesions.[20] In a recent study, enteroclysis correctly predicted the presence of obstruction in 100%, the absence of obstruction in 80%, the level of obstruction in 89%, and the cause of obstruction in 86% of patients undergoing surgery.[12]

Small bowel studies, however, are inferior to CT in the detection of closed-loop or strangulated obstruction, and gut ischemia. As a result, some radiologists currently recommend CT as the first investigation after plain films in difficult-to-diagnose bowel obstructions,[23–26] although to some extent this depends not only on local expertise but also on clinical circumstances.[27] In patients with suspected SBO but with normal or equivocal plain films, enteroclysis is helpful in excluding lower grades of partial obstruction, compared to CT,[28] and may also guide surgical treatment (adhesiolysis) in adhesive obstruction. In contrast, in patients with probable SBO on plain film, SBE may be appropriate if simple mechanical obstruction is suspected, and CT in those patients with signs of peritonitis or suspected strangulation. In patients with a history of malignancy, CT and enteroclysis may be complementary.[20] In elderly, frail patients with SBO, CT may be more appropriate, easier to perform, often diagnostic, and less time-consuming compared with enteroclysis.

Computed tomography

Computed tomography (CT) has the advantage of demonstrating not only the presence, level, and severity of SBO, but also the cause and potential complications (closed-loop or strangulation, ischemia).[29] CT may help in characterizing SBO from extrinsic causes (adhesions, hernia, or extrinsic masses), intrinsic causes (small bowel adenocarcinoma or lymphoma, Crohn's disease, tuberculosis, radiation enteropathy, intramural hemorrhage, bezoars, or intussus-ception), or intestinal malrotation. For CT, dilute barium or water-soluble contrast is usually given either orally or via a nasogastric tube approximately 30–120 minutes prior to scanning, together with intravenous contrast. The diagnosis of obstruction is made when there is a discrepancy in the caliber of proximal and distal small bowel[11]; often a point of transition can be demonstrated. Absence of air or fluid in the distal small bowel or colon denotes complete obstruc-tion. Intestinal pneumatosis and hemorrhagic mesenteric changes can be seen in advanced strangulation. Prospective studies have demonstrated that the accuracy of CT in diagnosing bowel obstruction is higher than 95% and that its sensitivity and specificity are each higher than 94%.[29,30] In patients with partial, recurrent SBO without a history of previous abdominal surgery, CT should be considered the initial investigation of choice, followed by small bowel series if inconclusive, and in some cases barium enema.[31] Adhesions may not be detectable by CT scan.[11]

Magnetic resonance imaging

Fast magnetic resonance imaging (MRI) with T_2-weighted images is reported to be more accurate, sensitive, and specific compared to contrast-enhanced helical CT scanning in establishing the location and cause of bowel obstruction.[32] In a prospective study of 44 patients with suspected small and large bowel obstruction, the accuracy, sensitivity, and specificity of fast MRI for diagnosing obstruction were 96%, 95%, and 100% respectively compared to 71%, 71%, and

71% for contrast, helical CT. The negative predictive values of fast MRI and helical CT for excluding the presence of obstruction were 80% and 56%, respectively. Fast MRI was able to differentiate all cases of benign obstruction from obstruction due to malignancy. The advantages of fast MRI over helical CT scanning are (1) that image acquisition time is short (1–2 seconds per slice), which means that images can be acquired in the space of a single breath-hold (12 slices), and (2) that no contrast agents are required. In addition, because of its multiplanar capability, MRI is also more effective at demonstrating the transition point of the obstruction. Unlike CT, MRI is not limited by the presence of barium in patients initially undergoing a small bowel series. The limitations of fast MRI include comparatively poor anatomic definition and limited soft tissue characterization compared to CT, and the traditional limitations of MRI scanning and local expertise.[32] When helical CT scanning is non-diagnostic in a patient with suspected SBO and fast MRI is not available, a small bowel follow-through examination is often useful.[23]

MR enteroclysis, using gadolinium-based contrast agents and methylcellulose, has been shown to demonstrate the intestinal and extra-intestinal features of Crohn's disease with results comparable to those of SBE.[33]

Ultrasonography

Abdominal ultrasonography is more sensitive and specific than plain films for the diagnosis of small bowel obstruction[34,35] but is not as accurate as CT or small bowel radiology. In a study comparing plain films, ultrasound, and CT in 32 patients presenting with a clinical suspicion of intestinal obstruction, the reported sensitivity and specificity of CT for the diagnosis of SBO was 93% and 100%, respectively, compared to 83% and 100% for ultrasound, and 50% and 75% for plain radiography.[36] The level of obstruction was correctly predicted in 93% on CT compared to only 70% and 60% for ultrasound and plain films, respectively. CT was also superior to ultrasound and plain films for determining the cause of the obstruction (87% vs. 23% vs. 7%, respectively). However, abdominal ultrasound has been shown to be useful in demonstrating strictures in patients with known Crohn's disease with a reported sensitivity and specificity of 79–90% and 98–100%, respectively.[37] Although not as helpful as CT for diagnosis of location, cause, and possible strangulation, ultrasound may be appropriate as a bedside test in critically ill patients with suspected SBO.

Radio-opaque markers

In some patients with adhesive obstruction, false negative enteroclysis examination results may occur, particularly when obstruction is intermittent. In some cases, partial obstruction may only become apparent after ingesting solid foods and indigestible particles, or high-fibre foods (roughage). Radio-opaque markers, normally used for assessing colonic transit times, have been used to simulate partial small bowel obstruction caused by food.[38] In a study of four patients, two of whom had previously normal SBE,

20 solid 4 mm radio-opaque markers were used to challenge suspected partial small bowel obstruction. Serial plain abdominal x-rays showed initial dispersal of markers leaving the stomach followed by subsequent coalescence of markers at sites of partial obstruction. In all four cases, the sites of obstruction were confirmed at surgery.

Video capsule endoscopy (VCE)

As with CT and small bowel series, wireless video capsule endoscopy (VCE) is capable of imaging the entire small bowel but with the advantage of high-resolution, 'villous' views of the small intestinal mucosa. For the most part, VCE has been used to investigate patients with overt or occult gastrointestinal bleeding in whom previous endoscopic and radiologic investigations have been negative. In such patients, VCE has been shown to be superior to both push enteroscopy[39–43] and small bowel studies,[44] with a significantly higher diagnostic yield. Capsule endoscopy also appears to be more sensitive in detecting small bowel mucosal disease than barium small bowel studies. In one of the first studies, 20 patients with suspected small bowel disease underwent both VCE and small bowel follow-through.[44] VCE was considered diagnostic in 45% compared with just 20% of patients for SBFT. Video capsule endoscopy identified suspicious lesions in 50% of patients in whom SBFT was normal. Hara et al reported on 52 patients who underwent VCE, predominantly for obscure GI bleeding, of which 42 of 52 patients (81%) had 36 SBFT examinations, 4 enteroclysis, and 19 conventional CT, within 6 months of VCE.[45] SBFT was positive in only 1 of 40 patients (3%) compared with VCE, which demonstrated positive findings in 22 patients (55%). Similarly, CT was positive in 4 of 19 patients (21%) compared with VCE, which was positive in 12 of 19 patients (63%). Although the most common finding was angioectasia, VCE detected significantly more ulcers than either SBFT or CT. In addition, VCE detected 3 of 5 surgically confirmed masses (carcinoid, intussusception, lymphangioma) compared to SBFT, which detected none, and CT, which demonstrated 1 of 4 masses. In a separate retrospective cohort analysis of 72 patients investigated for small bowel disease, VCE was demonstrated to have a significantly higher diagnostic yield than SBFT (83% vs. 41%), irrespective of the type of small bowel lesion detected.[46] VCE also appears to be more sensitive than dedicated small bowel enteroclysis for the detection of small bowel ulcers.[47] Two patients with multiple small bowel ulcers (up to 1 cm in diameter) in the jejunum and previous negative small bowel radiology were referred after VCE for repeat 'state of the art' enteroclysis by two experienced GI radiologists, who were told in advance of the VCE findings. Despite being ideal technically perfect examinations, both studies failed to detect any ulcers.

VCE has also been shown to be superior to SBFT for the diagnosis of suspected Crohn's disease. VCE has been shown to detect small intestinal lesions consistent with Crohn's disease in 43–71% of patients, when conventional tests, including flexible endoscopy and SBFT, have been negative.[48–52] In a comparative study of VCE, SBFT, and ileoscopy in patients with known or suspected CD, without stricture, VCE demonstrated lesions in 56% of patients, whereas SBFT revealed diagnostic findings in 19%, and ileoscopy in 44%.[50] In a separate study comparing VCE, SBFT, and entero-CT in patients with suspected Crohn's disease, VCE demonstrated lesions consistent with Crohn's disease in 77% of patients compared to diagnostic yields of 23% and 20% for SBFT and CT, respectively.[53] Furthermore, capsule endoscopy detected all of the lesions diagnosed by SBFT and CT. Other comparative studies of VCE and CT enteroclysis have reached similar conclusions.[54]

VCE is clearly more sensitive than traditional radiological methods for detecting perhaps the early stages of Crohn's disease. In addition, there is also supporting evidence that VCE may be more sensitive than small bowel series for the detection of Crohn's disease strictures, as well as strictures due to other causes. Kastin et al. reported on a patient with suspected Crohn's disease in whom multiple ileal strictures were found by VCE.[55] Prior to VCE, the patient had undergone numerous investigations including multiple SBFT examinations and repeated CT examinations as well as flexible endoscopy and push enteroscopy, all of which were negative. Because of capsule impaction, surgery was performed and revealed nine ileal strictures. Other authors have described similar experiences of capsule retention in unsuspected strictures in patients with either known or suspected Crohn's disease.[51,56-59] Overall, the rate of capsule retention in patients investigated for known or suspected Crohn's disease is reported to be 1.7% (3 out of 177 patients).[60] In all three patients, SBFT was entirely normal and elective surgery was performed resulting in symptom relief. In addition to Crohn's disease strictures, capsule retention has also been reported in patients with strictures or diaphragm-like lesions secondary to NSAIDs,[61-63] radiation-induced enteritis,[64] small bowel tumours,[65] Meckel's diverticulum,[59] and post-surgical anastomotic ulceration with stenosis,[66] despite a normal small bowel study. It is for the above reasons that current recommendations are that VCE should be used with caution in patients with known or suspected partial small bowel obstruction or stricture, or those at risk of developing small bowel strictures. Despite the reported insensitivity of small bowel series for the detection of strictures, in such patients it is recommended that a small bowel study be performed (ideally SBE) to exclude significant luminal narrowing before VCE.[67-69] However, with the advent of the Patency Capsule, a self-dissolvable 'dummy' capsule, the need for SBFT or SBE may become relatively obsolete in the investigation of patients with suspected partial small bowel obstruction, prior to VCE.

Capsule retention

Capsule retention may be suspected in patients in whom the battery runs out before the capsule is seen to pass the ileocecal valve, or when there is retention of the capsule above a stricture or mass (endoluminal lesion) that may be visible on review of the recorded capsule images. In such cases, patients rarely experience symptoms of mechanical obstruction, but plain abdominal x-ray (supine and oblique films) should be performed 1–2 weeks after the procedure to

determine whether the capsule has been excreted or retained in the small bowel (Figure 11.1). The average small bowel passage time is 4 hours 26 minutes 3 seconds with a range of 17 minutes 24 seconds to 12 hours 34 minutes 56 seconds.[70] The capsule is usually expelled naturally after an average of 72 hours (range 24 to 222 hours),[70] although Taylor et al[71] described a patient in whom there was retention of the capsule endoscope above a stricture for 3 months, without adverse effect.

Non-migration or retention of the capsule endoscope has been reported to occur in 1.25–13% of patients in reported case series.[58,59,62,72] In the first worldwide report of capsule retention during VCE, the incidence rate of surgical intervention was 0.75% (7 of 934 patients studied).[73] Six of the seven patients had a normal small bowel series and in all seven cases an endoluminal pathologic process was found that explained the patient's symptoms. Other authors have described similar cases where capsule retention led to the diagnosis of partial small bowel obstruction from either endoluminal[74,75] or extraluminal causes.[76] With one exception,[74] all of the patients remained asymptomatic despite capsule impaction.

Because of the attendant risks of emergency exploratory laparotomy, careful consideration should be given to any patient in whom there is the potential for capsule retention, and in such cases the decision to perform VCE should always be made in conjunction with the surgical team. If the capsule is seen to remain in the small bowel on follow-up abdominal films, then exploratory laparotomy and intraoperative enteroscopy should be advised (Figure 11.2). In the majority of cases surgery can be performed electively; however, VCE should not be performed in patients who are not candidates for surgery or who refuse surgery.

The Given Patency Capsule®

Because of the problems associated with unexpected capsule retention in patients with partial small bowel obstructing lesions, the manufacturers of the capsule endoscope developed a self-dissolvable capsule that could be used as a "sham" test to assess the degree of small intestinal luminal narrowing prior to performing VCE.

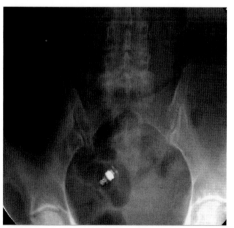

FIGURE 11.1 Retention of the PillCam video capsule on plain x-ray.

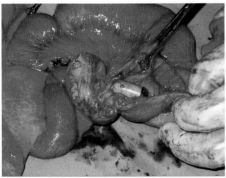

FIGURE 11.2 Retained video capsule at laparotomy. In this case a carcinoid tumour was found to be the cause of partial small bowel obstruction.

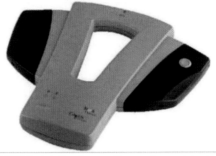

FIGURE 11.4 The detector (Patency Scanner) that is used in conjunction with the Given Patency Capsule to confirm either retention or excretion of the Patency Capsule. The Patency Scanner works by activating the radiofrequency identification tag (RFID), and receives a radiofrequency signal that is re-transmitted by the RFID tag.

Patency Capsule design

The Given Patency Capsule is composed of two parts: (a) a disintegrating "patency" capsule with the same dimensions as the standard small video capsule (11 mm × 26 mm), and (b) a radiofrequency identification tag within the capsule (Figure 11.3). The Given Patency Capsule is designed to remain intact in the gastrointestinal tract for approximately 100 hours, following which, if still present within the body, the capsule will disintegrate spontaneously. The body of the capsule is composed of compressed lactose, which readily dissolves in contact with gastrointestinal fluids, and 10% barium sulfate powder, making the capsule radio-opaque. Thus, it is possible to view the Given Patency Capsule using fluoroscopy. Attached to the body of the capsule is a "plug" composed of wax, which acts as "a time-pacer" for the disintegration of the capsule. The entire unit is then coated with a very thin layer of a liquid impermeable polymer, Parylene C. Surface erosion caused by gastric juice and intestinal fluids forms a hole in the plug over the designated time period. Through this hole, intestinal fluids penetrate to reach the body of the capsule, dissolving the lactose–barium mixture and leaving behind the Parylene C coating.

Tracking of the Given Patency Capsule is based on a radiofrequency identification tag incorporated into the capsule. The tag consists of two components: (a) a metal coil that is activated by radiofrequency waves emitted by the Patency Scanner (Figure 11.4), and which acts as a two-way antenna, and (b) a silicon chip that is, in turn, activated by radiofrequency energy emitted by the metal coil, transmitting a unique identification signal that is subsequently detected by the Patency Scanner.

Preliminary clinical evaluation of the Given Patency Capsule

In January 2002, we conducted a pilot study to assess the feasibility and safety of VCE in patients with known or suspected small bowel strictures, following initial assessment of small bowel luminal patency using the Given Patency Capsule. Small bowel strictures were identified on follow-through examinations in the 6 months preceding study enrollment. In all, seven centers partici-pated (Costamagna G, Rome; Herrerias J, Seville, Spain; Lochs H, Berlin, Germany; Schreiber S, Kiel, Germany; Reddy N, Hyderabad, India; Rutgeerts P, Leuven, Belgium; Warwick W, Sydney, Australia) in a multi-center study which completed enrollment in September 2004.

Study protocol

During the first visit, patients swallowed the Given Patency Capsule and subsequently fluoroscopy was performed on Day 2, 8–10 hours after ingestion, to document the position of the capsule. In those patients where the Given Patency Capsule had not been excreted, further x-rays were performed at 24 hours after ingestion and repeated where necessary until capsule excretion had been confirmed. Immediate fluoroscopy was performed if patients experienced abdominal pain, or where there was clinical suspicion of gastrointestinal obstruction, or gastrointestinal related adverse events. Patients were asked, where possible, to retrieve the capsule and/or its components from the stool, and to return to the study investigators.

Study results

In total, 91 patients (46 female; mean age 39 years (range 20–85 years)) were enrolled into the study. In all patients, an SBFT had been performed within the 6 months preceding enrollment. On review of the small bowel films, in 18/91 patients (20%) there was suspicion of a stricture; these were patients with familial adenomatous polyposis (FAP), postoperative adhesions, and ischemic enteritis. In the remaining 73 patients (80%) there was a definite, confirmed stricture, which was due to, in decreasing frequency, Crohn's

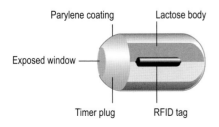

Parylene coating   Lactose body

Exposed window

Timer plug   RFID tag

FIGURE 11.3 Cross-sectional view of the Given Patency Capsule.

disease (54/73), tuberculosis (11/73), suspected adhesions (4/73), and other causes (4/73).

All of the patients ingested the capsule without any difficulty. The mean capsule excretion time was 53 hours (range 5–439); the capsule was retrieved intact in 46 patients (51%), totally or partially disintegrated in 40 patients (44%), and could not be retrieved in 5 patients. A single patient withdrew consent during the study period, and, in this case, a record of whether the capsule was retrieved was not available.

Adverse events

Adverse events were reported in 22 patients (24%). Seventeen patients complained of abdominal pain that resolved within 24 hours of ingestion of the capsule. Three patients were hospitalized due to severe abdominal pain, but all were managed conservatively with symptomatic treatment and corticosteroids, with symptom resolution within 24 hours. Two patients underwent surgery. One patient developed intestinal obstruction with plain abdominal films showing an intact Given Patency Capsule and dilated small bowel loops. At surgery, an intact capsule was found retained within a 25 cm length Crohn's stricture. The second patient underwent elective surgery within 30 days of ingestion of the Given Patency Capsule, for an unrelated cause.

Interestingly, no correlation was found between the radiological features of the small bowel strictures and the capsule transit time. Surprisingly, in some patients with tight strictures the capsule was excreted intact within a very short time — less than 6 hours. This suggested that the Given Patency Capsule could be used to assess the degree of luminal patency of the small intestine before ingestion of the PillCam video capsule endoscope. We therefore extended the study to a second phase in which patients in whom the Given Patency Capsule had been excreted intact within 72 hours, without any ill effects, were invited to ingest the PillCam capsule.

Safety of the PillCam video capsule after use of the Given Patency Capsule

In this second phase of the study, 67 patients were enrolled, of which 29 fulfilled the inclusion criteria, having had an intact Given Patency Capsule excreted 72 hours after ingestion (Figure 11.5). The etiology of the underlying small bowel stricture was Crohn's disease in 15 patients, suspected stricture in 10, tuberculosis in 2, and other causes in 2 patients. Thirty-eight patients (56.8%) were excluded, due to retrieval of a non-intact capsule in 29 patients, adverse events in 5, and failure to retrieve the Given Patency Capsule in 4 cases. The results of this study showed that the PillCam capsule endoscope passed through all 29 strictures without any adverse events reported, confirming our clinical suspicion that the Given Patency Capsule could be safely used to assess small bowel luminal patency prior to performing VCE in patients with known small bowel strictures. The mean transit time of the PillCam was also found to correlate well with the mean transit time of the Given Patency Capsule — 27 hours (SD = 22) PillCam vs. 26 hours (SD = 18) Given Patency Capsule; Pearson rho coefficient, $r = 0.7$, $p = 0.0015$.

Conclusion

Recurrent small bowel obstruction is a common problem encountered in clinical practice. Traditionally, this has been investigated by way of small bowel radiology, ultrasonography, and CT scanning. VCE provides high-resolution images of the entire small bowel, and has been shown to be more sensitive than the traditional radiological investigations, not only for the detection of early small bowel mucosal disease but also for "occult" small bowel strictures. The event of capsule retention above an unsuspected small bowel stricture is rare, but in many cases may lead to a curative surgical resection. The newly developed Given Patency Capsule has been shown to be a promising tool for assessing the degree of small intestinal luminal narrowing prior to performing VCE. The use of a self-dissolvable patency capsule should in the future reduce the risk of capsule retention in patients with suspected small bowel strictures, and may avoid the need to perform a small bowel series in such patients. Since the original pilot study, the manufacturers of the Given Patency Capsule have modified the design of the capsule to include two wax plugs rather than one. Further clinical studies using this new patency capsule are eagerly awaited.

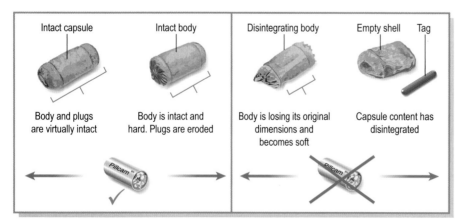

FIGURE 11.5 Images of the Given Patency Capsule excreted intact, and after capsule disintegration, leaving behind the Parylene C coating (shell) and RFID tag. In those patients in whom the Patency Capsule is excreted intact, performance of VCE using the PillCam video capsule appears to be safe.

References

1. Onwudike M, Sundaresan M, Melville D, Wood JJ. Diaphragm disease of the small bowel — a case report and literature review. Dig Surg 2002;19:410–3.

2. Ray NF, Denton WG, Thamer M. Abdominal adhesiolysis: inpatient care and expenditures in the United States in 1994. J Am Coll Surg 1998;186:1–9.

3. Beck DE, Opelka FG, Bailey HR. Incidence of small-bowel obstruction and adhesiolysis after open colorectal and general surgery. Dis Colon Rectum 1999;42:241–8.

4. Zbar RI, Crede WB, McKhann CF, Jekel JF. The postoperative incidence of small bowel obstruction following standard, open appendectomy and cholecystectomy: a six-year retrospective cohort study at Yale-New Haven Hospital. Conn Med 1993;57:123–7.

5. Renz BM, Feliciano DV. Unnecessary laparotomies for trauma: a prospective study of morbidity. J Trauma 1995;38:350–6.

6. Barkan H, Webster S, Ozeran S. Factors predicting the recurrence of adhesive small-bowel obstruction. Am J Surg 1995;170:361–5.

7. Landercasper J, Cogbill TH, Merry WH. Long-term outcome after hospitalization for small-bowel obstruction. Arch Surg 1993;128:765–70.

8. Miller G, Boman J, Shrier I. Natural history of patients with adhesive small bowel obstruction. Br J Surg 2000; 87:1240–7.

9. Murray MJ, Gonze MD, Nowak LR, Cobb CF. Serum D-lactate levels as an aid to diagnosing acute intestinal ischaemia. Am J Surg 1994;167:575–8.

10. Lange H, Jackel R. Usefulness of plasma lactate concentration in the diagnosis of acute abdominal disease. Eur J Surg 1994;160:381–4.

11. Megibow AJ, Balthazar EJ, Cho KC. Bowel obstruction: evaluation with CT. Radiology 1991;180:313–8.

12. Shrake PD, Rex DK, Lappas JC. Radiographic evaluation of suspected SBO. Am J Gastroenterol 1991;86:175–8.

13. Khaleghian R. The small bowel enema in the management of small-bowel obstruction. Australas Radiol 1983;27:154–9.

14. Dunn JT, Halls JM, Berne TV. Roentgenographic contrast studies in acute small-bowel obstruction. Arch Surg 1984; 119:1305–8.

15. Brolin R. Partial small bowel obstruction. Surgery 1984; 95:145–9.

16. Maglinte DDT, Peterson LA, Vahey TN. Enteroclysis in partial small bowel obstruction. Am J Surg 1984;147:325–9.

17. Maglinte DDT, Hall R, Miller RE. Detection of surgical lesions of the small bowel by enteroclysis. Am J Surg 1984;127:225–9.

18. Anderson C, Humphry W. Contrast radiography in small bowel obstruction: a prospective randomized trial. Mil Med 1997;162:749–52.

19. Fevang BT, Jensen D, Fevang J. Upper gastrointestinal contrast study in the management of small bowel obstruction — a prospective randomised study. Eur J Surg 2000;166:39–43.

20. Caroline DF, Herlinger H, Laufer I. Small bowel enema in the diagnosis of adhesive obstructions. AJR Am J Roentgenol 1984;142:1133–9.

21. Abbas S, Bissett I, Parry B. Oral water soluble contrast for the management of adhesive small bowel obstruction. Cochrane Database Syst Rev, CD004651, 2005.

22. Chen SC, Chang KJ, Lee PH. Oral urografin in postoperative small bowel obstruction. World J Surg 1999;23:1051.

23. Peck JJ, Milleson T, Phelan J. The role of computed tomography with contrast and small bowel follow-through in management of small bowel obstruction. Am J Surg 1999;177:375–8.

24. Balthazar E. For suspected small-bowel obstruction and an equivocal plain film, should we perform CT or a small-bowel series? AJR Am J Roentgenol 1994;163:1260–1.

25. Daneshmand S, Hedley C, Stain S. The utility and reliability of computed tomography scan in the diagnosis of small bowel obstruction. Am Surg 1999;65:922–6.

26. Donckier V, Closset J, Van Gansbek D. Contribution of computed tomography to decision making in the management of adhesive small bowel obstruction. Br J Surg 1998;85:1071–4.

27. Maglinte DDT, Herlinger H, Turner WW Jr. Radiologic management of small-bowel obstruction: a practical approach. Emerg Radiol 1994;1:138–49.

28. Maglinte DD, Gage SN, Harmon BH, et al. Obstruction of the small intestine: accuracy and role of CT in diagnosis. Radiology 1993;188:61–4.

29. Balthazar EJ. CT of small-bowel obstruction. AJR Am J Roentgenol 1994;162:255–61.

30. Megibow A, Megibow A. Bowel obstruction: evaluation with CT. Radiol Clin North Am 1994;32:861–70.

31. Stelmach W, Cass A. Small bowel obstructions: the case for investigation for occult large bowel carcinoma. Aust NZ J Surg 1989;59:181–3.

32. Beall DP, Fortman BJ, Lawler BC. Imaging bowel obstruction: a comparison between fast magnetic resonance imaging and helical computed tomography. Clin Radiol 2002;57:719–24.

33. Maglinte DDT, Siegelman ES, Kelvin FM. MR Enteroclysis: the future of small-bowel imaging? Radiology 2000; 215:639–41.

34. Ogata M, Mateer J, Condon R. Prospective evaluation of abdominal sonography for the diagnosis of bowel obstruction. Ann Surg 1996;223:237–41.

35. Grunshaw N, Renwick IG, Scarisbrick G, et al. Prospective evaluation of ultrasound in distal ileal and colonic obstruction. Clin Radiol 2000;55:356–62.

36. Suri S, Gupta S, Sudhakar PJ. Comparative evaluation of plain films, ultrasound and CT in the diagnosis of intestinal obstruction. Acta Radiol 1999;40:422–8.

37. Nakstad B, Naess PA, de Lange C, Schistad O. Complications of umbilical vein catheterization: neonatal total parenteral nutrition ascites after surgical repair of congenital diaphragmatic hernia. J Pediatr Surg 2002; 37:E21.

38. Johnson PA, Miner PB Jr, Geier D, Harrison LA. Value of radiopaque markers in identifying partial small bowel obstruction. Gastroenterology 1996;110:1958–63.

39. Ell C, Remke S, May A, Helou L, Henrich R, Mayer G. The first prospective controlled trial comparing wireless capsule endoscopy with push enteroscopy in chronic gastrointestinal bleeding. Endoscopy 2002;34:685–9.

40. Mylonaki M, Fritscher-Ravens A, Swain P. Wireless capsule endoscopy: a comparison with push enteroscopy in patients with gastroscopy and colonoscopy negative gastrointestinal bleeding. Gut 2003;52:1122–6.

41. Mata A, Bordas JM, Feu F, et al. Wireless capsule endoscopy in patients with obscure gastrointestinal bleeding: a comparative study with push enteroscopy. Aliment Pharmacol Ther 2004;20:189–94.

42. Lewis BS, Swain P. Capsule endoscopy in the evaluation of patients with suspected small intestinal bleeding: results of a pilot study. Gastrointest Endosc 2002;56:349–53.

43. Adler DG, Knipschield M, Gostout C. A prospective comparison of capsule endoscopy and push enteroscopy in patients with GI bleeding of obscure origin. Gastrointest Endosc 2004;59:492–8.

44. Costamagna G, Shah SK, Riccioni ME, et al. A prospective trial comparing small bowel radiographs and video capsule endoscopy for suspected small bowel disease. Gastroenterology 2002;123:999–1005.

45. Hara AK, Leighton JA, Sharma VK, Fleischer DE. Small bowel: preliminary comparison of capsule endoscopy with barium study and CT. Radiology 2004;230:260–5.

46. Friedman S. Comparison of capsule endoscopy to other modalities in small bowel. Gastrointest Endosc Clin N Am 2004;14:51–60.

47. Liangpunsakul S, Chadalawada V, Rex DK, Maglinte D, Lappas J. Wireless capsule endoscopy detects small bowel ulcers in patients with normal results from state of the art enteroclysis. Am J Gastroenterol 2003;98:1295–8.

48. Fireman Z, Mahajna E, Broide E, et al. Diagnosing small bowel Crohn's disease with wireless capsule endoscopy. Gut 2003;52:390–2.

49. Herrerias JM, Caunedo A, Rodriguez-Tellez M, Pellicer F, Herrerias JM Jr. Capsule endoscopy in patients with suspected Crohn's disease and negative endoscopy. Endoscopy 2003;35:564–8.

50. Bloom PD, Rosenberg MD, Klein SD. Wireless capsule endoscopy (CE) is more informative than ileoscopy and SBFT for the evaluation of the small intestine (SI) in patients with known or suspected Crohn's disease [Abstract]. Gastroenterology 2003;124 Suppl 1:A203.

51. Ge ZZ, Hu YB, Xiao SD. Capsule endoscopy in diagnosis of small bowel Crohn's disease. World J Gastroenterol 2004;10:1349–52.

52. Arguelles-Arias F, Caunedo A, Romero J, et al. The value of capsule endoscopy in pediatric patients with a suspicion of Crohn's disease. Endoscopy 2004;36:869–73.

53. Eliakim R, Suissa A, Yassin K, Katz D, Fischer D. Wireless capsule video endoscopy compared to barium follow-through and computerised tomography in patients with suspected Crohn's disease — final report. Dig Liver Dis 2004;36:519–22.

54. Voderholzer WA, Beinhoelzl J, Rogalla P, et al. Small bowel involvement in Crohn's disease: a prospective comparison of wireless capsule endoscopy and computed tomography enteroclysis. Gut 2005;54:369–73.

55. Kastin DA, Buchman AL, Barrett T, Halverson A, Wallin A. Strictures from Crohn's disease diagnosed by video capsule endoscopy. J Clin Gastroenterol 2004;38:346–9.

56. Fork FT, Toth E, Sato S. Capsule enteroscopy in patents with Crohn's disease. First Given conference on capsule endoscopy [Abstract], Rome, A43, 2002.

57. Lo SK. Capsule endoscopy in the diagnosis and management of inflammatory bowel disease. Gastrointest Endosc Clin N America 2004;14:179–93.

58. Chong AK, Taylor AC, Miller AM, Desmond PV. Initial experience with capsule endoscopy at a major referral hospital. Med J Aust 2003;178:537–40.

59. Fireman Z, Eliakim R, Adler S, Scapa E. Capsule endoscopy in real life: a four-centre experience of 160 consecutive patients in Israel. Eur J Gastroenterol Hepatol 2004; 16:927–31.

60. Eliakim R, Adler SN. Capsule video endoscopy in Crohn's disease — the European experience. Gastrointest Endosc Clin N Am 2004;14:129–37.

61. Yousfi MM, De Petris G, Leighton JA, et al. Diaphragm disease after use of nonsteroidal anti-inflammatory agents: first report of diagnosis with capsule endoscopy. J Clin Gastroenterol 2004;38:686–91.

62. Sears DM, Avots-Avotins A, Culp K, Gavin MW. Frequency and clinical outcome of capsule retention during capsule endoscopy for GI bleeding of obscure origin. Gastrointest Endosc 2004;60:822–7.

63. Manetas M, O'Loughlin C, Kelemen K, Barkin JS. Multiple small-bowel diaphragms: a cause of obscure GI bleeding diagnosed by capsule endoscopy. Gastrointest Endosc 2004;60:848–51.

64. Lee DW, Poon AO, Chan AC. Diagnosis of small bowel radiation enteritis by capsule endoscopy. Hong Kong Med J 2004;10:419–21.

65. Hartmann D, Schilling D, Rebel M, et al. Diagnosis of a high-grade B-cell lymphoma of the small bowel by means of wireless capsule endoscopy. Z Gastroenterol 2003;41:171–4.

66. De Franchis R, Avesani EM, Abbiati C, et al. Unsuspected ileal stenosis causing obscure GI bleeding in patients with previous abdominal surgery — diagnosis by capsule endoscopy: a report of two cases. Dig Liv Dis 2003; 35:577–84.

67. American Society of Gastrointestinal Endoscopy. Wireless capsule endoscopy. Gastrointest Endosc 2002;56:621–4.

68. Faigel DO, Fennerty MB. "Cutting the cord" for capsule endoscopy. Gastroenterology 2002;123:1385–8.

69. O'Loughlin C, Barkin JS. Wireless capsule endoscopy: summary. Gastrointest Endosc Clin N Am 2004;14:229–37.

70. Barkin JS, O'Loughlin C. Capsule endoscopy contraindications: complications and how to avoid their occurrence. Gastrointest Endosc Clin N Am 2004;14:61–5.

71. Taylor A, Miller A, Woods R, Desmond P. Long-term retained capsule without ill effects in a patient with ileal ulceration and undiagnosed stricture. In: Jacob H, ed. Proceedings of the first Given conference on capsule endoscopy, Rome, 2002. Rochash Printing, Haifa, Israel, 2003, p. 115.

72. Ang TL, Fock KM, Ng TM, Teo EK, Tan YL. Clinical utility, safety and tolerability of capsule endoscopy in urban Southeast Asian population. World J Gastroenterol 2003;9:2313–6.

73. Barkin JS, Friedman S. Wireless capsule endoscopy requiring surgical intervention: the world's experience [Abstract]. Am J Gastroenterol 2002;97:S298.

74. Mergener K, Schembre DB, Brandabur JJ, Smith MA, Kozarek RA. Clinical utility of capsule endoscopy — a single center experience. Am J Gastroenterol 2002;97:S299.

75. Sears DM, Avots-Avotins A, White J, Culp K. Fortuitous M2A obstruction leads to localization of unsuspected vascular stricture. Am J Gastroenterol 2002;97:S128.

76. Keuchel M, Thaler CH, Csomos G. Technical and medical problems associated with M2A video capsule endoscopy. In: Jacob H, ed. Proceedings of the second Given Conference on capsule endoscopy, 2003, p. 145.

CHAPTER **12**

Approach to the Pediatric Patient

Victor L Fox

KEY POINTS

1. Pediatric indications for capsule endoscopy are similar to adult indications, although investigation for neoplasia is rare.

2. Gastrointestinal bleeding is the most common indication for young children, and inflammatory bowel disease is the most common indication for older children and adolescents.

3. Endoscopic capsule placement is generally required for children under 10 years of age.

4. Minimum age thresholds for safety and efficacy have not been established but capsule endoscopy has been conducted in children as young as 2 years of age without complication.

5. Special bowel preparations and prokinetic medications may enhance but are not essential for complete small bowel examination.

Introduction

Complete small bowel enteroscopy in children prior to the advent of video capsule endoscopy (VCE) required laparotomy with manual advancement of the bowel over an endoscope, typically a small-diameter colonoscope. While this approach is still frequently necessary for therapeutic enteroscopy, the wireless capsule endoscope now enables nonoperative diagnostic endoscopic imaging of the entire small bowel in the majority of children, at least as young as 2–3 years of age. This is possible because of the small caliber of the capsule and the portability of the battery-powered data recorder.

In 2001, the United States Food and Drug Administration (FDA) issued approval of the M2A capsule (Given Imaging, Yoqneam, Israel) for use in adult patients over the age of 18 years, and in 2003 this approval was expanded for pediatric application in children age 10–18 years. To date, most pediatric VCE examinations have, therefore, been performed in children over the age of 10 years. Although children under 10 years of age are certainly capable of swallowing a device of this dimension, as illustrated by a rich medical literature on foreign body ingestion by infants and children, they are rarely willing to cooperate on demand. And just as there are exceptionally cooperative children as young as 7 or 8 years of age, so are there adolescents and even young adults who will refuse to swallow a capsule.

Although some pediatric gastroenterologists take exception to the FDA ruling, others remain reluctant to introduce the device endoscopically into small children where the risk of impaction and potential need for operative removal has not been carefully assessed. Published pediatric data have been limited to a small number of case reports[1-4] and small series.[5-9] The largest series of children under 10 years included 20 patients ranging in age from 2 to 9 years (mean 5.9) and in weight from 13 to 32 kg (mean 22).[9] A minimum age and size limit for safe and clinically effective VCE using current devices is still unknown.

Indications

The indications for VCE in children are comparable in spectrum to those in adults but differ in frequency due to the relative rarity of certain diagnoses such as small bowel tumors, refractory sprue, acquired angiodysplasia, and Barrett's esophagus. General indications common to both adults and children include obscure gastrointestinal bleeding, suspected Crohn's disease or other inflammatory or ulcerating disease, non-inflammatory enteropathies, polyposis disorders, and vascular lesions, both congenital and acquired, such as gastroesophageal and small bowel varices and vascular malformations.

Gastrointestinal bleeding

Gastrointestinal bleeding (GIB) was the primary indication for VCE in 17 of 20 (85%) children less than 10 years of age studied at Children's Hospital Boston.[9] Bleeding may be either occult or overt from an obscure source (Figure 12.1) or in the context of a known diagnosis such as inflammatory bowel disease (Figure 12.2) or polyposis (Figure 12.3), or a known vascular anomaly (Figure 12.4) for which complete intestinal mapping is sought to plan for appropriate intervention.[10] Capsule endoscopy is more sensitive than angiography for detecting vascular anomalies involving the small intestine,[11] especially when investigating small venous malformations (Figure 12.5) and in the absence of brisk bleeding.

Inflammatory bowel disease

Inflammatory bowel disease (IBD) is currently the predominant indication for VCE in older children and adolescents. Two small pediatric series have demonstrated the added diagnostic value of VCE after performing routine contrast radiography and esophagogastroduodenoscopy (EGD) with colonoscopy including examination of the terminal ileum. Arguelles-Arias et al[5] studied 12 children between the ages of 12 and 16 years who were suspected of

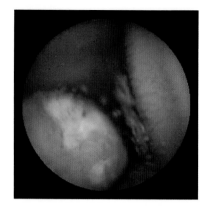

FIGURE 12.3 Large ulcerated small bowel polyp in a 16-year-old male with familial juvenile polyposis.

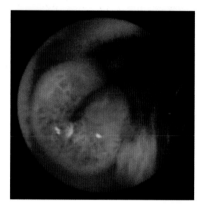

FIGURE 12.4 One of many polypoid venous malformations found throughout the small bowel in a 6-year-old female with blue rubber bleb nevus syndrome.

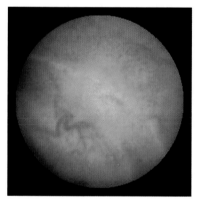

FIGURE 12.5 One of multiple serpiginous small-caliber vessels found in the small bowel of an 8-year-female with Turner's syndrome.

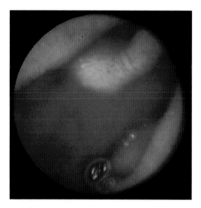

FIGURE 12.1 Fresh bleeding associated with focal villous drop-out in the proximal small bowel of a 7-year-old female who presented with profound anemia, occult blood positive stool, and negative EGD, ileocolonoscopy, Meckel scan, UGI and small bowel barium examination, and abdominal CT.

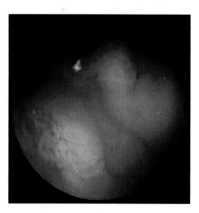

FIGURE 12.2 One of several ulcers found in the small bowel of a 15-year-old male with a prior history of ulcerative colitis who presented with acute melena.

having Crohn's disease but had inconclusive radiographic and endoscopic findings. Capsule endoscopy identified lesions compatible with Crohn's disease in 7 of 12 (58.3%) children. Sant'Anna et al[7] found Crohn's-like lesions in 10 of 20 (50%) children age 10–18 years who were studied by VCE after negative or non-diagnostic radiographic and endoscopic examinations.

Incidental aphthous ulcers of the small bowel are not uncommon in adult patients, presumably due to NSAID exposure, although they may be idiopathic. These lesions can be difficult to distinguish from Crohn's-related ulcers. Such lesions appear to be rare in children, so that the finding of focal small bowel ulcers in a child with other clinical indications of IBD is highly suggestive of Crohn's disease. VCE may help to distinguish ulcerative colitis or indeterminate colitis from Crohn's disease by either excluding or detecting characteristic ulceration of the small bowel (Figure 12.6). This distinction assumes critical importance when colectomy followed by ileal pouch with anal anastomosis (IPAA) is being considered in a patient with suspected ulcerative colitis. Negative small bowel findings in a child with chronic or recurrent pouchitis following colectomy and IPAA also provides added reassurance that the original diagnosis of ulcerative colitis is correct and that Crohn's disease remains unlikely. VCE is also useful in the diagnostic evaluation of a patient with an atypical presentation of IBD such as isolated oral (Figure 12.7), anogenital, or cutaneous lesions. Glycogen storage disease type 1b and Behçet's syndrome[12] are rare disorders that can present during childhood years and also manifest Crohn's disease-like ulcerations optimally assessed by VCE.

The primary concern about using VCE in patients with IBD is the increased risk of capsule retention or impaction due to an inflammatory or fibrotic stricture leading to unplanned surgical intervention. Prior screening with contrast radiography can reduce but not completely eliminate this risk. Prescreening with a self-dissolving "patency capsule" should fully eliminate this risk. FDA approval for this device in the USA was given in 2006 for adults. Capsules may be transiently retained at occult sites of stenosis (Figure 12.8) without causing obstructive symptoms and later pass spontaneously, sometimes after initiating anti-inflammatory therapy.[7]

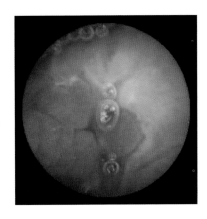

FIGURE 12.8 Ulcerated stricture in a 20-year-old male with Crohn's disease with negative small bowel barium examination. The capsule was retained at this site on the video recording but passed spontaneously without pain several days later.

Polyposis

VCE is an ideal modality for investigating patients with known or suspected polyposis given its greater sensitivity and lack of radiation exposure compared with barium contrast radiography. The three most important polyposes of childhood are Peutz–Jeghers syndrome (PJS), familial adenomatous polyposis (FAP), and juvenile polyposis syndrome (JPS). Each is inherited as an autosomal dominant condition with variable phenotypic expression, and new spontaneous mutations are relatively common. Each is associated with an increased risk of gastrointestinal or colorectal cancer during adult years. Colorectal cancer during childhood has rarely been reported with FAP and JPS.

Children with Peutz–Jeghers syndrome often present with intermittent abdominal pain due to small bowel intussusceptions induced by one or more polyps. VCE is indicated if barium contrast radiography of the small bowel fails to detect polyps in a symptomatic child with typical freckling of the lips and buccal mucosa (Figure 12.9a, b) or a positive family history. Once a diagnosis is established, VCE may be preferable to contrast radiography for repeated surveillance. Advances in therapeutic endoscopy should allow patients with PJS to avoid or delay laparotomy for polypectomy. The size and location of polyps identified by VCE can direct the endoscopic approach. For example, large polyps (> 1–1.5 cm) in the proximal small bowel may be reached by peroral push enteroscopy, while mid or distal small bowel lesions may require double balloon enteroscopy (adolescent) or laparotomy-assisted enteroscopy (young child). Nearly all polyps can be removed safely endoscopically if proper techniques are employed.

Familial adenomatous polyposis (FAP) may present in childhood with diarrhea, bleeding, or abdominal pain, although most often the condition is asymptomatic in young children. While the colon is predominantly affected, the stomach and small bowel are also frequently involved. Gastric polyps are typically fundic gland type but also may be wholly comprised or contain foci of adenoma. The diagnosis may be detected by screening colonoscopy in children known to be genetically at risk because of an affected parent or sibling, or in children with conditions associated with FAP such as osteomas of the jaw or skull, congenital hypertrophy of retinal pigmented epithelium,

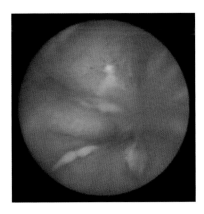

FIGURE 12.6 Linear Crohn's-like ulcers found in the terminal ileum of a 15-year-old female with indeterminate colitis.

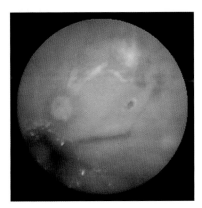

FIGURE 12.7 Aphthous ulceration in the small bowel of a 14-year-old male with chronic granulomatous chellitis.

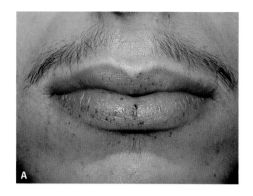

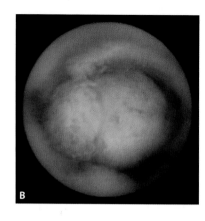

FIGURE 12.9 Peutz–Jeghers syndrome: (a) pigmented macules on the lips of an adolescent male (courtesy of Dr. Marilyn Liang); (b) distal small bowel polyp detected in a 12-year-old male with abdominal pain and negative small bowel barium examination.

desmoid tumor, glioblastoma (Turcot's syndrome), or hepatoblastoma. The earliest mucosal change cannot be visually identified by conventional endoscopy and consists of focal adenoma with low-grade dysplasia detected microscopically in random forceps biopsies. As lesions continue to grow, they form small nodules easily mistaken for normal lymphoid tissue but with subtly different epithelium. Larger typical adenomatous polyps are more often seen in adolescents. The prevalence of small bowel adenoma in children detected by VCE has not been reported and the advantage of such early detection is unproven.

Juvenile polyposis syndrome is among the most rare of the hereditary polyposis syndromes. The cumulative risk of developing colorectal cancer is considerable, estimated at 68% by 60 years of age.[13] The incidence of JPS is difficult to determine because of overlapping findings with solitary or sporadic juvenile polyps, which are frequently found in the colons of children presenting with painless rectal bleeding. Patients with JPS may form polyps in the stomach and small bowel (Figure 12.10), although systematic evaluation with contrast radiography or VCE has not been reported in children.

Intestinal malabsorption

Important chronic intestinal malabsorption disorders of childhood include gluten-sensitive enteropathy (GSE, celiac disease), protein allergy enteropathy, and intestinal lymphangiectasia. In contrast with the pattern of long, delicate villi in healthy mucosa (Figure 12.11), variable degrees of fold thickening and villous atrophy are typically seen with GSE and allergic enteropathy (Figure 12.12a, b) and peculiar thick, white-tipped villi are seen with lymphangiectasia (Figure 12.13), particularly after ingestion of a fat-laden meal. These conditions are usually definitively diagnosed by duodenal biopsies obtained during upper GI endoscopy. However, VCE may be considered for children with strongly positive serology (endomysial or tissue transglutaminase antibodies) for GSE who are able to swallow the capsule. Endoscopic biopsies will remain necessary for children who are unable to swallow the capsule, who have ambiguous endoscopic findings, or whose condition requires histologic examination to characterize epithelial cell morphology or the specific types of infiltrating inflammatory cells.

Other enteropathies

Other enteropathies potentially investigated by VCE in children include idiopathic eosinophilic gastroenteritis, ischemic injury due to vasculitides such as Henoch–Schönlein purpura (HSP)[14] or idiopathic autoimmune vasculitis, autoimmune enteropathy, graft versus host disease, and intestinal graft rejection. In these cases, VCE might be used to assess the gross extent or detect recurrence of a known condition rather than to establish a primary diagnosis.

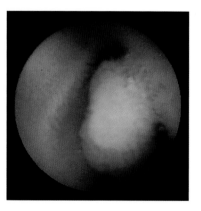

FIGURE 12.10 Juvenile polyp found in the small bowel of a 16-year-old male with juvenile polyposis after a negative small bowel barium examination.

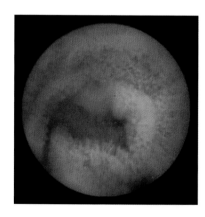

FIGURE 12.11 Long, thin villi in normal small bowel mucosa.

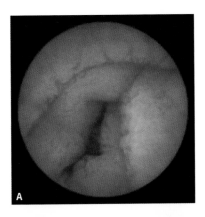

FIGURE 12.12 Thickened and notched folds with shortened villi in the proximal small bowel (a) and thickened, shortened villi in a more distal portion of small bowel (b) in a 3-year-old male with food allergy-induced protein-losing enteropathy presenting with anemia and hypoalbuminemia.

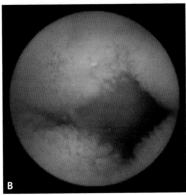

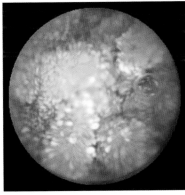

FIGURE 12.13 Thickened, white-tipped villi in a 12-year-old male with protein-losing enteropathy and biopsy-confirmed intestinal lymphangiectasia associated with repaired complex congenital heart disease.

an attractive alternative to EGD with sedation as a diagnostic screen for esophageal varices in patients with portal hypertension. Children with cystic fibrosis (CF) who have chronic lung disease and coexistent liver disease would be appropriate candidates for this approach given the increased risk of sedation in this population. Children with other chronic liver diseases such as biliary atresia, primary sclerosing cholangitis, autoimmune hepatitis, chronic HBV and HCV infection, and α_1-antitrypsin deficiency might also benefit by capsule screening for esophageal varices to determine timing of primary medical prophylaxis for bleeding (Figure 12.14). Capsule esophagoscopy could also be used in children to monitor outcome of initial endoscopic ablation of esophageal varices and for delayed recurrence of varices in patients who remain at long-term risk, such as those with portal hypertension due to extra-hepatic portal vein obstruction or slowly progressive liver disease.

Columnar epithelium or metaplasia of the esophagus is occasionally detected in children and may consist of specialized intestinal-type epithelium (Barrett's esophagus), gastric-type epithelium, or a mixture of both. Children at highest risk for metaplasia of the esophagus have long-standing gastroesophageal reflux disease (GERD) and may include patients with CF, with severe cerebral palsy, or with other neuromuscular or structural disorders (e.g. hiatal hernia or repaired esophageal atresia) associated with impaired gastroesophageal motility and excessive acid exposure. Screening capsule esophagoscopy might be practical to detect columnar metaplasia in cooperative older children who are at increased risk for the condition and are safely able to ingest the capsule.

Chronic esophagitis in childhood is typically characterized by pale, thickened, non-eroded mucosa, diminished or non-visible vascularity, and sometimes by areas of exudate most prominently seen in allergic esophagitis. Erosive or ulcerating esophagitis is uncommon and generally occurs in children with exceptionally severe GERD. Since normal esophageal mucosa appears pale with indistinct vascularity when the lumen is not fully distended, visual inspection by VCE might lead to an erroneous diagnosis of esophagitis. Erosive and exudative esophagitis are more likely to be correctly diagnosed by VCE.

Abdominal pain

Abdominal pain alone is not an appropriate indication for VCE in a child. However, when combined with one or more clinical signs and symptoms such as diarrhea, fever, weight loss, vomiting, anemia, or suspicious radiography, the yield of abnormal findings will increase and justify the examination. VCE may in such cases identify ulceration, stenosis, polyps or tumors that were not detected by small bowel contrast radiography or CT.

Emerging indications

Esophagoscopy

Capsule endoscopy of the esophagus is possible in any child capable of swallowing the capsule. This approach is

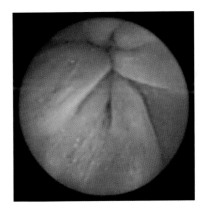

FIGURE 12.14 Small blue varices at the gastroesophageal junction in a 10-year-old male who underwent a Kasai procedure (portoenterostomy) as an infant for biliary atresia. Splenomegaly and paraesophageal varices were noted on abdominal ultrasonography.

Colonoscopy

Partial views of the colon may be obtained during VCE when performed in a child after a colon cleansing preparation (Figure 12.15). Although the technique remains unproven, VCE might be used to screen highly selected children for conditions such as diffuse colitis (Figure 12.16), colonic polyposis, or diffuse vascular anomalies of the colon, where findings from a partial survey of the colon might be sufficient to direct further diagnostic testing or therapy. Adequate bowel cleansing would be a prerequisite, and use of a colonic stimulant such as bisacodyl would likely be necessary to enhance capsule migration through the colon. Additional prokinetic agents might be needed to accelerate delivery of the capsule to the colon by enhancing gastric and small bowel transit.

Special techniques

The approach to VCE in an older adolescent is the same as for most adult patients. Young adolescents are sometimes less cooperative with swallowing the capsule, and most children under the age of 8–10 years require endoscopic placement. Children may be encouraged to practice swallowing large vitamin capsules or candies such as jellybeans prior to arrival for testing. This avoids the inconvenience and cost of a failed or rescheduled test. When ingestion is unsuccessful, the capsule may be returned to the magnetized packaging, which inactivates the battery,

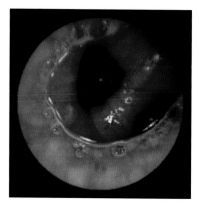

FIGURE 12.15 Normal colonic mucosa and haustral fold pattern in a 9-year-old female.

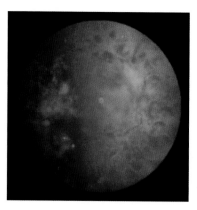

FIGURE 12.16 Erythematous and ulcerated cecal mucosa in a 17-year-old female with ulcerative colitis.

and reserved for endoscopic placement in the same child at a later time. Techniques for capsule placement and application of recording leads are easily adaptable for most children. The capsule should be delivered into the duodenum when placed endoscopically to avoid prolonged gastric retention. Endoscopic placement has been reported in children as young as 2 years without complication[9] and it may be possible to perform studies in even smaller children using currently available equipment, although redesigned equipment would make the process easier and potentially safer.

Endoscopic placement

Endoscopic capsule placement in a child requires moderate to deep sedation or general anesthesia. Depending on the technique or device used for capsule delivery, protection of the airway with an endotracheal tube may be preferred to avoid accidental airway obstruction by a dislodged device.

Once the child has been adequately sedated or anesthetized, a screening EGD should be performed to exclude strictures or other anatomic impediments to endoscopic delivery or new findings that might eliminate the need for a capsule examination. Diagnostic biopsies should be avoided so that post-biopsy bleeding does not obscure findings. The antennae leads are most easily applied with the child supine on the examining table. Soft gauze-like material may be used to wrap the redundant antennae wires against the body for added comfort and to prevent willful detachment by young children (Figure 12.17a, b). Placing the patient in the left lateral decubitus position allows easy manipulation of the head and neck during intubation of the esophagus.

The AdvanCE™ capsule delivery device (US Endoscopy, Mentor, Ohio) is the only commercially released device specifically designed for endoscopic capsule delivery (Figure 12.18a–c). It is a single-use device that consists of a plastic shell with opaque side walls and transparent butt end into which the capsule snaps in place and is held securely. The shell, which measures 13 mm in outside diameter and extends the length of the capsule, is screwed onto the tip of a 2 mm diameter flexible catheter that is advanced through the operating channel of the endoscope. The capsule is released from the delivery device by a stiff wire plunger that is driven by a simple handle attached to the opposite end of the catheter. Successful capsule release is confirmed by viewing the transparent end of the holding shell. The catheter is sufficiently stiff that the shell containing a loaded capsule can be positioned several centimeters in front of the tip of the endoscope to allow unobstructed viewing and still maintain adequate axial alignment for advancement through areas of resistance, such as the esophageal and pyloric sphincters. This device has major advantages over other basket and snare devices that lack stiffness, obstruct the endoscopic view, induce mucosal trauma, or fail to ensure controlled release of the capsule.

A lower cost technique that has worked adequately utilizes a Roth net catheter (US Endoscopy) and a reusable clear plastic ligation adaptor or suction cap[6] (Figure 12.19).

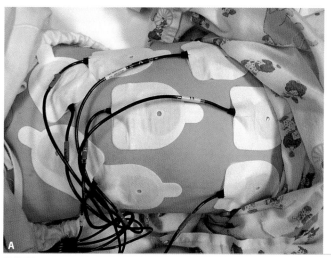
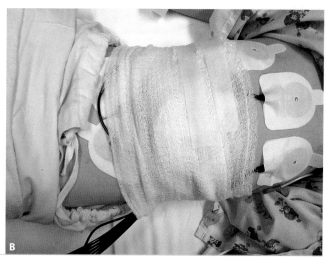

FIGURE 12.17 Antennae leads (a) and gauze wrapping (b) to cover wires and prevent detachment of antennae from a 5-year-old child.

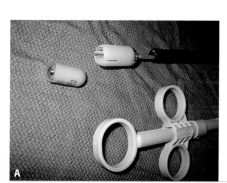
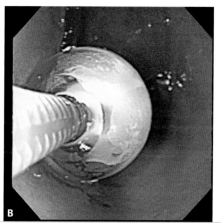
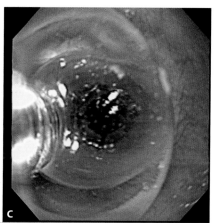

FIGURE 12.18 (a) AdvanCE™ capsule deployment catheter (US Endoscopy). Endoscopic view during (b) and after (c) capsule deployment.

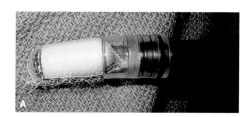
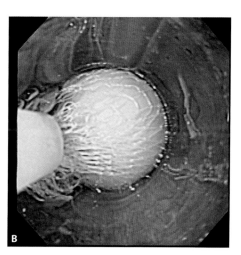

FIGURE 12.19 (a) Capsule held in Roth net basket and seated against transparent ligation adaptor at tip of endoscope. (b) Endoscopic view of front-loaded capsule in distal pharynx. (From Gastrointest Endosc 2004;60:881–921 with permission.)

The capsule is retained within the net and held with one end seated against the plastic ligation adaptor to maintain axial alignment and provide unobstructed viewing. The net is opened within the duodenum to release the capsule. If the capsule fails to release easily from the net, a firm pull on the net catheter will shear the net against the ligation adaptor and release the capsule. Other reported techniques have employed an overtube and Roth net basket alone[15] or wire basket.[16]

Advancing the capsule through the pylorus in a very small child can be difficult. If maintaining steady pressure alone fails, a small dose of intravenous glucagon (0.5 mg) to relax smooth muscle or balloon dilation of the pylorus can be used.

Shorter antennae wires and a smaller size vest are marketed by Given Imaging, Inc., for pediatric application. However, the diameter of the antennae has not been reduced so that crowding and overlap of leads occurs in very small children. Customized vests for the data recorder can be made for small children, or parents can carry the standard vest alongside the child or place it on a stroller or cart.

Bowel preparation and prokinetic agents

Optimal regimens for bowel preparation have not been studied in children. A clear liquid diet beginning the afternoon before a study followed by an overnight fast generally results in adequate clearing of gastric and small bowel contents and reasonable quality imaging. In adult patients, ingestion of a polyethylene glycol (PEG) solution[17] or simethicone[18] prior to capsule ingestion has independently improved the quality of images by purging debris, wetting the mucosal surface, and reducing foamy bubbles. Although simethicone might be easily administered, most bowel purging agents are poorly tolerated or accepted by children and interfere with compliance. However, a flavorless salt-free PEG solution (Miralax, Braintree Laboratories, Braintree, MA) has been used with great success in children treated for constipation, and a recent study demonstrated safety and efficacy as a bowel preparation for children undergoing colonoscopy.[19] A modified version of this protocol that includes oral bisacodyl to enhance purging has been used at Children's Hospital Boston for colonoscopy with excellent results in both tolerability and quality of cleansing.

While addition of prokinetic agents such as metoclopramide[20] in adult patients appears to shorten gastrointestinal transit and increase the rate of complete small bowel imaging to cecum, comparable studies have not yet been performed in children. The relatively narrow bowel lumen, pyloric channel, and ileocecal valve in children might be expected to impede capsule transit and result in a higher rate of incomplete small bowel examinations. Yet preliminary experience at Children's Hospital Boston (unpublished data) has shown that approximately 80% of ingested capsules enter the cecum and 90% reach the distal ileum within an 8-hour recording without prior bowel cleansing or prokinetic agents. This is comparable to published results in adult patients that have not received prokinetic agents or modified bowel preparations. However, this rate of complete small bowel examination dropped significantly in young children when the capsule was introduced endoscopically.[9] Sedatives or anesthetic agents as well as extensive endoscopic manipulation during combined EGD and colonoscopy may transiently diminish small bowel motility. A single dose of intravenous erythromycin (1–3 mg/kg) may be used to counteract this effect. Erythromycin not only stimulates gastric emptying but also induces migrating motor complexes that may enhance movement of the capsule through the small intestine. While other prokinetic drugs such as metoclopramide and tegaserod have not yet been tested in children undergoing VCE, they too are likely to improve the rate of complete small bowel examination.

Future design considerations

Ideal capsules for infants and young children would have a smaller diameter in the range of 5–6 mm, a shorter length of about 12–15 mm, and lighter weight. Cooperation with ingestion by young children might be enhanced, and capsules of this dimension should easily pass spontaneously through the pylorus and ileocecal valve in any full-term neonate or young child. Faster frame rates (already available in the esophageal capsule) would improve the sensitivity of detecting sparse lesions in patients of any age. Pediatric antennae should have smaller diameters, and vests used to hold the data recorder should be scaled to fit a greater range of young children more comfortably. Interrupted real-time monitoring will increase efficiency of testing by earlier recognition of completed studies.

Summary

Capsule endoscopy has dramatically enhanced the process of noninvasive diagnostic small bowel imaging in children by improving the sensitivity and specificity of detection of vascular, inflammatory, and polyposis lesions. Young patients benefit by reduced exposure to ionizing radiation and less frequent laparotomy-assisted enteroscopy. Current technology permits examination of all age groups, except very young infants, with either capsule ingestion or endoscopic placement and only minor modifications in standard adult protocols. Continued clinical experience and data from clinical trials will determine the place for VCE in pediatric algorithms for management of GI bleeding, IBD, vascular anomalies, and polyposis syndromes.

Acknowledgement

The author thanks Dr Richard Grand for critical review of this manuscript.

References

1. Stiffler HL. Capsule endoscopy: a case study of an 11-year-old girl. Gastroenterol Nurs 2003;26:38–40.

2. Aabakken L, Scholz T, Ostensen AB, Emblem R, Jermstadd T. Capsule endoscopy is feasible in small children. Endoscopy 2003;35:798.

3. Wu JF, Liou JH, Lien HC, et al. Bleeding from ileal nodular lymphoid polyposis identified by capsule endoscopy. J Pediatr Gastroenterol Nutr 2004;39:295–8.

4. Barkay O, Moshkowitz M, Reif S. Crohn's disease diagnosed by wireless capsule endoscopy in adolescents with abdominal pain, protein-losing enteropathy, anemia and negative endoscopic and radiologic findings. Israel Medical Association Journal 2005;7:216–8.

5. Arguelles-Arias F, Caunedo A, Romero J, et al. The value of capsule endoscopy in pediatric patients with a suspicion of Crohn's disease. Endoscopy 2004;36:869–73.

6. Barth BA, Donovan K, Fox VL. Endoscopic placement of the capsule endoscope in children. Gastrointest Endosc 2004;60:818–21.

7. Sant'Anna AM, Dubois J, Miron MC, Seidman EG. Wireless capsule endoscopy for obscure small-bowel disorders: final results of the first pediatric controlled trial. Clin Gastroenterol Hepatol 2005;3:264–70.

8. Mow WS, Lo SK, Targan SR, et al. Initial experience with wireless capsule enteroscopy in the diagnosis and management of inflammatory bowel disease. Clin Gastroenterol Hepatol 2004;2:31–40.

9. Fox VL. Capsule endoscopy in children less than 10 years of age [abstract]. J Pediatr Gastroenterol Nutr 2005;41:528.

10. Fishman SJ, Smithers CJ, Folkman J, et al. Blue rubber bleb nevus syndrome: surgical eradication of gastrointestinal bleeding. Ann Surg 2005;241:523–8.

11. Barth BA, Fishman SJ, Fox VL. Wireless capsule endoscopy for gastrointestinal bleeding due to intestinal vascular anomalies [abstract]. J Pediatr Gastroenterol Nutr 2003;37:331.

12. Gubler C, Bauerfeind P. Intestinal Behçet's disease diagnosed by capsule endoscopy. Endoscopy 2005;37:689.

13. Jass JR, Williams CB, Bussey HJR, Morson BC. Juvenile polyposis — a precancerous condition. Histopathology 1988;13:619–30.

14. Skogestad E. Capsule endoscopy in Henoch-Schönlein purpura. Endoscopy 2005;37:189.

15. Carey EJ, Heigh RI, Fleischer DE. Endoscopic capsule endoscope delivery for patients with dysphagia, anatomical abnormalities, or gastroparesis. Gastrointest Endosc 2004;59:423–6.

16. Seidman EG, Sant'Anna AM, Dirks MH. Potential applications of wireless capsule endoscopy in the pediatric age group. Gastrointest Endosc Clin North Am 2004;14:207–17.

17. Dai N, Gubler C, Hengstler P, Meyenberger C, Bauerfeind P. Improved capsule endoscopy after bowel preparation. Gastrointest Endosc 2005;61:28–31.

18. Albert J, Gobel CM, Lesske J, Lotterer E, Nietsch H, Fleig WE. Simethicone for small bowel preparation for capsule endoscopy: a systematic, single-blinded controlled study. Gastrointest Endosc 2004;59:487–91.

19. O'Connor J. Polyethylene glycol 3350 without electrolytes: a new safe, effective, and palatable bowel preparation for colonoscopy in children. J Pediatr Gastroenterol Nutr 2004;39:105–6.

20. Selby W. Complete small-bowel transit in patients undergoing capsule endoscopy: determining factors and improvement with metoclopramide. Gastrointest Endosc 2005;61:80–5.

Section THREE

Diseases of the Small Bowel

CHAPTER **13**

Use of Capsule Endoscopy for the Evaluation of Inflammatory Bowel Disease

Stuart L Triester and Jonathan A Leighton

KEY POINTS

1. Video capsule endoscopy by providing complete imaging of the small intestine provides useful information in patients with known or suspected inflammatory bowel disease.

2. Video capsule endoscopy may establish a primary diagnosis of Crohn's disease in patients for whom there is a high degree of suspicion, even if other tests are not diagnostic.

3. In patients with known Crohn's diesease, video capsule endoscopy may be useful for detecting recurrence and establishing the extent of small bowel involvement.

4. In patients with indeterminate colitis, a positive video capsule endoscopy may establish a diagnosis of Crohn's disease.

Introduction

For many years, the small intestine has been the least accessible portion of the gastrointestinal tract for endoscopic evaluation. Since being introduced in 2001, wireless video capsule endoscopy (Given Pillcam®, Given Imaging, Yoqneam, Israel) (VCE) has given endoscopists easy access for direct mucosal investigation of the small intestine, and as a result has revolutionized the management of multiple small bowel disorders. Thus far, VCE is best established as an effective tool in the investigation of obscure gastrointestinal bleeding (see Chapter 8). However, a number of clinical trials have been undertaken to evaluate the role of VCE in other disorders affecting the small bowel, most frequently that of Crohn's disease (CD). CD is an inflammatory disease associated with both mucosal and transmural inflammation of the gastrointestinal tract. While any segment can be affected, the small intestine is involved in approximately 70% of patients. Up to 30% of patients will have disease limited to the small bowel, particularly the distal ileum.[1]

At present, there is no gold standard for the diagnosis of small bowel CD. A diagnosis of CD is made using a combination of clinical, endoscopic, radiologic, histologic, and biochemical evaluations. The lack of a gold standard testifies to the heterogeneous presentation of CD as well as the difficulty of small bowel evaluation. Due to these issues, the diagnosis of small bowel CD can be challenging and is often delayed. When small intestinal CD is suspected clinically, a small bowel barium radiographic study has traditionally been performed along with colonoscopy with ileoscopy. However, barium studies are limited by their poor sensitivity for early lesions of CD, and endoscopic evaluation is confined to only the most distal regions of the small bowel. Newer radiographic techniques such as computed tomography (CT) enterography and magnetic resonance (MR) enteroclysis appear promising, but are not yet well established.

VCE offers a number of potential advantages compared with current modalities in the evaluation of these challenging patients. The examination is usually painless, involves no radiation exposure, and minimizes patient inconvenience. Because it directly images the entire small bowel mucosa, it may offer the prospect of earlier diagnosis in patients with mild to moderate symptoms and normal ileoscopy and/or imaging. Its primary drawback in the setting of possible small bowel CD is its relative contraindication in patients with known or suspected strictures, a common problem in this patient population. Additionally, as VCE has no capacity for biopsy at present, histologic confirmation of visualized abnormalities is only possible when they are reachable by other endoscopic means.

This chapter summarizes the experience with VCE for patients with known or suspected small intestinal CD, with particular attention to prospective trials comparing VCE with alternative diagnostic modalities. In addition, use of VCE to assist in definitive diagnosis of patients with indeterminate colitis will be discussed. The authors will also review in detail the limitations of applying present capsule technology to the study of CD as well as technical issues regarding the use of VCE in CD. Finally, future goals for clinical research in this area will be explored.

Appearance of Crohn's disease on capsule endoscopy

While efforts have been made to develop a minimum standard terminology for reporting of findings on VCE,[2] no system is presently in routine use in either research or clinical practice. As a result, a variety of capsule findings have been reported as consistent with the diagnosis of CD. Minor findings described include villous denudation, mucosal nodularity, scattered erosions, and occasional aphthae. More advanced lesions such as linear, stellate, or serpiginous ulcerations, circumferential ulcerations, and ulcers associated with stenosis or stricture may also be seen (Figure 13.1). While the most severe visualized lesions are fairly convincing as a source of clinical symptoms and consistent with a diagnosis of CD, the lesser findings are harder to interpret in the absence of outcomes data. Additionally, other disorders such as NSAID-induced enteropathy must remain in the differential diagnosis even in the most advanced lesions (Figure 13.2).

Capsule endoscopy in patients with suspected small bowel Crohn's disease

Early reports on the use of VCE for establishing a diagnosis of suspected small bowel CD have involved limited case reports and retrospective series. More recently, an increasing number of abstracts and full publications have prospectively evaluated VCE versus comparative diagnostic modalities in patients in whom CD is clinically suspected. In many cases, these prospective trials have also included patients with established CD in whom a suspected recurrence is being evaluated.

Initial peer-reviewed studies evaluating VCE in suspected non-stricturing CD focused on the yield of VCE when conventional endoscopy and small bowel follow-through (SBFT) were normal (Table 13.1). Fireman et al[3] studied 17 patients with suspected CD based on the presence of clinical symptoms (iron deficiency anemia, diarrhea, abdominal pain, weight loss) with VCE. Exclusion criteria included a history of small bowel obstruction, small bowel strictures seen on x-ray, "major" abdominal surgery, or use of non-steroidal anti-inflammatory drugs (NSAIDs) in the preceding year. Twelve of the 17 patients (71%) were diagnosed with CD based on VCE findings described as "mucosal erosions, ulcers, and strictures," with lesions mainly identified in the

Table 13.1 Yield of capsule endoscopy in case series for patients with suspected Crohn's disease

Authors	Reference	n	VCE yield
Fireman et al	3	17	71%
Herrerias et al	4	21	43%
Arguelles-Arias et al	5	12 (pediatric)	58%
Ge et al	6	20	65%
Mow et al	7	8	37.5%
Scapa et al	8	13	46%
Kalantzis et al	9	22	36%

distal small bowel. Importantly, only 6 of the 17 patients had undergone successful ileoscopy, all of which were negative. Patients were recruited from a nationwide search (in Israel) and as such may not be representative of those seen in general clinical practice. All 12 patients diagnosed with CD were treated with mesalamine and "short-term steroids," with either "good" or "some" clinical improvement reported, but no additional detail was provided on clinical followup.

Herrerias et al[4] reported on 21 patients with "clinical and biochemical suspicion" of CD. All patients had negative stool studies, SBFT, and colonoscopy. Ileoscopy was successful in 17/21 patients, with no endoscopic abnormalities seen and either no or minimal histologic abnormalities. None of the patients were using NSAIDs. VCE revealed lesions compatible with CD in 9/21 patients (43%), with aphthous ulcers, linear ulcers, and mucosal fissures described. All patients diagnosed with CD had ileal lesions, including 6 of the 17 patients with prior negative ileoscopy, and 5 of the patients had proximal small bowel lesions as well. Patients diagnosed with CD were treated with "standard therapy with prednisone and mesalazine," and all were in clinical or "analytical" remission at 3-month followup, but no further clinical detail was provided. These authors also performed a similar study in 12 pediatric patients,[5] finding a 58% yield in diagnosing small bowel CD, with all diagnosed patients clinically improved with therapy at 3 months.

Ge et al[6] studied 20 patients with suspected CD and negative prior endoscopic and small bowel radiographic evaluation. No patient was on NSAIDs or had any clinical or radiographic history of small bowel obstruction. CD was diagnosed by VCE in 13/20 patients (65%) with "mucosal erosions, aphthae, nodularity, large ulcers, and ulcerated stenosis" seen. Three patients had capsule retention at stenoses thought to be caused by Crohn's disease, but no information regarding eventual capsule passage or need for surgical intervention was provided. All diagnosed patients with CD were treated with "5-ASA and short term steroid treatment" with 11 showing "good clinical improvement."

Mow et al[7] evaluated 8 patients out of the large referral population at Cedars-Sinai Medical Center for suspected CD

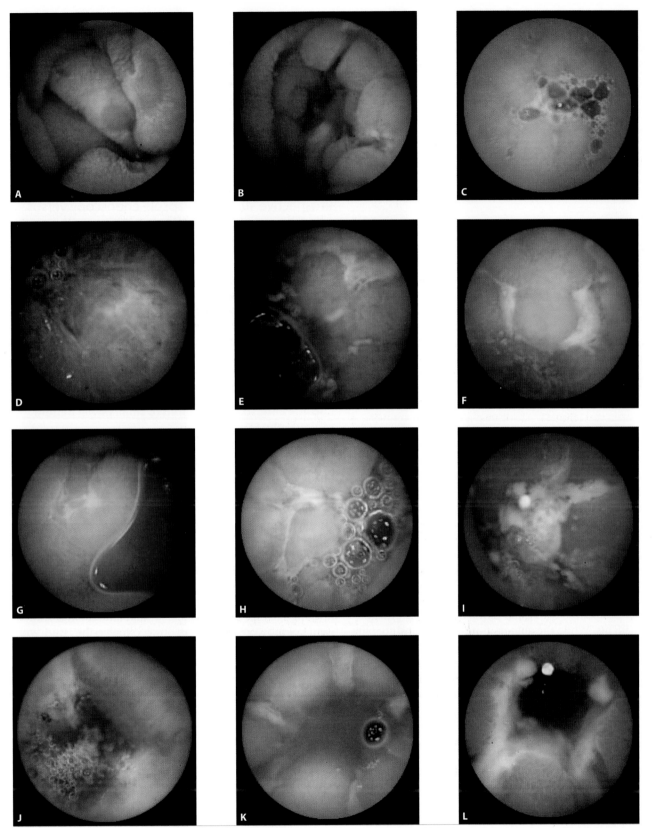

FIGURE 13.1 Spectrum of capsule endoscopic images described in patients with suspected or established Crohn's disease. Minor findings include (a) focal villous denudation, (b) mucosal nodularity, or (c, d) focal erosions and mucosal granularity. More advanced findings include (e, f) serpiginous, (g) stellate, and (h) linear ulcerations, (i, j) confluent or circumferential ulcerations, or (k, l) ulceration with associated luminal strictures.

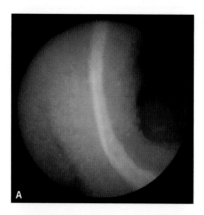

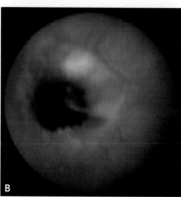

FIGURE 13.2 Examples of NSAID-induced enteropathy ("diaphragm disease"): (a) band-like ulceration; (b) circumferential ulceration with stricture.

for CD was added for these 6 patients, no information on clinical outcome is provided.

Kalantzis et al[9] recently published their experience as the first facility in Greece to employ VCE in the evaluation of small bowel disease, including 22 patients with suspected CD. They report VCE findings consistent with CD in 8/22 patients (36%), but with no further information provided. They also note CD being diagnosed by VCE in 7/108 patients with obscure gastrointestinal bleeding as well as 4/32 patients with chronic diarrhea, and note histologic confirmation of the diagnosis in 4 of these 11 total patients.

Prospective studies of capsule endoscopy versus other diagnostic modalities in patients with suspected Crohn's disease

Eight prospective studies have been published comparing VCE with one or more alternative diagnostic modalities in patients with suspected small bowel CD; five as peer-reviewed manuscripts and three in abstract form only. Seven studies compared VCE with small bowel barium radiography (either SBFT or enteroclysis), four studies compared VCE with colonoscopy with ileoscopy, two compared it with push enteroscopy, two compared it with CT enterography, and one study compared it with MR enteroclysis.

Capsule endoscopy compared to small bowel barium radiography (Table 13.2)

with VCE. Three of 8 patients (37.5%) had multiple small bowel ulcerations consistent with CD seen on VCE and responded to therapy. However, two of these three patients also had ileal ulcerations on ileoscopy, and the third had unsuccessful ileoscopy but evidence of ileal edema on small bowel series. As a result, the additional information provided by VCE in these patients is somewhat limited. As part of a larger series evaluating the use of VCE for a variety of suspected small bowel pathology, Scapa et al[8] studied 13 patients with "clinically suspected CD" who had normal upper endoscopy, colonoscopy, and SBFT. They report findings compatible with small bowel CD in 6/13 (46%) of these patients. While the authors note that medical therapy

Eliakim et al[10] compared VCE to SBFT in 35 patients with clinical suspicion for CD secondary to diarrhea (83% of patients), abdominal pain (89%), and/or weight loss (69%). Patients taking NSAIDs were excluded, as were any patients in whom a stricture was seen on SBFT (none was seen). Findings on VCE identified as "medically significant or explained the patient's reason for referral" were found in 27/35 (77%) patients versus 8/35 (23%) with SBFT, a statistically significant difference. VCE findings included ulcers and erosions (36%), erythema (22%), aphthae (17%), and nodular lymphoid hyperplasia (20%). Patients in whom imaging studies and VCE had discordant findings underwent colonoscopy with ileoscopy to resolve the issue, with

Table 13.2 Prospective yield of capsule endoscopy versus barium radiography in patients with suspected Crohn's disease

Authors	Reference	Publication type	n	Type of barium radiography	Yield of VCE	Yield of barium radiography
Eliakim et al	10	Manuscript	35	SBFT	77%	23%
Chong et al	11	Manuscript	21	EC	9%	0%
Hara et al	12	Manuscript	8	SBFT	37.5%	12.5%
Costamagna et al	13	Manuscript	1	SBFT	0%	0%
Toth et al	14	Abstract	29	SBFT	28%	10%
Dubcenco et al	15	Abstract	8	SBFT	50%	12.5%

SBFT, small bowel follow-through; EC, enteroclysis.

normal ileoscopy found in patients with positive radiologic imaging but normal VCE. However, it is not clear that all reported VCE findings (e.g. erythema and lymphoid hyperplasia) truly represent CD, and no clinical followup data are provided.

Recently, Chong et al[11] reported on 21 non-NSAID-using patients with suspected CD (as well as 22 with known CD) studied with VCE versus enteroclysis. VCE visualized the cecum in 17/21 patients; the remaining 4 patients were reported to have had negative ileoscopy within the preceding 6 months. Four of the 21 patients had erosions or ulcers detected by VCE versus no findings consistent with CD on enteroclysis or SBFT (4 patients). However, only 2 of the 4 VCE-positive patients (9% of total) were felt to truly have CD, and the difference in yield between VCE and enteroclysis was not significant. The authors corresponded with referring physicians following the study, with a mean followup of 8.4 months. Physicians reported a change in the management plan for 14 of the 21 patients, often with treatment geared towards presumed irritable bowel syndrome. Eight of the 21 patients, including both patients diagnosed with CD, reported symptomatic improvement.

Hara et al[12] from our institution compared VCE and SBFT in 17 patients (8 suspected CD, 9 established CD). VCE identified small bowel ulcers and erosions consistent with CD in 3/8 patients (37.5%) with suspected CD versus 1/8 patients (12.5%) with SBFT. As part of a larger study evaluating VCE versus SBFT in the diagnosis of small bowel disorders (primarily obscure gastrointestinal bleeding), Costamagna et al[13] evaluated a single patient with suspected CD. They reported flattened proximal jejunal mucosa on VCE, but subsequent endoscopic biopsies were normal and SBFT in this patient was negative as well.

Toth et al[14] evaluated 47 patients (29 suspected CD, 18 established CD) with VCE versus SBFT. In patients with suspected CD, VCE had a 28% yield (8/29) for lesions consistent with CD (multiple erosions, ulcerations, and/or strictures) compared to a 10% (3/29) yield for SBFT (E. Toth, personal communication). Dubcenco et al[15] reported positive findings on VCE in 4/8 patients with suspected CD versus 1/8 for SBFT (E. Dubcenco, personal communication). Bloom et al[16] reported a higher yield with VCE (58%) than with SBFT (21%) in 19 patients with either suspected or established CD, but no subgroup breakdown data were presented (omitted from Table 13.2).

Capsule endoscopy compared to colonoscopy with ileoscopy

Hara et al[12] also compared VCE to colonoscopy with ileoscopy in their series, finding a 50% yield (4/8 patients) with ileoscopy versus 37.5% (3/8) with VCE. Three abstracts have also studied VCE versus colonoscopy with ileoscopy. Toth et al[14] found a 21% yield (6/29 patients) for ileoscopy for lesions consistent with CD versus 28% (8/29) for VCE (E. Toth, personal communication). Dubcenco and colleagues[15] described positive findings in 2/8 patients with ileoscopy versus 4/8 with VCE. As previously mentioned, Bloom et al[16] studied 19 patients with suspected or established CD, but did not provide subgroup data. In their

population, yields of ileoscopy (53%) and VCE (58%) were similar.

Capsule endoscopy compared to other diagnostic modalities

Two reports compared VCE with push enteroscopy. As CD less commonly involves the proximal small bowel, authors used push enteroscopy as a complementary modality to other endoscopic and/or radiologic studies rather than as a primary modality to diagnose suspected CD. Chong et al[11] reported no findings consistent with CD on push enteroscopy in 21 patients versus 2/21 (9%) on VCE. Toth et al[14] found a 10% yield (3/29 patients) with push enteroscopy versus 28% (8/29) for VCE (E. Toth, personal communication).

CT enterography, a technique using negative oral contrast along with thin cut imaging to maximize small bowel detail, has demonstrated superiority over SBFT for the detection of extraluminal findings and complications of CD.[17–19] Eliakim et al[10] studied CT enterography versus VCE in patients with suspected CD. CT enterography was felt to be positive in only 7/35 patients (20%) versus 27/35 for VCE (77%). The yield for CT enterography was essentially the same as for SBFT (8/35 patients). This likely reflects the limited ability of CT enterography to identify early mucosal lesions, as studied patients did not have advanced disease and as such were unlikely to have significant extraluminal complications of CD which may have been better visualized on CT. Hara et al[12] also compared VCE to CT enterography in their smaller series, reporting findings consistent with CD in 3/8 patients (37.5%) with VCE versus 2/8 (25%) with CT enterography.

A final report compared VCE to MR enteroclysis, another new diagnostic imaging tool. Golder et al[20] have recently published on 18 patients, though most (16/18) are patients with established CD rather than suspected CD (2/18 patients). Of these two patients, one patient with intermittent diarrhea whose symptoms resolved without treatment was found to have only angiodysplasias on VCE and had a negative MR, and the other patient had no findings with either study and was ultimately found to have *Clostridium difficile* colitis.

Capsule endoscopy in patients with established Crohn's disease

Abdominal pain in patients with CD is a common problem. However, multiple potential etiologies for such pain exist in this patient population, particularly that of overlapping functional bowel disease. In patients with medical or surgical remissions, development of abdominal pain or alarm symptoms leads to endoscopic and radiologic evaluation for either small bowel recurrence or extension of established colonic CD. Increasingly, investigators have become interested in the use of VCE to establish or disprove the diagnosis of recurrent small bowel CD when standard evaluation is unrevealing, or in some cases to use VCE as an initial diagnostic modality.

As part of their larger series, Mow et al[7] evaluated 20 patients with established CD to determine the extent of small bowel disease in patients with recurrent or ongoing symptoms. Most patients had SBFT prior to undergoing VCE, and no episode of capsule retention occurred. Eight of 20 patients (40%) had findings considered diagnostic on VCE (diffuse or > 3 small bowel ulcerations), 6/20 (30%) had findings considered suspicious (= 3 ulcerations), and 6/20 (30%) had findings considered normal or nonspecific (erythema only). In 12/14 patients with diagnostic or suspicious findings, VCE results led to an increase in medical therapy, with clinical improvement reported in 11/12 patients.

In the recent series by Kalantzis et al,[9] 6 patients were studied with VCE for "further evaluation of diagnosed Crohn's disease." They report VCE findings compatible with CD in 5 of the 6 patients (83%), but no further details on the nature of the VCE findings or subsequent clinical followup were presented.

Prospective studies of capsule endoscopy versus other diagnostic modalities in patients with established Crohn's disease

Ten prospective trials have been published comparing VCE with one or more alternative diagnostic modalities in patients with established CD being evaluated for a small bowel recurrence or extension of known small bowel disease. Six studies are available as peer-reviewed manuscripts, with an additional four studies in abstract form only. Eight studies compared VCE with SBFT or enteroclysis, three studies compared VCE with colonoscopy with ileoscopy, two compared it with push enteroscopy, two compared it with CT enterography/enteroclysis, and one study compared it with MR enteroclysis.

Capsule endoscopy compared to small bowel barium radiography (Table 13.3)

Chong et al[11] compared VCE to enteroclysis in 22 patients with previously diagnosed CD (11 patients with isolated small bowel disease, 5 colonic disease, 4 colonic/small bowel disease, 1 perianal disease, 1 gastric/cecal disease) who were suspected to have recurrent CD. Seventeen of 22 patients (77%) had mucosal changes consistent with CD on VCE versus 4/22 (18%) with enteroclysis, and all patients with positive enteroclysis had positive VCE. As expected, the majority of positive findings were in the distal small bowel. A change in management occurred in 16/22 patients as a result of either positive or negative findings on VCE, and 9 patients reported symptomatic improvement at followup.

Buchman et al[21] studied 30 patients with established CD without prior surgery who presented with clinical evidence of recurrent disease (abdominal pain, diarrhea, anemia, peripheral arthralgias). An additional 12 screened patients were excluded due to strictures seen on SBFT. A scoring system (grade 1–3) was devised for both SBFT and VCE findings. Findings consistent with CD were identified in 21/30 patients with VCE (70%) versus 20/30 patients with SBFT (67%), a non-significant difference. Grading scores between the two modalities were significantly correlated ($r = 0.65$). VCE identified disease in 6 patients with normal SBFT, but SBFT noted disease (grade 1) in 5 patients with normal VCE. Despite normal SBFT, two capsules were retained and eventually required stricturoplasty for removal. The yield with SBFT in this study is higher than would be predicted from the literature. This may be due to the images being interpreted by a gastrointestinal specialty radiologist, or to a false positive SBFT in patients with normal or minor findings on VCE, as utilization of a grading system may have biased the interpreter towards making a "grade 1" diagnosis on SBFT rather than reporting normal results on equivocal studies. As these patients had never undergone surgery, findings on SBFT related to scarring from previously active CD cannot be ruled out. Additionally, use of NSAIDs was not listed as an exclusion criterion in the study.

Hara et al's series[12] included 9 patients with established CD comparing VCE and SBFT for the diagnosis of recurrent

Table 13.3 Prospective/retrospective studies of capsule endoscopy versus barium radiography in patients with established Crohn's disease

Authors	Reference	Study type	Publication type	Type of barium radiography	n	Yield of VCE	Yield of barium radiography
Mow et al	7	Retrospective	Manuscript	NA	20	70%	NA
Kalantzis et al	9	Retrospective	Manuscript	NA	6	83%	NA
Chong et al	11	Prospective	Manuscript	EC	22	77%	18%
Buchman et al	21	Prospective	Manuscript	SBFT	30	70%	67%
Hara et al	12	Prospective	Manuscript	SBFT	9	100%	33%
Costamagna et al	13	Prospective	Manuscript	SBFT	2	100%	50%
Marmo et al	22	Prospective	Abstract	EC	19	74%	21%
Toth et al	13	Prospective	Abstract	SBFT	18	78%	17%
Dubcenco et al	14	Prospective	Abstract	SBFT	23	87%	17%

SBFT, small bowel follow-through; EC, enteroclysis.

CD. Yield for VCE was 100% (9/9 patients) versus 33% (3/9) for SBFT. As part of their larger series, Costamagna et al[13] evaluated 2 patients with suspicion for recurrent CD. Both patients had small bowel ulcerations consistent with CD on VCE, while SBFT revealed ileal nodularity in one patient consistent with CD but was normal in the other patient.

A number of recent abstracts have also compared VCE to barium radiography in patients with established CD. Marmo and colleagues[22] reported on 19 patients with newly diagnosed non-stricturing CD who were prospectively evaluated with VCE and enteroclysis. VCE had a 74% yield (14/19 patients) for small bowel lesions versus 21% (4/19) with enteroclysis. Toth et al's series[14] included 18 patients with previously diagnosed CD. VCE identified small bowel Crohn's lesions in 14/18 patients (78%) compared with 3/18 (17%) with SBFT (E. Toth, personal communication). All cases with positive SBFT also had positive VCE. Dubcenco et al[15] evaluated 23 patients with known CD for recurrent small bowel disease by VCE and SBFT. Yield for VCE was 87% (20/23 patients) versus 17% (4/23) for SBFT (E. Dubcenco, personal communication). Bloom et al's series[16] did not provide subgroup data and was discussed earlier.

Capsule endoscopy compared to colonoscopy with ileoscopy

Hara et al's series[12] also evaluated colonoscopy with ileoscopy versus VCE in patients with established CD and suspected recurrent disease of the small bowel. They reported a yield of 100% for VCE (9/9 patients) compared with 78% for ileoscopy (7/9), but ileoscopy was unsuccessful in one patient. Three abstracts compared VCE with ileoscopy as well. Toth et al[14] found evidence of CD in 14/18 patients (78%) with VCE versus 11/18 (61%) with ileoscopy (E. Toth, personal communication). Three cases with positive ileoscopy had negative VCE exams due to the capsule not reaching the cecum during the examination. Dubcenco et al[15] reported an 87% yield (20/23 patients) for VCE compared with 52% (12/23) for ileoscopy, including a number of findings in the proximal small bowel beyond the reach of ileoscopy. Bloom et al's series[16] has been previously discussed.

Capsule endoscopy compared to other diagnostic modalities

Two studies compared VCE with CT enterography/enteroclysis. Voderholzer et al[23] studied 56 patients with established CD with VCE and CT enteroclysis. Sixteen patients had undergone prior ileocecal or small bowel resection and none were using NSAIDs. Fifteen patients were found to have stenoses with a diameter of < 1 cm on CT enteroclysis and were excluded from the trial, leaving 41 patients for comparison (33 active CD, 8 "quiescent"). The yield of VCE for "small bowel" lesions (defined by the authors as jejunum or proximal ileum) was 61% (25/41) versus 29% (12/41) for CT enteroclysis, a statistically significant difference (p = 0.004). Yield reported in the ileocecal/neoterminal ileal region was similar for VCE and CT enteroclysis. Hara et al's series[12] found a 78% yield (7/9 patients) for CT enterography versus 100% (9/9) for VCE in their small sample of 9 patients.

Two studies compared VCE with push enteroscopy in patients with established CD. Chong et al[11] reported a 14% yield (3/22 patients) for push enteroscopy compared with a 77% yield (17/22) for VCE. Toth et al[14] described findings consistent with CD on push enteroscopy in only 1/18 patients (6%) versus 14/18 (78%) with VCE. As previously mentioned, yield of push enteroscopy in this setting would be predicted to be low due to the relatively infrequent involvement of the proximal small bowel in CD.

Golder et al[20] evaluated 16 patients with established CD with VCE and MR enteroclysis. They reported findings compatible with CD in 12/18 patients (67%) with VCE compared with 9/18 (50%) for MR enteroclysis. VCE detected significantly more lesions than MR in the proximal and mid small bowel (p = 0.016). An equal number of lesions were detected by each technique in the distal small bowel. The authors reported that there were no changes in patient management as a result of diagnostic findings in the study.

Summary of capsule endoscopy in patients with suspected Crohn's disease or suspected small bowel recurrence of established Crohn's disease

VCE is a promising new tool for the study of patients in whom a clinical suspicion of small bowel CD is raised. Nearly all described studies show it to be a superior diagnostic modality to SBFT and colonoscopy with ileoscopy, and limited studies suggest it may be superior to newer cross-sectional imaging modalities as well. However, sample sizes in these trials have invariably been small. Our group has recently performed a meta-analysis of available prospective trials comparing VCE with one or more alternate diagnostic modalities for the diagnosis of suspected initial presentation of CD or suspected small bowel recurrence of established CD.[24] We found an incremental yield of 43% (95% confidence interval (CI) = 29–56%) for VCE over SBFT for the diagnosis of small bowel CD, with a number needed to test of only 2 patients for an additional positive finding with VCE. Subgroup analysis revealed no statistically significant difference in yield between VCE and SBFT for patients with suspected initial CD (incremental yield with VCE = 24%, 95% CI = (–8%)–55%), but a highly significant difference in patients with suspected recurrent CD (incremental yield with VCE = 53%, 95% CI = 33–74%). The number of patients and overall positive findings with either modality in the suspected initial CD arm was small (total n = 89 patients) and heterogeneous between studies, and thus a larger sample may have revealed a significant difference (type II error). Analysis of VCE versus colonoscopy with ileoscopy (incremental yield with VCE = 16%, 95% CI = 3–30%) and CT enterography/enteroclysis (incremental yield with VCE = 32%, 95% CI = 3–61%) also found a significantly improved yield with VCE.

While VCE compares favorably to these alternate diagnostic modalities, patients in clinical trials are highly selected and may not adequately represent the spectrum of patients seen in general practice. As such, criteria that distinguish patients with a higher pre-test probability of CD would be helpful in order to maximize the benefit of VCE and avoid the diagnostic confusion of minor clinically insignificant abnormalities seen on capsule examination. Typical "alarm" symptoms and signs used to identify patients for the clinical studies reviewed in this chapter have included abdominal pain along with diarrhea, weight loss, iron deficiency anemia or extra-intestinal manifestations suggestive of active CD. A number of studies have evaluated the yield of VCE in patients with chronic abdominal pain in the absence of these additional findings, with consistently poor results. Bardan and colleagues[25] used VCE to study 20 patients with chronic abdominal pain without alarm symptoms. Fourteen of 20 exams were completely normal, and the other 6 studies had clinically insignificant findings that did not change management. Fireman et al[26] evaluated 24 patients with chronic abdominal pain or symptoms suggestive of irritable bowel syndrome with VCE. Only 1/24 patients (4%) had clinically significant findings, with an appearance on VCE suggestive of CD. Mele et al[27] reported a much higher yield of 45% (9/20) in patients with chronic abdominal pain, but included transit abnormalities, non-bleeding vascular ectasias, and nonspecific erythematous lesions as positive findings. Though the erythematous lesions could possibly represent early CD, they are of questionable clinical significance without long-term followup.

Our group has retrospectively reviewed VCE findings in 64 patients with Rome II-defined chronic abdominal pain (35 patients), diarrhea of > 6 weeks' duration (14 patients) or both (15 patients) without alarm symptoms and with negative conventional endoscopic and radiographic investigation.[28] The cecum was identified in 81% (52/64) of the examinations. Six of the 64 patients (9%) had findings on VCE that explained the patient's symptoms (3 patients with findings consistent with CD confirmed by biopsy or CT enterography, 2 with NSAID-induced enteropathy, and 1 with a submucosal mass later determined to be a carcinoid tumor). Yield was lowest in patients with chronic abdominal pain (6%) but higher in patients with diarrhea (14%) or both abdominal pain and diarrhea (13%). Capsule retention occurred in both patients with NSAID-induced enteropathy despite previously normal SBFTs. All 6 patients with positive capsule findings clinically improved with directed therapy. Though overall yield with VCE was low, the percentage of positive studies may prove to be significant due to the large number of patients who present with chronic abdominal pain and/or diarrhea. However, this is a relatively small study and the data are subject to the inherent limitations of retrospective series.

Based on the significantly decreased yield of VCE for the diagnosis of suspected CD in the absence of alarm symptoms, the authors' current practice is to reserve VCE for those patients with symptoms or laboratory evaluation suggestive of organic disease despite negative results on conventional endoscopy and imaging studies (Table 13.4). These criteria also apply to patients with a suspected small bowel recurrence of established CD, though the pre-test probability of CD is certainly much higher. Prospective studies with clinical

Table 13.4 "Alarm" criteria that raise clinical suspicion for Crohn's disease

Abdominal pain and/or diarrhea plus at least one of the following: Symptoms
Weight loss
Fevers
Extra-intestinal manifestations (arthralgias, uveitis, erythema nodosum, etc.)
Symptoms suggestive of obstruction
Gastrointestinal bleeding
Family history of inflammatory bowel disorder
Abnormal laboratory studies
Iron deficiency anemia
Elevation in erythrocyte sedimentation rate (ESR) or C-reactive protein (CRP)
Hypoalbuminemia
Leukocytosis

followup will be required to fully confirm these strategies. A proposed algorithm for patients in whom small intestinal CD is suspected based on these criteria is presented in Figure 13.3. While CT enterography may be a superior imaging modality to SBFT (or enteroclysis) for suspected CD, the test has limited availability at present and as such SBFT remains a first-line study in general practice. For those patients with a negative SBFT and colonoscopy with ileoscopy in whom obstructive symptoms raise concern for possible capsule impaction, CT enterography or use of the patency capsule may be the next best option.

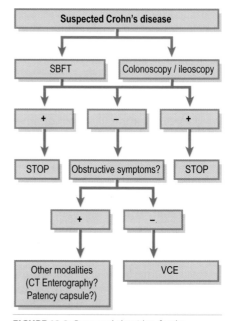

FIGURE 13.3 Proposed algorithm for the evaluation of patients with suspected small intestinal Crohn's disease.

Ultimately, in order for VCE to be fully implemented into diagnostic pathways for CD, it must demonstrate a beneficial effect on patient outcomes as well as prove to be a cost-effective intervention. Preliminary data from the studies reviewed in this article suggest improved outcomes after VCE due to targeted medical therapy for those patients found to have lesions consistent with CD, as well as a change in therapeutic strategy in those patients with normal VCE examinations. These data are promising but will require significantly larger controlled trials than have been published to date to confirm these salutary effects.

Goldfarb and colleagues[29] have recently published an economic analysis comparing VCE to traditional modalities for the diagnosis of suspected small bowel CD. Based on average diagnostic yields in the literature of 69.59% for VCE versus 53.87% for a combined approach with SBFT and colonoscopy with ileoscopy, the analysis determined VCE to be a less costly strategy as long as its yield was 64.1% or greater. The authors also report VCE to be less costly as a first-line test in this setting. These data are provocative but present VCE and SBFT/colonoscopy as mutually exclusive strategies, which may not translate into clinical practice. In addition, the included trials were not subjected to a systematic analysis to evaluate for study heterogeneity.

In summary, many small trials suggest that VCE is poised to emerge as a significant tool in the diagnosis and management of patients with suspected or established CD. However, clinicians must await larger controlled trials with adequate outcomes data to solidify VCE's place in the diagnostic armamentarium.

Capsule endoscopy in patients with indeterminate colitis

Indeterminate colitis (IC) is defined as a chronic inflammatory bowel disease (IBD) confined to the colon without endoscopic, radiologic or pathologic features diagnostic for either CD or ulcerative colitis. The diagnosis is generally made after two sequential exams where mucosal biopsies from different segments of the colon (involved and uninvolved) are non-diagnostic for either form of IBD, and once other forms of colitis which may resemble IBD have been excluded.[30] Up to 10% of patients with IBD are classified as IC.[31] In most cases of IC, identification of small bowel lesions would lead to a change in the diagnosis to CD and likely alter clinical management. As VCE offers the potential for mucosal evaluation of the entire small bowel, a number of preliminary studies have examined the role of VCE in potentially reclassifying a diagnosis of IC as CD.

As part of the case series described earlier, Mow et al[7] utilized VCE to evaluate 3 patients with IC and 19 patients diagnosed as ulcerative colitis in whom clinical suspicion for small bowel involvement had been raised. Of the 3 patients with IC, one had multiple small bowel ulcerations on VCE and "improved on mesalamine," while the other

2 patients had normal studies. Of the other 19 patients, 8 had lesions diagnostic for CD, including 3 patients with prior ileal pouch anal anastomosis. Five of these patients had subsequent histologic confirmation of CD by ileoscopy. Seven of the 8 patients diagnosed with CD were reported as improved with increased medical therapy.

Many of these same investigators reported on the utility of VCE versus serologic markers for the diagnosis of small bowel CD in 23 patients with IC.[32] Serologic markers have been found to be specific (> 90%) but less sensitive (50–70%) tests for the diagnosis of IBD.[33] In this report, VCE identified small bowel lesions (multiple discrete erosions or ulcerations) in 52% (14/23) of the patients. VCE was more sensitive than CD-like serologic markers (ASCA or OMP-C) for the diagnosis of small bowel CD in these patients (61% vs. 30%, p < 0.05). The authors' conclusion was that VCE and serologic markers may be complementary studies that together will allow for improved confirmation of CD in patients diagnosed with IC. Larger studies are clearly necessary to confirm this hypothesis.

Mascarenhas-Saraiva et al[34] used VCE to evaluate 27 patients with IC. Six patients (22%) had findings diagnostic for CD (multiple small bowel ulcerations), and 2 others (7%) had findings considered suspicious for the diagnosis (= 3 ulcerations). The capsule did not reach the cecum in 3 patients included in the analysis. Hume et al[35] studied 10 patients with clinically active IC (pain, diarrhea, elevated inflammatory markers), 4 of whom had previously undergone proctocolectomy, and all of whom had non-diagnostic ileoscopy. VCE identified small bowel CD (multiple serpiginous ulcers with mucosal inflammation) in 4/10 patients (40%). It was noted that 5/10 patients had incomplete small bowel examinations secondary to prolonged small bowel transit, a finding that may possibly reflect underlying inflammation.

In summary, VCE may have a role to play in the setting of IC. However, the present data are limited and come from highly selected tertiary referral populations. Many of these patients were considered to have medically refractory disease, thus warranting additional evaluation. As such, the frequency of small bowel findings in this series may be higher than what might be found in general clinical practice. It is not yet clear that small bowel lesions seen with VCE in these patients definitively represent CD. It is also unknown whether patients diagnosed with ulcerative colitis might have a higher prevalence of small bowel lesions than the general population. At the present time, then, a cautious recommendation to consider VCE as an additional diagnostic modality in patients with refractory IC seems reasonable. Prospective data including longer-term outcomes on this topic are eagerly awaited.

Limitations to the study of small bowel Crohn's disease with present capsule technology

Although VCE is a promising technology for the evaluation of patients with CD, there are a number of concerns with its use in this population. One significant problem is the potential for capsule retention proximal to CD-related strictures. The rate of capsule retention in the largest published series of VCE for obscure gastrointestinal bleeding was 0.75% (7/934 patients) despite negative SBFT in 6/7 patients.[36] All patients underwent surgical resection, and pathology explaining the reason for each patient's symptoms was found at the site of capsule impaction (a so-called "therapeutic complication"). Due to the stenosing nature of CD, however, a higher rate of capsule retention may be expected if VCE is performed in these patients. In the studies reviewed in this chapter, rates of capsule retention ranged from 0 to 6.7% despite small bowel imaging being performed prior to VCE in nearly all patients.

The capsule manufacturer has attempted to address the risk of capsule retention through the development of a "patency capsule" (Given® Patency System, Given Imaging, Yoqneam, Israel) to be given prior to the standard capsule in patients with suspected luminal stenoses. This device has identical dimensions to the standard capsule and contains a radiofrequency transponder that can be detected by an external scanner. If not excreted intact, the capsule dissolves within 40–70 hours into small fragments which can be more easily passed through stenoses.

A number of abstracts have been published evaluating the patency capsule in clinical use. The largest series by Spada et al[37] evaluated 85 patients with suspected (5 patients) or confirmed (80 patients) small bowel strictures on conventional radiology who received the patency capsule. The capsule was excreted intact in 39/80 patients with confirmed strictures (49%) and in all 5 patients with suspected strictures. Twenty patients experienced abdominal pain during the examination. Thirty-three patients with intact patency capsule excretion underwent evaluation with VCE with no adverse events. While these results seem promising, a series by Gay et al[38] raises some concern. They evaluated 22 patients with suspected small bowel stenosis with the patency capsule, and describe 3 patients with symptomatic intestinal occlusion, 2 of whom required emergency surgery for resolution. They suggest that the present dissolution rate of the patency capsule may be too slow to be safely administered to patients with a high likelihood of stricture. Larger studies on this topic are awaited. In the meantime, the authors' practice is to perform small bowel imaging on the majority of patients being considered for VCE evaluation for suspected CD, particularly any patients with symptoms potentially representing obstruction.

In addition to the risk of capsule retention, a second shortcoming is the possibility of inadequate visualization of small bowel mucosa due to either limited battery life or debris obscuring the capsule's view. The present capsule has a battery life of approximately 8 hours. However, it is possible that the inflammation associated with CD may lead to slower transit times. In the series reviewed earlier by Mow et al,[7] the colon was reached in only 32/50 VCE examinations (64%). A larger series of 197 patients undergoing VCE for various indications noted visualization of the entire small bowel in 70% of patients (138/197).[39] This may result in inadequate visualization of the distal ileum, a critical component of the capsule examination in patients with suspected small bowel CD.

In an effort to eliminate small bowel debris and improve visualization, some recent trials have evaluated the effect of bowel preparation or prokinetics on the quality of capsule images. Viazis et al studied 40 patients prepared for VCE with a 2 liter polyethylene glycol (PEG)-based solution versus 40 patients with no bowel preparation.[40] Blinded examiners graded the visualization as "adequate" in 90% of PEG patients versus 60% of controls (p = 0.004). Importantly, a diagnosis was established in 65% of PEG patients versus only 30% of controls (p = 0.003). Another study confirms these findings, also noting a significantly decreased small bowel transit time in patients undergoing bowel preparation with 4 liters of PEG, leading to improvement in the rate of cecal visualization (97% vs. 76%).[41] Other recent trials have suggested decreased transit time with the use of prokinetics such as erythromycin[42,43] or metoclopramide.[44] Based on the available data, the authors' institution now utilizes a 2 L PEG-based bowel preparation the evening prior to VCE. A review of the 111 VCE examinations performed at our institution since initiation of the bowel preparation compared with an equal number of examinations prior to its use reveals a subjective improvement in reader visualization, but surprisingly an identical rate of cecal visualization (83.8%).

The evolution of these safety and technical issues is critical to the development of VCE as a clinical tool in the diagnosis and management of CD. However, a discussion of the limitations of the available data is equally important to determine how best to use this exciting new device. One clear issue pertains to the relevance of study populations to clinical practice. All comparative studies between VCE and an alternative diagnostic modality exclude patients with demonstrated strictures to avoid retained capsules, thereby selecting against the patients most likely to have positive studies with the alternate modality. This restricts the impact of study results to a smaller subgroup of patients with non-stricturing CD.

Perhaps the most significant issue facing VCE in the evaluation of CD is its inability to provide pathologic confirmation of observed findings. In clinical studies, a variety of findings encompassing a broad range of severity have been described as potentially consistent with the diagnosis of CD, and thereby a positive result with VCE. As a diagnosis of CD has far-reaching effects on the psychological and financial health of patients as well as their physical health, caution in making this diagnosis based on subtle VCE findings is appropriate. The long-term clinical significance of finding occasional mucosal lesions in the small bowel on VCE is presently unclear, and will require prospective studies to clarify the issue.

There are presently no standardized criteria for the diagnosis of CD with VCE, and as a result the yield of VCE between clinical trials may not be fully comparable. As previously noted, a Minimum Standard Terminology (MST) system has been devised,[2] but has not yet been adopted in clinical research. Lewis has recently developed a VCE scoring system incorporating aspects of the MST and based on the previously validated Crohn's disease Endoscopic Index of Severity, which emphasizes the distribution and longitudinal extent of VCE findings[45] (Table 13.5). However, this model has yet to be independently validated.

In the absence of a gold standard for pathologic diagnosis, the specificity of lesions (e.g. mucosal breaks) seen on VCE for the diagnosis of CD is unknown. For example, NSAIDs are a well-known cause of small bowel ulceration. A landmark autopsy study in 1985 found an 8.4% prevalence of small bowel ulceration in patients who had been using NSAIDs versus only 0.6% of nonusers.[46] Two recent studies evaluating the frequency of small bowel lesions in healthy controls undergoing VCE have shed substantial new light on this issue as well. Graham et al[47] studied 21 chronic NSAID users and 20 controls with VCE. They reported a 71% incidence of small bowel injury in NSAID users, but surprisingly a 10% incidence (2/20 patients) in controls as well. However, lesions in controls were limited to red spots in one patient and minor erosions in another, and the sample size was small. In another larger trial using VCE to assess small bowel injury with celecoxib, naproxen plus omeprazole, or placebo, Goldstein et al prospectively evaluated 422 healthy patients with VCE at baseline and after 2 weeks of treatment[48]: 13.8% of the cohort was excluded from the study due to the presence of small intestinal lesions at baseline VCE, the majority of these lesions were mucosal breaks. After 2 weeks, 7% of placebo-treated patients were found to have new mucosal breaks as compared to 55% and 16% for the naproxen and celecoxib groups, respectively. As the North American prevalence of

CD ranges from 26 to 198.5 per 100 000 persons,[49] clearly most if not all of the lesions seen in these healthy control patients do not represent CD. As such, the results of these two trials suggest that the positive predictive value of an individual mucosal lesion seen on VCE for the diagnosis of CD is poor. These findings emphasize the challenges of VCE research in the evaluation of CD, and these issues need to be kept in mind when reviewing the present literature.

The future of capsule endoscopy in the evaluation of Crohn's disease

Investigators have only scratched the surface of VCE's potential use in the diagnosis and management of CD. VCE may provide answers to a host of clinical questions regarding the heredity, natural history, response to therapy, and prediction of the postoperative course of this chronic disorder. The increasing number of proximal small bowel findings found with VCE may lead to a reassessment of the distribution of CD lesions as well as a critical look at the true benefit of site-specific therapy. A number of studies have recently been initiated in an effort to answer some of these questions.

The issue of whether VCE might be used to evaluate relatives of index patients with CD is a fascinating one. Might these patients have a higher incidence of small bowel lesions than the general population, and will the presence of such lesions predict the development of CD?

Table 13.5 Lewis Capsule Endoscopy Scoring Table

	Duodenum	Jejunum	Regions* Proximal ileum Lesions	Distal ileum	
	Number	Distribution pattern	Longitudinal extent	Shape	Size (by circumference)
Erythema		Localized, 1 Patchy, 2 Diffuse, 3	Short segment, 1 Long segment, 2 Whole region, 3		
Edema		Localized, 1 Patchy, 2 Diffuse, 3	Short segment, 1 Long segment, 2 Whole region, 3		
Nodularity	Single, 1 Few, 2 Multiple, 3	Localized, 1 Patchy, 2 Diffuse, 3	Short segment, 1 Long segment, 2 Whole region, 3		
Ulcer	Single, 3 Few, 5 Multiple, 7	Localized, 3 Patchy, 5 Diffuse, 7	Short segment, 3 Long segment, 5 Whole region, 7	Circular, 3 Linear, 5 Irregular, 7	< 14, 3 1/4–1/2, 5 > 1/2, 7
Stenosis	None, 0 Single, 10 Multiple, 20	Traversed, 10 Not traversed, 20	Nonulcerated, 5 Ulcerated, 10		

*Score by region by adding points listed.

Will earlier identification of such patients translate into therapy for pre-clinical disease? Central to these issues will be additional data regarding the prevalence of small bowel lesions in the normal population as well as long-term data on the persistence of such lesions. Perhaps a future version of the capsule may have biopsy capabilities, offering histologic confirmation of visualized abnormalities.

What can VCE offer to the patient with active CD? Could VCE function as a tool to demonstrate response to therapy? The present treatment paradigm in CD focuses more on clinical improvement than endoscopic healing, but perhaps this is because small bowel lesions not visualized by conventional modalities could lead to discordance between endoscopic and clinical findings. If lesions were found throughout the small bowel on VCE, this might dictate a change in therapeutic strategy. Multiple studies evaluating mucosal healing with VCE after institution of medical therapy are likely to be undertaken in the next few years.

An additional focus of VCE research will be to both assist with preoperative planning and aid in the postoperative prediction of recurrence in patients requiring surgical intervention for IBD. Will there be utility in performing VCE prior to ileal pouch anal anastomosis in ulcerative colitis patients to ensure no significant small bowel abnormalities exist to suggest CD? Might the presence or absence of such abnormalities predict the likelihood of pouchitis or proximal CD postoperatively? The answers to such questions could have far-reaching effects on surgical practice in IBD.

The advent of capsule endoscopy represents an extraordinary opportunity for clinicians and investigators to improve the care of patients with inflammatory bowel disease. While early data are promising, much work remains to be done, and many clinical questions remain unanswered. The coming years should yield further advances in the capsule itself along with its contributions to the management of these often challenging patients.

References

1. Lashner BA. Clinical features, laboratory findings, and course of Crohn's disease. In: Kirsner JB, ed. Inflammatory bowel disease, 5th edn. Saunders, Philadelphia, 2000, pp. 305–14.

2. Delvaux M, Friedman S, Cave DR, et al. Minimum standard terminology for capsule endoscopy (CE-MST): development and validation of a comprehensive thesaurus, based on the analysis of 766 procedures examining the small bowel. Gastrointest Endosc 2003;57:M1857.

3. Fireman Z, Mahajna E, Broide E, et al. Diagnosing small bowel Crohn's disease with wireless capsule endoscopy. Gut 2003;52:390–2.

4. Herrerias JM, Caunedo A, Rodriguez-Tellez M, Pellicer F, Herrerias JM Jr. Capsule endoscopy in patients with suspected Crohn's disease and negative endoscopy. Endoscopy 2003;35:564–8.

5. Arguelles-Arias F, Caunedo A, Romero J, et al. The value of capsule endoscopy in pediatric patients with a suspicion of Crohn's disease. Endoscopy 2004;36:869–73.

6. Ge Z-Z, Hu Y-B, Xiao S-D. Capsule endoscopy in diagnosis of small bowel Crohn's disease. World J Gastroenterol 2004;10:1349–52.

7. Mow WS, Lo SK, Targan ST, et al. Initial experience with wireless capsule enteroscopy in the diagnosis and management of inflammatory bowel disease. Clin Gastroenterol Hepatol 2004;2:31–40.

8. Scapa E, Jacob H, Lewkowicz S, et al. Initial experience of wireless-capsule endoscopy for evaluating occult gastrointestinal bleeding and suspected small bowel pathology. Am J Gastroenterol 2002;97:2776–9.

9. Kalantzis N, Papnikolaou IS, Giannakoulopoulou E, et al. Capsule endoscopy: the cumulative experience from its use in 193 patients with suspected small bowel disease. Hepatogastroenterology 2005;52:414–9.

10. Eliakim R, Suissa A, Yassin K, Katz D, Fischer D. Wireless capsule video endoscopy compared to barium follow-through and computerised tomography in patients with suspected Crohn's disease — final report. Dig Liver Dis 2004;36:519–22.

11. Chong AKH, Taylor A, Miller A, Hennessy O, Connell W, Desmond P. Capsule endoscopy vs. push enteroscopy and enteroclysis in suspected small-bowel Crohn's disease. Gastrointest Endosc 2005;61:255–61.

12. Hara AK, Leighton JA, Heigh RI, et al. Crohn's disease of the small bowel: preliminary comparison of CT enterography, capsule endoscopy, small-bowel follow-through and ileoscopy. Radiology 2006;238:128–34.

13. Costamagna G, Shah SK, Riccioni ME, Foschia F, Mutignani M, Perri V. A prospective trial comparing small bowel radiographs and video capsule endoscopy for suspected small bowel disease. Gastroenterology 2002;123:999–1005.

14. Toth E, Fork FT, Almqvist P, et al. Wireless capsule enteroscopy: A comparison with enterography, push enteroscopy and ileo-colonoscopy in the diagnosis of small bowel Crohn's disease. Gastrointest Endosc 2004;59(5, Suppl. S):AB 173.

15. Dubcenco E, Jeejeebhoy KN, Petroniene R, et al. Diagnosing Crohn's disease of the small bowel: Should capsule endoscopy be used? CE vs. other diagnostic modalities. Gastrointest Endosc 2004;59(5, Suppl. S):AB 174.

16. Bloom P, Rosenberg M, Klein S, et al. Wireless capsule endoscopy is more informative than ileoscopy and SBFT for the evaluation of the small intestine in patients with known or suspected Crohn's disease. International Conference on Capsule Endoscopy (abstract); 2003.

17. Raptopoulos V, Schwartz RK, McNicholas MM, Movson J, Pearlman J, Joffe N. Multiplanar helical CT enterography in patients with Crohn's disease. Am J Roentgenol 1997;169:1545–50.

18. Wills JS, Lobis IF, Denstman FJ. Crohn's disease: state of the art. Radiology 1997;202:597–610.

19. Pompili GG, Damiani G, Mariani P, Matacena G, Ardizzone S, Bianchi Porro G, Cornalba G. Computerized tomography in the diagnosis of Crohn's disease [Italian]. Radiol Med (Torino) 1994;88:44–8.

20. Golder SK, Schreyer AG, Endlicher E, et al. Comparison of capsule endoscopy and magnetic resonance (MR) enteroclysis in suspected small bowel disease. Int J Colorectal Dis 2006;21:97–104.

21. Buchman AL, Miller FH, Wallin A, Chowdhry AA, Ahn C. Videocapsule endoscopy versus barium contrast studies for the diagnosis of Crohn's disease recurrence involving the small intestine. Am J Gastroenterol 2004;99:2171–7.

22. Marmo R, Rotondano G, Bianco MA, Piscopo R, Cipolletta L. Wireless capsule endoscopy vs. small bowel enteroclysis in the detection of ileal involvement in Crohn's disease: A prospective controlled trial. Gastrointest Endosc 2004;59(5, Suppl. S):AB177.

23. Voderholzer WA, Beinhoelzl J, Rogalla P, et al. Small bowel involvement in Crohn's disease: A prospective comparison of wireless capsule endoscopy and computed tomography enteroclysis. Gut 2005;54:369–73.

24. Triester SL, Leighton JA, Leontiadis GI, et al. A meta-analysis of the yield of capsule endoscopy compared to other diagnostic modalities in patients with non-stricturing small bowel Crohn's disease. Am J Gastroenterol 2006;101:954–64.

25. Bardan E, Nadler M, Chowers Y, Fidder H, Bar-Meir S. Capsule endoscopy for the evaluation of patients with chronic abdominal pain. Endoscopy 2003;35:688–9.

26. Fireman Z, Eliakim R, Adler S, Scapa E. Capsule endoscopy in real life: a four-centre experience of 160 consecutive patients in Israel. Eur J Gastroenterol Hepatol 2004; 16:927–31.

27. Mele C, Infantolino A, Conn M, Kowalski T, Cohen S, DiMarino A. The diagnostic yield of wireless capsule endoscopy in patients with unexplained abdominal pain. Am J Gastroenterol 2003;98:S298.

28. Fry LC, Carey EJ, Shiff AD, et al. The yield of capsule endoscopy in patients with abdominal pain or diarrhea. Endoscopy 2006;38:498–502.

29. Goldfarb NI, Pizzi LT, Fuhr JP, et al. Diagnosing Crohn's disease: an economic analysis comparing wireless capsule endoscopy with traditional diagnostic procedures. Dis Manag 2004;7:292–304.

30. Domizio P. Pathology of chronic inflammatory bowel disease in children. Baillière's Clin Gastroenterol 1994; 8:35–63.

31. Sands BE. Crohn's disease. In: Feldman M, Friedman LS, Sleisenger MH, eds. Sleisenger & Fordtran's Gastrointestinal and liver disease, 7th edn. Saunders, Philadelphia, 2002, pp. 2005–38.

32. Lo SK, Zaidel O, Tabibzadeh S, et al. Utility of wireless capsule enteroscopy (WCE) and IBD serology in re-classifying indeterminate colitis (IC). Gastroenterology 2003;124:S1310.

33. Lo SK. Capsule endoscopy in the diagnosis and management of inflammatory bowel disease. Gastrointest Endosc Clin N Am 2004;14:179–93.

34. Mascarenhas-Saraiva M, Baldaque-Silva F, Villas-Boas G, Soares J. Capsule endoscopy: A valuable help for the differential diagnosis of indeterminate colitis? Gastroenterology 2003;124:M1888.

35. Hume G, Whittaker D, Radford-Smith G, Appleyard M. Can capsule endoscopy (CE) help differentiate the aetiology of indeterminate colitis (IC)? Conference proceedings of 3rd International Conference on Capsule Endoscopy, Miami, Florida, 2004; 38A.

36. Barkin JS, Friedman S. Wireless capsule endoscopy requiring surgical intervention: the world's experience. Am J Gastroenterol 2002;97:S298.

37. Spada C, Spera G, Riccioni ME, Biancone L, Pallone F, Costamagna G. Given(®) patency system is a new diagnostic tool for verifying functional patency of the small bowel. Conference proceedings of the 4th International Conference on Capsule Endoscopy, Miami, Florida, 2005; 38.

38. Gay G, Ben Soussan E, Laurent V, Lerebours E, Delvaux M. Clinical evaluation of the "M2A patency capsule" system before a capsule endoscopy procedure (VCE), in patients with suspected intestinal stenosis. Conference proceedings of the 4th International Conference on Capsule Endoscopy, Miami, Florida, 2005; 81.

39. Mergener K, Enns R, Bradabur JJ, Schembre DB, Smith M. Complications and problems with capsule endoscopy: results from two referral centers. Gastrointest Endosc 2004;57:AB 170.

40. Viazis N, Sgouros S, Papxoinis K, et al. Bowel preparation increases the diagnostic yield of capsule endoscopy: a prospective, randomized, controlled study. Gastrointest Endosc 2004;60:534–8.

41. Dai N, Gubler C, Hengstler P, Meyenberger C, Bauerfeind P. Improved capsule endoscopy after bowel preparation. Gastrointest Endosc 2005;61:28–31.

42. Fireman Z, Mahajna E, Fish L, Kopelman Y, Sternberg A, Scapa E. Effect of erythromycin on gastric and small bowel (SB) transit time of video capsule endoscopy (VCE). Gastrointest Endosc 2003;57:M1859.

43. Kim YS, Chun JH, Kim KO, et al. Effect of erythromycin on the transit time of capsule endoscope through small intestine. Gastrointest Endosc 2003;57:M1880.

44. Selby W. Complete small-bowel transit in patients undergoing capsule endoscopy: determining factors and improvement with metoclopramide. Gastrointest Endosc 2005;61:80–5.

45. Lewis B, Legnani P, Galnek I, Kornbluth A, Brennan M, Spiegel R. The Crohn's disease capsule endoscopic scoring index: a new disease activity scale. Gastroenterology 2004;126:880.

46. Langman MJ, Morgan L, Worrall A. Use of anti-inflammatory drugs by patients admitted with small or large bowel perforations and haemorrhage. BMJ 1985;290:347–9.

47. Graham DY, Opekun AR, Willingham FF, Qureshi WA. Visible small-intestinal mucosal injury in chronic NSAID users. Clin Gastroenterol Hepatol 2005;3:55–9.

48. Goldstein JL, Eisen GM, Lewis B, Gralnek IM, Zlotnick S, Fort JG. Video capsule endoscopy to prospectively assess small bowel injury with celecoxib, naproxen plus omeprazole, and placebo. Clin Gastroenterol Hepatol 2005;3:133–41.

49. Goldfarb NI, Pizzi LT, Fuhr JP, et al. Diagnosing Crohn's disease: An economic analysis comparing wireless capsule endoscopy with traditional diagnostic procedures. Dis Manag 2004;7:292–304.

CHAPTER **14**

NSAIDs, Radiation and Foreign Bodies

Neal J Schamberg and Felice Schnoll-Sussman

KEY POINTS

1. Overview of the pathogenesis, clinical presentation, diagnosis, and management of NSAID-induced enteropathy.

2. Overview of the pathogenesis, clinical presentation, diagnosis, and management of radiation-induced enteropathy.

3. Role of imaging modalities in the diagnosis of these disease states prior to the advent of capsule endoscopy.

4. Discussion of the role of capsule endoscopy in the diagnosis of these disease states.

5. Role of capsule endoscopy in identifying the location of an ingested foreign body.

Introduction

The small bowel may be damaged by the use of non-steroidal anti-inflammatory drugs, radiation therapy or the ingestion of foreign objects. Capsule endoscopy is useful for the identification of these problems and their subsequent management. This chapter will review the pathogenesis, clinical presentation, diagnosis, and management of NSAID- and radiation-induced enteropathy, discuss other imaging modalities, and describe the role of capsule endoscopy.

NSAIDs and the small intestine

Non-steroidal anti-inflammatory drugs (NSAIDs) are widely used because of their beneficial effects in controlling acute and chronic pain and inflammation. However, they may cause potentially life-threatening complications secondary to the damage they can induce in the gastrointestinal tract. Most attention is paid to the potential adverse effects of NSAIDs on the gastroduodenal mucosa, which may lead to peptic ulceration or inflammation manifesting potentially as gastrointestinal bleeding, perforation or death.[1] However, the potential impact of NSAIDs on the gastrointestinal tract does extend beyond the gastroduodenal mucosa. In an autopsy study of NSAID users, although ulcers of the stomach and duodenum were found in 21.7% of patients, 8.4% of patients were found to have nonspecific ulceration of the small intestine, nearly three times the rate of small intestine ulceration found in non-users of NSAIDs.[2] These ulcerations were clinically significant since three of the patients died of small intestinal perforation at the site of ulceration. However, NSAID damage to the intestine is not limited to ulceration; thus, the term "NSAID-induced enteropathy" has come to encompass a clinical syndrome that can manifest as ulceration, strictures, hypoalbuminemia, malabsorption, ileal dysfunction, and bleeding.[3,4] In the review on the effects of NSAIDs on the small and large intestine by Bjarnason et al, it was estimated that up to 60–70% of NSAID users have asymptomatic enteropathy.[3] Tibble et al showed that the effect of NSAIDs on the small intestine was not dependent on the specific drug or dosage administered.[4]

Pathogenesis of NSAID-induced injury to the small intestine

NSAIDs may cause specific damage to the mitochondria of enterocytes lining the mucosa of the small intestine. The enterocytes become depleted of their adenosine triphosphate (ATP) stores within hours of NSAID administration. Intercellular junctions are maintained by an ATP-dependent process and the loss of ATP stores results in loss of integrity of intercellular junctions, thereby increasing the permeability of the mucosa.[3] Increased intestinal permeability allows bile acids, proteolytic enzymes, and bacteria to enter the intestinal wall. These substances attract neutrophils to the site of increased permeability and initiate an inflammatory cascade that can be measured clinically in patients taking NSAIDs.[3,5,6] It appears that the inflammation within the mucosa mediates the clinical sequelae of NSAID-induced enteropathy. Using radio-labeled white and red blood cells it has been shown that sites of inflammation in the mucosa correlate to the areas of malabsorption, ulceration, stricture formation, and bleeding.[5,7]

Clinical manifestations of NSAID-induced enteropathy

Bleeding from the small intestine

It is difficult to assess the exact magnitude and prevalence of clinically significant small intestinal bleeding secondary to NSAID use. The rate of bleeding is often slow and not readily apparent to the patient.[3] It is estimated that the rate of blood loss from NSAID-induced mucosal erosions and ulceration is 2–10 mL/day whereas normal blood loss is estimated to be < 1 mL/day. The amount of blood loss is much lower than is necessary to become visible in the stool.[3] For these reasons, small intestinal bleeding from NSAIDs typically manifests as chronic iron deficiency anemia detected by laboratory testing rather than overt visible bleeding. Much of the research in this area has focused on the rheumatoid arthritis population, which is often on chronic NSAID therapy. Although many patients with rheumatoid arthritis have anemia of chronic disease, a significant portion have iron deficiency anemia associated with chronic occult blood loss. The prevalence of iron deficiency anemia in rheumatoid arthritis patients may be as high as 50%.[8]

Another challenge in defining the exact prevalence of small intestinal bleeding in NSAID users is that the source of blood loss is not always easy to detect by conventional endoscopic techniques, i.e. upper gastrointestinal endoscopy and colonoscopy. Only 45% of anemic NSAID users will have sources found in the upper gastrointestinal tract by endoscopy, and a significant portion have bleeding distal to the gastroduodenal mucosa.[9] NSAID users make up a large percentage of patients who present with gastrointestinal blood loss without a source detectable by upper endoscopy or colonoscopy, so-called "occult" or "obscure gastrointestinal bleeding."[10]

The clinically significant prevalence of small intestinal bleeding from ulcers caused by NSAID therapy necessitates an effective method to detect these lesions to identify the problem as NSAID-related and rule out other sources of small bowel bleeding (Table 14.1). Based on the source of bleeding, the treatment may vary. Once NSAIDs are identified as the cause of bleeding, their use can be stopped or mucosal protective agents such as misoprostol can be

Table 14.1 Frequency of lesions found in the workup of obscure gastrointestinal bleeding

Angiodysplasia	70–80%

Miscellaneous
  Medications (mainly NSAIDs)
  Radiation enteritis
  Infections (tuberculosis)
  Crohn's disease
  Chronic mesenteric ischemia
  Zollinger–Ellison syndrome
  Vasculitis
  Meckel's diverticulum
  Jejunal diverticula
	10–25%

Tumors	5–10%

added to therapy, although with varying results.[3] Methods typically available to the clinician prior to the advent of capsule endoscopy have included small bowel enteroscopy, intraoperative endoscopy, small bowel barium enema (enteroclysis), angiography, and tagged red blood cell scans (scintigraphy). To detect bleeding, scintigraphy and angiography require the presence of higher rates of bleeding (up to 0.5–6 mL/minute) than those caused by NSAID-induced small bowel ulcers and have therefore typically proven less useful diagnostic tools in this type of clinical setting.[11] Intraoperative enteroscopy can have a high diagnostic yield in the evaluation of occult gastrointestinal bleeding[11]; however, this procedure often requires laparotomy and therefore would not be ideal to locate an NSAID-induced ulcer that could resolve with cessation of therapy. Small bowel or push enteroscopy, introduced in the 1990s, is a technique whereby a long endoscope (up to 250 cm long) is advanced past the proximal digestive tract into the small intestine. For anatomical reasons, the enteroscope can typically only reach 50–150 cm of the small intestine.[11] Various methods and endoscopes have been used to increase the efficacy of this procedure, and the reported duration and patient comfort between techniques appears to vary. An advantage to this procedure over others is the potential ability to treat bleeding lesions at the time of enteroscopy, using injections and cautery through the enteroscope.[11] A disadvantage of this diagnostic method is the need for sedating medications throughout the procedure.

The diagnostic yield of push enteroscopy in the evaluation of obscure gastrointestinal bleeding is estimated to be 35–70% based on several case series and summation of the literature.[9–13] In these series, the yield of enteroscopy can be impacted by the indication for the procedure, with lower yields for small mucosal defects typical of NSAID-induced ulcers and larger yield for lesions previously seen by radiographs.[13] Reports of case series of NSAID users with chronic gastrointestinal bleeding have demonstrated that 40–66% of patients on NSAIDs with occult gastrointestinal bleeding from a source not identified by upper endoscopy or colonoscopy have an identifiable lesion detected in the small bowel by enteroscopy.[9,10] Morris et al reported a success rate for enteroscopy for localizing bleeding sources in patients taking high-dose NSAIDs; however, the average duration of the procedure was 6 hours and they were unable to visualize one third of the small bowel lumen.[9]

A typical small bowel series using plain radiographic images of contrast-enhanced loops of small intestine has a poor diagnostic yield for finding sources of occult gastrointestinal bleeding.[14] Small bowel enteroclysis, which uses double contrast under pressure to enhance radiographic imaging of the small bowel, is a better test for locating bleeding lesions than a small bowel series[11]; however, the diagnostic yield for small bowel enteroclysis appears to be only as high as 14–20%.[15,16] Double-balloon enteroscopy uses a scope specifically designed to navigate the entire small bowel lumen. This procedure is more effective at identifying small bowel bleeding sources than conventional enteroscopy, however it is still not widely available in the United States.

In recent years, the ability to visualize the small intestinal mucosa and find previously undetectable lesions has been greatly enhanced by the advent of capsule endoscopy as a diagnostic imaging tool. In comparison to the previously discussed technologies, capsule endoscopy provides the only means by which the entire bowel mucosa can be directly viewed in a noninvasive fashion. Capsule endoscopy was approved by the U.S. Food and Drug Administration in 2001 for the evaluation of obscure gastrointestinal bleeding (Figure 14.1).

Several studies have been performed to test the diagnostic yield of capsule endoscopy in comparison to previous standard techniques used to image the small bowel.[17–19] In two studies capsule endoscopy was shown to be more effective than push enteroscopy in finding bleeding sources in patients with chronic occult gastrointestinal bleeding.[18,19] Results were similar in both studies as capsule endoscopy identified bleeding sources in 66% and 68% of patients versus 28% and 32% success for push enteroscopy, respectively, in each study. Some of the patients were on NSAID therapy, and capsule endoscopy appeared to be more effective than enteroscopy in identifying small intestinal ulcers.[18]

Capsule endoscopy also appears to be superior to small bowel radiographic imaging for the diagnosis of chronic gastrointestinal bleeding sources. In the study by Eli et al that compared capsule endoscopy to push enteroscopy,[18] each patient had had a negative small bowel barium study.

Hara et al showed a diagnostic yield of 48–66% for capsule endoscopy in identifying small bowel lesions, most of which were investigated for symptoms of bleeding.[19] In this study, the positivity rates of small bowel follow-through, enteroclysis, and contrast tomography (CT) were 3%, 0%, and 21%, respectively. Another study done in 40 patients, most with iron deficiency anemia and all with negative small bowel enteroclysis, found that capsule endoscopy was able to identify small bowel ulcers in 44% of patients.[20] These studies support the limited utility of small bowel radiographic exams with contrast enhancement for the diagnosis of occult bleeding lesions in the small bowel and the potential for improvement on these limitations by capsule endoscopy (Figures 14.2 and 14.3).

Recently, a randomized prospective study was completed evaluating the ability of capsule endoscopy to detect small bowel mucosal injuries in healthy volunteers taking either naproxen along with a proton pump inhibitor, the cyclooxygenase-2 (COX-2) specific inhibitor celecoxib, or placebo[21] (Figure 14.4). The proton pump inhibitor omeprazole was added as therapy to naproxen to mitigate the known increased risk of gastroduodenal ulceration with nonspecific NSAIDs. Subjects underwent an initial capsule endoscopy prior to medication intake. Interestingly, 13.8% of healthy volunteers had small bowel mucosal injuries observed on capsule endoscopy without known exposure to any medication known to be toxic to the small bowel; these patients were eliminated from the treatment phase of the study. Three hundred and fifty-six patients were randomized

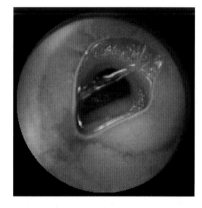

FIGURE 14.2 A 71-year-old with recurrent severe iron deficiency and transfusion requirement over a 3-year period. All previous procedures were negative. Prior chronic use of NSAIDs was the cause of this stricture. (Permission for use granted by Given® Imaging.)

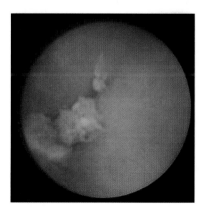

FIGURE 14.1 NSAID-related ulceration. (Permission for use granted by Given® Imaging.)

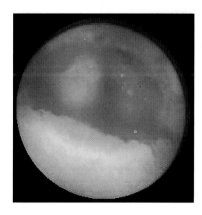

FIGURE 14.3 NSAID-related stricture and bleeding. (Permission for use granted by Given® Imaging.)

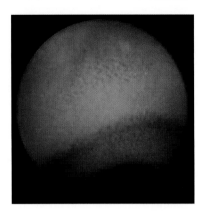

FIGURE 14.4 Small erosion in a patient on COX-2 inhibitors. The patient was not symptomatic from this lesion. (Permission for use granted by Given® Imaging.)

to celecoxib, naproxen plus omeprazole, or placebo for 2 weeks of therapy, after which time they underwent a second capsule endoscopy. The percentage of subjects with mucosal breaks detected by capsule endoscopy was 55%, 16%, and 7% for the naproxen/omeprazole, celecoxib, and placebo groups, respectively. There were 4.18, 0.50, and 0.14 mucosal breaks per average patient in each of the three groups respectively. The percentage of patients with blood visualized within the small bowel lumen in each of the three groups was 7%, 8%, and 1%, respectively. These results were statistically significant; however, no patient had symptoms attributable to the NSAID therapy such as bleeding or abdominal pain. The difference between the celecoxib and placebo groups was small but statistically significant, and the difference between celecoxib and naproxen/omeprazole was statistically significant in the percentage of patients with mucosal breaks and the number of mucosal breaks per patient.[21]

The study by Goldstein et al[21] was limited by short duration and the lack of correlation of the findings with clinically relevant parameters such as the prevalence of anemia within the study population. Given the relatively high percentage of healthy patients found to have mucosal breaks prior to therapy, it may be inferred that the sensitivity of capsule endoscopy for small bowel mucosal injury is high. However, it does also raise concern that the specificity of the test may be lower as many positive results were found in patients with no evidence of clinical sequelae. Although the sensitivity and specificity of capsule endoscopy in the diagnosis of NSAID-induced enteropathy is not yet known, Pennazio et al[22] reported a prospective outcomes study of capsule endoscopy in the evaluation of occult gastrointestinal bleeding. In their study of 100 patients with prior negative evaluations including upper endoscopy, colonoscopy, push enteroscopy, and enteroclysis, 92.3%, 12.9%, and 44.2% of patients had ongoing overt bleeding, previous overt bleeding, and hemoccult positive stools and iron deficiency anemia, respectively. The results of capsule endoscopy led to a definitive treatment that resolved the bleeding in 86.9% of patients. The sensitivity, specificity, positive predictive value, and negative predictive value of capsule endoscopy in this patient population were 88.9%, 95%, 97%, and 82.6%, respectively. Some of these patients were NSAID users, but most were not; however, it appears that capsule

endoscopy is a highly sensitive and specific diagnostic tool for identifying mucosal lesions that result in small bowel blood loss.

NSAID-induced small bowel strictures

Small bowel mucosal inflammation caused by NSAIDs, as previously discussed, can lead to ulceration and subsequent bleeding, but it may also lead to submucosal fibrosis which extends into the lumen causing stricture formation[3,23-25] (Figures 14.1 and 14.5). This entity is relatively rare and published experience is limited to case reports without any large studies or case series. Patients often present clinically with symptoms of intermittent intestinal obstruction which are often difficult to distinguish from the nonspecific abdominal symptoms found in 30–40% of patients using NSAIDs.[25] An entity called "diaphragm disease" is pathognomonic for NSAID-induced small bowel strictures, which are marked by multiple stenotic lesions that encroach on each other and narrow the lumen.[3,24-26] These strictures are typically found within the mid small intestine in patients on chronic NSAID therapy and can be mistaken for stricturing seen in Crohn's disease. The strictures can typically be identified by small bowel radiographic contrast exams and push enteroscopy. The treatment is typically cessation of NSAID therapy, with some patients becoming asymptomatic while others require surgical resection of the diseased segment of small bowel.[24,25]

Since the major potential complication of capsule endoscopy is retention of the capsule, requiring surgical removal, any suspicion of stricture in a patient warrants caution. Interestingly, a case report was published in which an NSAID-induced stricture was diagnosed by capsule endoscopy in a patient who had had a prior radiographic exam that failed to show a stricture.[26] The capsule identified the site of stricture and was unable to migrate past the narrowed segment. Surgery was performed to remove both the capsule and the strictured segment of bowel with the patient making an uneventful recovery without sequelae at 1 year of followup. Recently, the Agile Patency Capsule, a self-dissolving capsule that is the same size as the video capsule, has been developed. It dissolves over a 40-80 hour period after ingestion. Failure to pass this capsule is a contraindication to proceeding with a video capsule exam;

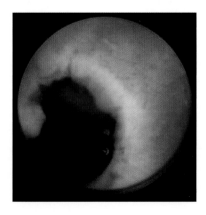

FIGURE 14.5 NSAID-induced small bowel stricture. (Permission for use granted by Given® Imaging.)

patients suspected of having a stricture may be initially evaluated with a patency study.

Other clinical sequelae of NSAID-induced enteropathy

Protein loss resulting in hypoalbuminemia and ileal dysfunction resulting in diarrhea or vitamin B_{12} deficiency are uncommon but well-identified clinical sequelae of NSAID-induced enteropathy. Diagnosis is usually confirmed when measuring levels of serum albumin or vitamin B_{12}. To date, the role for capsule endoscopy in the evaluation of these symptoms is unclear.

Radiation enteritis or radiation-induced enteropathy

Incidence

Radiation therapy plays an important role in the management of abdominal and pelvic malignancies, including urologic, gynecologic, colorectal, and anal cancers. The development of intestinal injury depends on the dose of radiation prescribed, with little damage being seen with 4000 centigray (cGy) or less, clinically significant bowel injury possibly occurring with 4500–5000 cGy, and increasing potential damage as the dose continues to rise.[27-31] Radiation damage to the small intestine causes both acute and chronic changes. Acute changes are common, but often transient.[28] Chronic radiation damage to the small intestine is known as "radiation-induced enteropathy" or "radiation enteritis." The incidence of radiation enteritis varies between 0.5% and 16.9% in the literature.[28] It is estimated that with 4500 cGy of radiation exposure, up to 5% of patients will develop radiation enteritis, whereas with 6500 cGy as many as 50% of patients will have clinical sequelae.[30]

Pathogenesis and clinical manifestations

Acute radiation changes depend on the rate and duration of time over which radiation is applied. The acute effect of radiation on the intestinal mucosa is suppression of cell proliferation in the crypts of the intestinal epithelium with resultant failure to keep up with normal turnover of intestinal epithelial cells. This results in denudation of the intestinal epithelium, shortening of the villi, and reduction of the total surface area of the epithelium.[28-32] With the damage to the epithelial surface, bacteria and other irritants within the bowel lumen can enter the mucosal layers, setting off an inflammatory cascade that leads to the influx of polymorphonuclear leukocytes and plasma cells with the formation of crypt microabscesses.[28-32] The inflammation and denudation of the epithelial layer of the intestinal mucosa allows for loss of electrolytes, water, and protein,[31] which leads to altered bowel transit time manifesting mainly as diarrhea. Accompanying symptoms can be abdominal pain, nausea, and vomiting.[28] These symptoms occur while the radiation treatment is ongoing, but usually the epithelial cells repair and clinical recovery is noted within 72 hours after the last radiation exposure.[28] All symptoms usually subside within a few weeks of therapy completion. Patients who experience severe acute radiation exposure may be at higher risk for developing chronic radiation enteritis. However, even patients who do not have any acute symptoms of radiation damage may go on to develop radiation enteritis.[31]

Late radiation effects occur far less frequently, but are considerably more serious. The effect on the intestinal mucosa is indirect and is the result of progressive occlusive vasculitis and diffuse collagen deposition causing fibrosis within the submucosa. The walls of arterioles supplying the mucosa become obliterated with loss of vessel lumen size and eventual ischemia of the mucosal surface. Long segments of intestine can be involved with diffuse narrowing, concentric fibrosis, and submucosal edema and fibrosis resulting in malabsorption, stenosis, stricture, obstruction, perforation, or fistula formation. Ulceration is also a common pathologic finding that can lead to fistulization or perforation, which may erode into vessel walls causing acute hemorrhage or chronic blood loss.[28,29]

Signs and symptoms of chronic radiation enteritis may appear as soon as 6 months or as long as 40 years after radiation therapy, with an average timeframe of 2–3 years.[28,29,31] There are multiple predisposing factors to radiation enteritis,[29,31] including prior abdominopelvic surgery in which the presence of adhesions fixes the intestinal segments in place and allows the same segments to be radiated excessively. Thin patients and elderly patients tend to have larger portions of their bowel lying in the pelvis and are at risk for receiving larger doses to these bowel segments. Patients with inflammatory bowel disease are at higher risk, as are patients with diseases that impair blood flow to the intestine, such as hypertension, arteriosclerosis, and diabetes. Chemotherapy following radiation therapy also increases the risk. Multiple strategies have been employed to reduce the risk of developing radiation enteritis, including reconstructing the perineum to exclude the intestinal loops from the pelvis during pre-radiation surgical resection of tumors, administering pharmaceutical radio-protectants, and improving abdominal imaging of the intestine prior to radiation, all with varying success.[32-35]

Prognosis and management of radiation enteritis

Deaths among patients with radiation enteritis are often due to recurrent malignancy or the late effects of radiation, estimates of 5-year survival for these patients being 40–60%.[28,31] Medical management of patients who develop clinically apparent radiation enteritis has been largely unsuccessful; however, patients who initially present with nausea, vomiting, abdominal pain or diarrhea should be managed conservatively if possible.[28] It has been estimated that about one third of patients who develop radiation enteritis will require a surgical procedure to treat their disease.[30] A significant number of these patients have suffered from intestinal malabsorption and are therefore nutritionally deficient, posing an increased peri-operative risk.[28,30,31] There are multiple surgical approaches to the treatment of this condition; however, full discussion of these approaches goes beyond the extent of this chapter. Morbidity and mortality after surgical management of this disease are significant and often depend on the nature of the radiation-induced complication that brought about the need for surgery. The presence of perforation or fistula usually signifies more extensive disease within the intestine and portends a worse prognosis for complete resolution of symptoms after surgery when compared to patients who undergo surgery for management of stricture or bleeding.[36] Operative morbidity can be as high as 30%[28] and postoperative mortality ranges from about 5% to 18%.[28,36] New complications from the original radiation therapy can occur in 23–39% of patients who have had surgery for an initial complication, which signifies that this is a progressive disease often difficult to cure.[28]

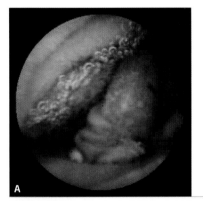

FIGURE 14.6 Area of jejunum showing erythema and fibrosis with some neovascularization. The patient had undergone radiation therapy in the past. (Permission for use granted by Given® Imaging.)

Diagnostic imaging for radiation enteritis and the role for capsule endoscopy

Establishing the diagnosis of chronic radiation enteritis is often difficult as symptoms start to manifest years after radiation exposure and are not specific to any particular intestinal disease. Laboratory tests for serum vitamin B_{12} and fecal fat excretion can hint at the cause and nature of the malabsorption, but abnormalities in these studies may be present in many diseases with associated ileal dysfunction and small bowel malabsorption. Findings on radiographic exams are often nonspecific, but can be helpful in establishing the diagnosis. Characteristic findings on barium studies include segmental sawtooth appearance of the small bowel, pooling of barium in the terminal ileum, and narrowing of the lumen; however, the appearance can be normal and the sensitivity and specificity of this technique are not completely known.[28] Additionally, barium studies can help localize a site of stenosis or fistula prior to surgery.[28,36] The reported experience with push enteroscopy for the diagnosis of radiation enteritis is limited. Willis et al[37] diagnosed radiation enteritis in 2 of 11 patients who presented with small bowel pathology seen on radiographic imaging, but the initial symptoms of these patients at presentation were not discussed.

Experience with capsule endoscopy in the diagnosis and management of radiation enteritis is also limited. This tech-nology appears promising in its ability to noninvasively identify radiation-related lesions throughout the small intestine early in the workup of patients with a history of radiation exposure. Affected areas typically present as erythematous edematous segments which may be complicated by fibrosis and subsequent stricturing (Figure 14.6).

Lee et al[38] reported their experience with capsule endoscopy in a patient who presented with gastrointestinal bleeding and a prior history of radiation treatment for cervical carcinoma 10 years earlier. The patient's bleeding site was found in the terminal ileum beyond the reach of the colonoscope. The small bowel barium enema was reported as normal; however, the capsule failed to pass beyond a stricture seen in the terminal ileum. Surgical resection of the diseased ileum revealed a stricture at the site of a bleeding ulcer and no other source of intestinal disease. Pathology confirmed radiation enteritis and the patient made a full recovery without further complications. This case highlights the potential risk of capsule retention in this patient population, but also shows the limitations of other diagnostic techniques in this disease. To prevent retention, any patient with suspected radiation enteritis or history of abdominal radiation, may be initially evaluated with the patency capsule prior to proceeding with a video capsule exam.

As it is known that the outcome is better for patients who undergo planned rather than emergent surgery,[30] it

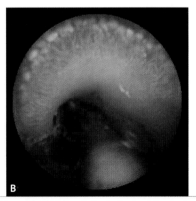
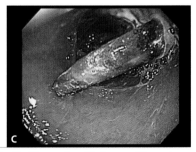

FIGURE 14.7 Foreign body. A 70-year-old female with recurrent abdominal pain 5 years after perforated diverticulitis was found to have an 18 cm piece of nasogastric tubing that had perforated the duodenal bulb posteriorly and re-entered the jejunum. Removal of the tubing led to complete resolution of pain. (a, b) Capsule endoscopic images of the tube within the small bowel lumen. (c) Endoscopic image of the tube in the duodenum. (Permission for use granted by Dr David R Cave.)

is essential to have a fast and safe way to make an early diagnosis with symptom onset.

Capsule endoscopy for the identification of foreign bodies

Foreign bodies are a rare cause of obscure gastrointestinal bleeding or abdominal pain. There has been limited reported experience in the identification of foreign bodies within the small bowel by capsule endoscopy. Ali et al presented 3 cases of foreign bodies identified by capsule endoscopy in 100 patients who presented with either obscure abdominal pain or gastrointestinal bleeding.[39] The first case was of a 70-year-old white female with recurrent abdominal pain 5 years after perforated diverticulitis. She was found by capsule endoscopy to have an 18 cm piece of nasogastric tube that had perforated the duodenal bulb posteriorly and re-entered the jejunum (Figure 14.7). Removal of the tube led to complete resolution of pain. In a second case, an erythematous and stenotic area was identified in the jejunum in an 82-year-old white male with epigastric pain. A 4 cm wood splinter was removed from that area by push enteroscopy. Additionally, capsule endoscopy was able to identify in a third case a metallic pin lodged in the wall of the jejunum that led to a hematoma and intussusception. The patient initially presented with severe periumbilical pain and anemia.

As evidenced by these cases, capsule endoscopy may prove to be a valuable diagnostic tool in the identification of foreign bodies in the small bowel presenting with abdominal pain and anemia.

References

1. Lewis JD, Bilker WB, Brensinger C, et al. Hospitalization and mortality rates from peptic ulcer disease and GI bleeding in the 1990s: relationship to sales of nonsteroidal anti-inflammatory drugs and acid suppression medications. Am J Gastroenterol 2002;97:2540–9.

2. Allison MC, Howatson AG, Torrance CJ, et al. Gastrointestinal damage associated with the use of nonsteroidal antiinflammatory drugs. N Engl J Med 1992;327:749–54.

3. Bjarnason I, Hayllar J, Macpherson AJ, et al. Side effects of nonsteroidal anti-inflammatory drugs on the small and large intestine in humans. Gastroenterology 1993;104: 1832–47.

4. Tibble JA, Sigthorsson G, Foster R, et al. High prevalence of NSAID enteropathy as shown by a simple faecal test. Gut 1999;45:362–6.

5. Sigthorsson G, Tibble J, Hayllar J, et al. Intestinal permeability and inflammation in patients on NSAIDs. Gut 1998;43:506–11.

6. Bjarnason I, Zanelli G, Smith T, et al. Nonsteroidal anti-inflammatory drug-induced intestinal inflammation in humans. Gastroenterology 1987;93:480–9.

7. Bjarnason I, Zanelli G, Prouse P, et al. Blood and protein loss via small intestinal inflammation induced by nonsteroidal anti-inflammatory drugs. Lancet 1987;2:711–4.

8. Vreugdenhil G, Wognum AW, van Eijk HG, et al. Anaemia in rheumatoid arthritis: the role of iron, vitamin B12, and folic acid deficiency, and erythropoietin responsiveness. Ann Rheum Dis 1990;49:93–8.

9. Morris AJ, Madhok R, Sturrock RD, et al. Enteroscopic diagnosis of small bowel ulceration in patients receiving non-steroidal anti-inflammatory drugs. Lancet 1991;337:520.

10. Morris AJ, Wasson LA, Mackenzie JF. Small bowel enteroscopy in undiagnosed gastrointestinal blood loss. Gut 1992;33:887–9.

11. Van Gossum A. Obscure digestive bleeding. Best Pract Res Clin Gastroenterol 2001;15:155–74.

12. Hayat M, Axon A, O'Mahony S. Diagnostic yield and effect on clinical outcomes of push enteroscopy in suspected small-bowel bleeding. Endoscopy 2000;32:369–72.

13. Landi B, Tkoub M, Gaudric M, et al. Diagnostic yield of push-enteroscopy in relation to indication. Gut 1998; 42:421–425.

14. Rabe R, Becker G, Begozzi, M. Efficacy study of the small-bowel examination. Radiology 1981;140:47–50.

15. Rex D, Lappas J, Maglinte, D. Enteroclysis in the evaluation of suspected small intestinal bleeding. Gastroenterology 1989;97:58–60.

16. Antes G, Neher M, Hiemeyer V. Gastrointestinal bleeding of obscure origin: role of enteroclysis. Eur Radiol 1996; 6:851–4.

17. Mylonaki M, Fritscher-Ravens A, Swain P. Wireless capsule endoscopy: a comparison with push enteroscopy in patients with gastroscopy and colonoscopy negative gastrointestinal bleeding. Gut 2003;52:1122–6.

18. Eli C, Remke S, May A, et al. The first prospective controlled trial comparing wireless capsule endoscopy with push enteroscopy in chronic gastrointestinal bleeding. Endoscopy 2002;34:685–9.

19. Hara AK, Leighton JA, Sharma VK, et al. Small bowel: Preliminary comparison of capsule endoscopy with barium study and CT. Radiology 2004;230:260–4.

20. Liangpunsakul S, Chadalawada V, Rex DK, et al. Wireless capsule endoscopy detects small bowel ulcers in patients with normal results from state of the art enteroclysis. Am J Gastroenterol 2003;98:1295–8.

21. Goldstein JL, Eisen GM, Lewis B, et al. Video capsule endoscopy to prospectively assess small bowel injury with celecoxib, naproxen plus omeprazole, and placebo. Clin Gastroenterol Hepatol 2005;3:133–41.

22. Pennazio M, Santucci R, Rondonotti E, et al. Outcome of patients with obscure gastrointestinal bleeding after capsule endoscopy: Report of 100 consecutive cases. Gastroenterology 2004;126:643–53.

23. Levi BS, de Lacey G, Price AB, et al. "Diaphragm-like" strictures of the small bowel in patients treated with non-steroidal anti-inflammatory drugs. Br J Radiol 1990;63:186–9.

24. Bjarnason I, Price AB, Zanelli G, et al. Clinicopathological features of nonsteroidal antiinflammatory drug- induced small intestinal strictures. Gastroenterology 1988; 94:1070–4.

25. Smale S, Tibble J, Sigthorsson G, et al. Epidemiology and differential diagnosis of NSAID-induced injury to the mucosa of the small intestine. Best Pract Res Clin Gastroenterol 2001;15:723–38.

26. Yousfi MM, De Petris G, Leighton JA, et al. Diaphragm disease after use of nonsteroidal anti-inflammatory agents: first report of diagnosis with capsule endoscopy. J Clin Gastroenterol 2004;38:686–91.

27. Sher BA, Bauer J. Radiation-induced enteropathy. Am J Gastroenterol 1990;85:121–8.

28. Kao MS. Intestinal complications of radiotherapy in gynecologic malignancy — clinical presentation and management. Int J Gynaecol Obstet 1995;49:S69–S75.

29. Regimbeau JM, Panis Y, Gouzi JL, et al. Operative and long term results after surgery for chronic radiation enteritis. Am J Surg 2001;182:237–42.

30. Galland RB, Spencer J. Natural history and surgical management of radiation enteritis. Br J Surg 1987; 74:742–7.

31. Macnaughton WK. Review article: new insights into the pathogenesis of radiation-induced intestinal dysfunction. Aliment Pharmacol Ther 2000;14:523–8.

32. Waddell BE, Rodriguez-Bigas MA, Lee RJ, et al. Prevention of chronic radiation enteritis. J Am Coll Surg 1999;189:611–24.

33. Green N. The avoidance of small intestine injury in gynecologic cancer. Int J Radiol Oncol Biol Phys 1983;9:1385–90.

34. Green N, Iba G, Smith WR. Measures to minimize small intestine injury in the irradiated pelvis. Cancer 1975; 35:1633–40.

35. Galland RB, Spencer J. The natural history of clinically established radiation enteritis. Lancet 1985;325:1257–8.

36. Mendelson RM, Nolan DJ. The radiologic features of chronic radiation enteritis. Clin Radiol 1985;36:141–8.

37. Willis JR, Chokshi HR, Zuckerman GR, et al. Enteroscopy-enteroclysis: experience with a combined endoscopic-radiographic technique. Gastrointest Endosc 1997; 45:163–7.

38. Lee DWH, Poon, AOS, Chan ACW. Diagnosis of small bowel radiation enteritis by capsule endoscopy. Hong Kong Med J 2004;10:419–21.

39. Ali T, Cave DR. Foreign bodies in the small bowel detected by capsule endoscopy. Am J Gastroenterol 2004; 99:S61–S62.

CHAPTER **15**

Vascular Abnormalities of the Small Bowel

Warwick Selby

Introduction

Traditionally, obscure gastrointestinal bleeding (OGIB) has presented a major clinical challenge because of the difficulty in investigating the small intestine where it was presumed that the blood loss originated. Obscure bleeding, defined as bleeding of unknown origin that persists or recurs after a negative initial endoscopy and colonoscopy, can be either overt, with melena or frank bleeding, or occult, the latter presenting as iron deficiency anemia or positive stool occult blood.[1] It represents approximately 5% of all patients presenting with gastrointestinal bleeding.[2,3] The development of capsule endoscopy has clearly shown that vascular abnormalities of the small bowel are the most frequent cause of OGIB. Because they are typically flat and small they have rarely been detected by radiology using standard contrast methods for the small intestine. Only if they are bleeding rapidly can they be detected by nuclear scan or angiography. Push enteroscopy is limited to the proximal small intestine. The new technique of double balloon enteroscopy offers diagnostic and therapeutic capability along the entire small bowel, and in many patients will avoid the need for surgical intervention.

Classification of vascular abnormalities (Table 15.1)

Congenital disorders

Hereditary hemorrhagic telangiectasia

Hereditary hemorrhagic telangiectasia (HHT; Osler–Rendu–Weber syndrome) is an autosomal dominant genetic disorder characterized by multiple arteriovenous malformations (AVM) in solid organs and telangiectases in skin and mucosal surfaces.[4] It has a prevalence of 1 in 10 000 or more. There is a wide ethnic and geographical distribution. Most cases result from mutations in one of two genes: the endoglin (*ENG*) gene on chromosome 9, or the activin receptor like kinase (*ALK1*) gene on chromosome 12. Histologically, the lesions are connections between arterioles and dilated post-capillary venules, with lymphocytic perivascular infiltration.[5] They may be small (telangiectases) or large (AVMs). AVMs are usually found in lungs, central nervous system, upper gastrointestinal tract, and/or liver. Smaller telangiectases are found on the skin, particularly lips, nose, and fingertips, and on oral mucosa (Figure 15.1). Telangiectases are also found in the gastrointestinal (GI) tract in over 80% of symptomatic patients.[5] Although uncommon in the esophagus, they are found not only in the stomach but along the full length of the small bowel. The number found

Table 15.1 Classification of small bowel vascular abnormalities

Congenital
    Hereditary hemorrhagic telangiectasia (Osler–Rendu–Weber syndrome)
    Blue rubber bleb nevus syndrome

Acquired
    Angioectasia
    Dieulafoy lesion
    Small bowel varices
    Venous ectasia
    Hemangioma

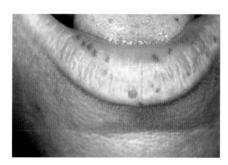

FIGURE 15.1 Multiple telangiectases on the lips of a patient with hemorrhagic hereditary telangiectases. (From Braverman IM. Skin signs of gastrointestinal disease. Gastroenterology 2003;124:1595–614, with permission of Elsevier.)

at endoscopy in the stomach and duodenum correlates directly with the number found in the jejunum and ileum.[6] The lesions are usually multiple, although the site and number vary between individuals (Figure 15.2).

The diagnosis of HHT can be made when an individual meets any three of the following criteria:

- Spontaneous recurrent epistaxis
- Mucocutaneous telangiectases, especially tongue, lips, mouth, fingers, nose
- Internal AVM (pulmonary, cerebral, hepatic, GI, spinal)
- Primary relative with HHT.

While recurrent nosebleeds are the most common feature of HHT, GI bleeding occurs in over 25% of patients. This does not usually present until 50–60 years of age. The severity of bleeding also tends to increase with age.[7] Once patients do start to bleed it can be a major clinical problem and lead to significant morbidity. GI bleeding may be overt or occult. Not unexpectedly, the greater the number of telangiectases in symptomatic patients the lower the hemoglobin and the greater the need for transfusion.[6]

Because the GI lesions are multiple, finding and treating the active bleeding point can be very difficult, and bleeding is likely to recur. Attempts to treat patients endoscopically are usually unsuccessful, and many end up on hormonal or other medical therapy if bleeding is recurrent.[8]

Blue rubber bleb nevus syndrome

Blue rubber bleb nevus syndrome is a rare condition characterized by multiple cutaneous and GI venous malformations.[9–11] The latter commonly produce recurrent GI bleeding, usually obscure. Patients usually present at

birth or in early childhood although adult presentations are reported. Most cases are sporadic but an autosomal dominant form has been described.

The lesions are dysplastic venous channels with flat endothelium and attenuated walls.[11] They are soft, blue nodules which are easily compressible. The skin lesions are usually multiple and vary in size from very small to a few centimeters. Their size tends to increase with age. They are found particularly on the upper limbs, trunk, and perineum. Apart from the skin, vascular lesions are found most commonly in the small intestine, although they can be found also in the upper GI tract and colon. Because of this, patients present commonly with obscure GI bleeding, either overt or with anemia. Diagnosis has been difficult because the lesions are beyond the reach of conventional endoscopy and are not visible on radiology unless they are large. However, they can be found at push enteroscopy and are readily visible at capsule endoscopy (Figure 15.3).[12,13] Once identified, bleeding lesions can be treated endoscopically by sclerotherapy, band ligation or coagulation.[11] Surgery may also be required.[14]

Acquired abnormalities

Angioectasias

Angioectasias are the most common of the acquired vascular abnormalities of the small bowel. They have also

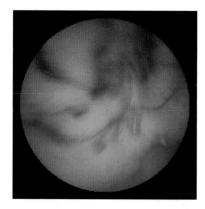

FIGURE 15.2 Two telangiectases in the jejunum seen at capsule endoscopy in a man with hereditary hemorrhagic telangiectasia. (Courtesy of Dr. Gregor Brown and Dr. Brian Saunders, Wolfson Unit for Endoscopy, St Mark's Hospital, Harrow, London, UK.)

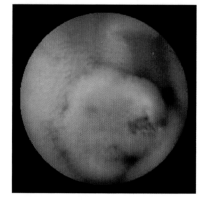

FIGURE 15.3 Blue rubber bleb nevus syndrome. Capsule endoscopy shows a typical large lesion in a 22-year-old woman requiring transfusion every 2–4 weeks. Once the extent of small bowel involvement was documented with capsule endoscopy she underwent intraoperative enteroscopy with removal and coagulation of multiple lesions. (Courtesy of Drs Gregor Brown and Brian Saunders, Wolfson Unit for Endoscopy, St Mark's Hospital, Harrow, London, UK.)

been referred to as angiodysplasias, AVMs, and telangiectasias. However, the latter terms are not strictly correct as there is no dysplastic element and in the majority there is no direct communication between artery and vein. Angioectasias initially consist of dilatation of normal pre-existing submucosal veins with later ectasia of overlying mucosal venules and capillaries (Figure 15.4). If competence of the precapillary sphincter is lost, an arteriovenous communication may develop.[15,16] Macroscopically, they are cherry red in color and often have a fern-like pattern. They vary in size from a few ectatic capillaries to 10 mm or more (Figures 15.5–15.8). The larger lesions are more likely to bleed while small lesions may not be clinically significant.[15]

Angioectasias can be found anywhere along the GI tract. They may be single or multiple (Figure 15.9). They are usually asymptomatic, being detected as an incidental finding in up to 3% of individuals over 65 years of age.[17] Most data relate to colonic angioectasias, which account for 2.6–6.2% of patients with GI bleeding.[16] Typically, they were described as being most common in the right side of the colon. However, with the advent of more effective endoscopic methods of examining the small intestine, and in particular capsule endoscopy, it has become apparent that their frequency in the small intestine is much greater than previously recognized.

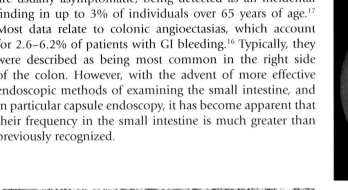

FIGURE 15.4 Dilated submucosal and mucosal vascular channels characteristic of angioectasia.

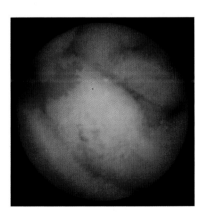

FIGURE 15.5 Large, fern-like angioectasia in a 72-year-old man with persistent iron deficiency anemia. There was also a gastric angioectasia. Both were treated endoscopically.

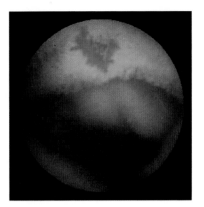

FIGURE 15.6 Large jejunal angioectasia seen at capsule endoscopy in a 71-year-old woman with 3 years of recurrent anemia. The lesion was ablated at push enteroscopy with a heater probe. There was no recurrence of anemia at 2 years.

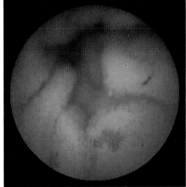

FIGURE 15.7 Ileal angioectasia in a 59-year-old man with iron deficiency anemia responding to iron therapy. No treatment was performed.

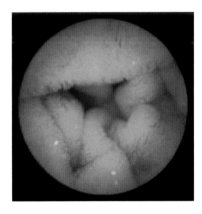

FIGURE 15.8 Duodenal angioectasia seen at capsule endoscopy in an 82-year-old with over 3 years of anemia. The lesion was adjacent to the ampulla of Vater but not seen at two previous upper GI endoscopies. It was ablated at push enteroscopy using argon plasma coagulation.

The etiology of acquired angioectasias is unknown. In most cases they are thought to be degenerative lesions. Their frequency rises with increasing age and the elderly are more likely to bleed from them. An association has been described with aortic stenosis (Heyde's syndrome),[18] chronic renal failure,[19] and von Willebrand disease.[20] The bleeding in patients with aortic stenosis is more likely to be obscure, presumably from the small bowel, than from the upper or lower GI tract (Figure 15.10).[21] This may explain why a prospective study of upper and lower endoscopy was unable to find an increased frequency of angioectasias in patients with aortic stenosis.[22] The link with aortic valve disease has been shown to be due to an acquired loss of high molecular weight multimers of von Willebrand factor, as a

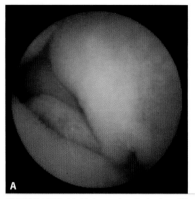
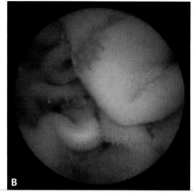
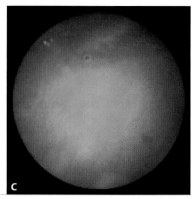

FIGURE 15.9 Multiple angioectasias in a 75-year-old man with chronic anemia. (a) Small duodenal angioectasia, (b) a large jejunal lesion, (c) a third small angioectasia in the ileum.

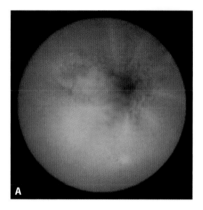
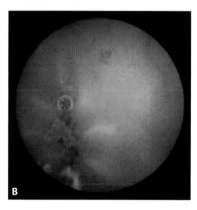

FIGURE 15.10 An 81-year-old woman with transfusion dependent anemia. Multiple angioectasias were found along the small intestine at capsule endoscopy, including two in the ileum (a) and (b). Endoscopic therapy failed to control bleeding. Investigation as part of her workup revealed asymptomatic severe aortic stenosis. Valve replacement has not been performed.

result of the high shear stress from the damaged valve.[16,18] Vincentelli reported skin or mucosal bleeding in 21% of patients with severe aortic stenosis (4 of which episodes were gastrointestinal).[18] These patients had loss of von Willebrand function which was proportional to the severity of their valvular stenosis. Von Willebrand factor and its function were restored quickly after valve replacement surgery. The long-term outcome has not been well studied, although anecdotal reports of long-term cessation of GI bleeding after aortic valve replacement have been described.[23]

Dieulafoy lesion

This abnormality is an uncommon cause of GI bleeding. It represents a tiny submucosal defect with fibrinoid necrosis at its base, overlying a large, tortuous, "persistent caliber" artery in the muscularis mucosae.[24,25] There is subintimal fibrosis of the artery and characteristically an absence of inflammation at the edge of the mucosal defect, which appears histologically normal (Figure 15.11). The fact that the mucosal defect is so small and not ulcerated means that Dieulafoy lesions are often overlooked at endoscopy if there is no active bleeding at the time. By far the majority of Dieulafoy lesions are in the stomach. However, in recent years it has become apparent that they occur in other parts of the GI tract as well, including the small bowel.[24–27] In one large series, 20% of all Dieulafoy lesions were in the small

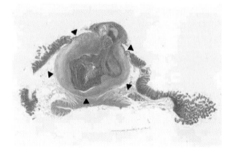

FIGURE 15.11 Histology of a Dieulafoy lesion shows a large submucosal vessel with a muscular wall eroding through the mucosa. (From Ueno N, Tada S, Nakamura T, et al. Bleeding jejunal Dieulafoy lesion. Gastrointest Endosc 2002;55:558, with

intestine.[26] Even this may be an underestimate of their true frequency.

Bleeding from Dieulafoy lesions is typically massive but intermittent. Diagnosis is difficult; if the lesion is not bleeding at the time of endoscopy, repeat procedures are often necessary. Even if the lesion is bleeding it is often obscured by blood. In the small intestine diagnosis is even harder because of the problems involved with access. Once again, capsule endoscopy has proven an excellent diagnostic modality for these abnormalities, particularly in the presence of active bleeding (Figure 15.12).

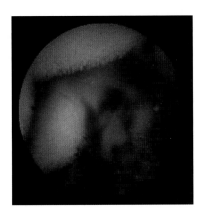

FIGURE 15.12 Active bleeding from a jejunal Dieulafoy lesion. No abnormality had been seen at prior push enteroscopy. The lesion was treated surgically.

Small bowel varices

Varices outside the esophagus and stomach are a rare cause of GI bleeding. They can be found in the small intestine or the colon. Small bowel varices may occur as part of hepatic portal hypertension, following abdominal surgery at a small intestinal anastomosis or in relation to adhesions in patients with underlying portal hypertension, after superior mesenteric vein thrombosis or spontaneously.[28] They should be considered in any patient with liver disease who presents with obscure GI bleeding. Diagnosis has been very difficult, though cases have been described using Sonde[29] or push[30] enteroscopy. Capsule endoscopy has facilitated the diagnosis, with varices reported in the jejunum and ileum (Figure 15.13).[28,31–33] They have a typical serpiginous, nodular appearance, with or without a bluish coloration. Therapy is the same as with other varices — local endoscopic treatment if possible, or decompression, either by transjugular intrahepatic portosystemic stenting (TIPS) or shunt surgery.

Small bowel ischemia

Ischemia of the small intestine may be acute or chronic. Acute ischemia results from spontaneous or therapeutic embolization or thrombosis of one or more mesenteric arteries, the celiac axis or superior mesenteric artery.[34] Presentation may be with acute abdominal pain, bleeding, and diarrhea. In extreme cases, an acute abdomen or perforation may occur. Chronic ischemia is more indolent.

It is the result of severe atherosclerotic narrowing of a major splanchnic vessel, with occlusion of one or two of the remaining vessels. It mostly affects the middle-aged and elderly with other risk factors for cardiovascular disease. The typical clinical triad is of post-prandial pain, weight loss, and fear of eating. Diarrhea or constipation may also occur. Diagnosis is by demonstration of the vascular narrowing, using Doppler ultrasound, contrast CT or angiography. Endoscopically, there may be ulceration and bleeding. Strictures may occur in patients with long-standing ischemia (Figure 15.14).

Venous ectasia

A finding commonly seen in patients undergoing capsule endoscopy for obscure GI bleeding is venous ectasia, also called phlebectasia. The significance of this possible abnormality is not clear, but it is not likely to be a major cause of bleeding. This lesion appears as a flat blue area which is not raised like either a small bowel varix or a blue rubber bleb nevus (Figure 15.15). It appears they are found more often with capsule endoscopy than push enteroscopy, presumably because of the lack of air insufflation with the former procedure. Phlebectasia is also found not uncommonly in patients with more significant pathology in the small bowel (Figure 15.16). There is generally no indication to treat these lesions when found, even when they are multiple.

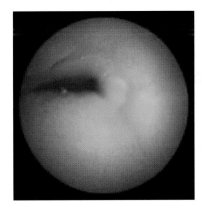

FIGURE 15.14 Ischemic ileal stricture in a 44-year-old man with Down's syndrome who had had previous laparotomy with colonic and small bowel resection for ischemia, probably secondary to torsion.

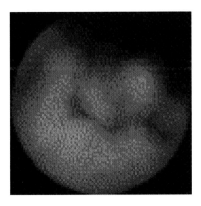

FIGURE 15.13 Serpiginous small bowel varices in a patient with mesenteric vein thrombosis. (From Tang SJ, Zanati S, Dubcenco E, et al. Diagnosis of small-bowel varices by capsule endoscopy. Gastrointest Endosc 2004;60:129–35, with permission of Elsevier.)

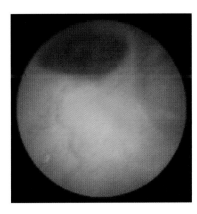

FIGURE 15.15 Large phlebectasia in a man of 80. Capsule endoscopy was otherwise normal.

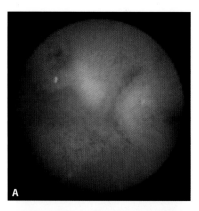

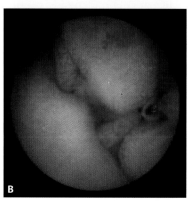

FIGURE 15.16 Phlebectasia (a) in an 84-year-old man with four episodes of melena over one year. This was an incidental finding in association with at least six large angioectasias, including one in the proximal jejunum (b). The angioectasias were ablated at push enteroscopy.

Hemangioma

Hemangiomas are uncommon vascular abnormalities of the GI tract. It is not clear whether they are congenital hamartomas or true benign neoplasms.[35] They represent 5–10% of benign small bowel tumors and < 0.5% of all tumors of the GI tract.[36] In the small intestine they are equally distributed along the jejunum and ileum but are less common in the duodenum. They typically present in young men and women, particularly in the third decade.

There are two histological types: capillary and cavernous. Capillary hemangiomas are made up of tiny vessels the size of capillaries, lined by a hyperplastic endothelium. In contrast, cavernous hemangiomas are comprised of large, thin-walled vascular spaces, also with a hyperplasic endothelium. Mixed forms also occur. Both types have been described in the small intestine.[37,38] Hemangiomas may be single or multiple and vary considerably in size from small to large.

Hemangiomas may be asymptomatic. If they do present, obscure GI bleeding is the most common manifestation. This is more likely to be occult with a capillary hemangioma and overt with a cavernous hemangioma. If large, they may rarely produce intussusception or intestinal obstruction.

Diagnosis has been very difficult because of their location and therefore hemangiomas have been largely overlooked as a cause of obscure GI bleeding. They are rarely large enough to be detected on small bowel radiology. If bleeding is brisk then angiography may show the bleeding point. However, they can now be readily detected by capsule endoscopy. The lack of air insufflation with this technique

may also make these abnormalities easier to see.[35] The appearance varies from small red nodules to large, bluish-pink vascular areas (Figure 15.17).

Treatment is generally by surgical resection. Endoscopic removal is hazardous, with a significant risk of massive bleeding or perforation.

Clinical features

Vascular abnormalities in the small bowel, by their location, present with obscure GI bleeding, either overt or occult. The severity of bleeding varies considerably from patient to patient. Overt bleeding is often recurrent and anemia is typically long-standing. There is typically no history of other symptoms such as abdominal pain or weight loss. Such patients produce a difficult challenge to the clinician. They may have had many admissions to hospital and multiple transfusions. The average duration of the bleeding history is typically around 24 months. At least 50% of patients have required transfusion at some stage of their illness. Multiple investigations have been performed, with an average of over 2 upper GI endoscopies and colonoscopies per patient, but often many more than this.[39,40] Small bowel follow-through, enteroclysis, CT scanning, ^{99}Tc red cell scan, Meckel's scan, angiography, and even surgery have often been performed without a diagnosis being reached.

As discussed above, a vascular abnormality as the cause for OGIB should be suspected in certain clinical situations. These include patients with aortic stenosis, chronic renal failure or von Willebrand disease. Telangiectases on the skin or mucous membranes should raise the suspicion of HHT, particularly if there is also a history of epistaxis, bleeding into other organs or a family history of the disease. In rare instances there may be blue rubber blebs on inspection of the skin. In patients with liver disease varices should be suspected, particularly if there is a history of previous abdominal surgery.

Diagnosis

Small bowel vascular lesions are the most common cause of obscure GI bleeding, whether overt or obscure. The traditional diagnostic methods of small bowel radiology, radioisotope scanning, and angiography are poor in their ability to detect small bowel bleeding. Push enteroscopy was a significant advance in diagnostic ability. However, it is the introduction of capsule endoscopy that has revolutionized the detection of vascular lesions of the small bowel.

Small bowel radiology

The yield of small bowel barium follow-through in the diagnosis of small bowel bleeding varies from 0.5% to 6%. Enteroclysis, which involves the instillation of contrast material directly into the proximal small intestine, has a higher yield, approximately 10–21%. However, neither

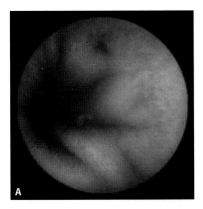

FIGURE 15.17 Large hemangioma in a 62-year-old with a 7-year history of iron deficiency anemia. Once identified at capsule endoscopy (a) it was removed at surgery (b). (c) Histology confirmed the diagnosis. (Courtesy of Dr Shehan Abey.)

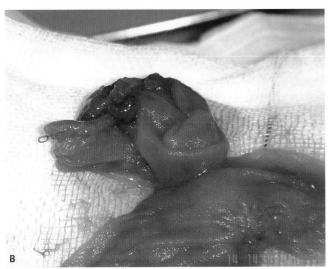

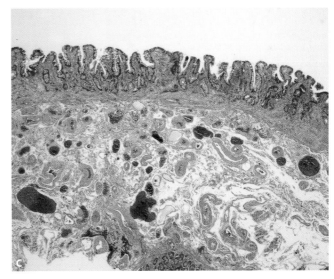

of these techniques is likely to detect angioectasias or other vascular lesions unless they are large. In one report, enteroclysis was suggestive of angioectasia in only 2% of 128 studies.[41]

The newer techniques of CT or MRI enteroclysis offer promise for improved radiological diagnosis in suspected small bowel disease. However, the limitations in finding vascular abnormalities are similar to other radiological methods.[42,43]

Red cell scanning

Isotopically labeled scanning using ^{99}Tc-labeled red cells is usually reserved for patients with active and rapid bleeding. It can only detect blood loss at a rate of at least 0.1–0.4 mL/min and as such is not very sensitive.[44] The most important finding is a blush of extravasated isotope seen immediately after scanning is commenced (Figure 15.18). Delayed scans are often made after 12–24 hours, but can be misleading because of pooling of blood distal to the bleeding site. Most experience with red cell scanning is with acute lower GI bleeding, where the yield in selected cases may be as high as 45%.[45] In general, its use is limited by false positive and false negative results. Of course, red cell scanning does not indicate the nature of the lesion that is bleeding. It has often been used as a precursor to mesenteric angiography, if the scan is positive.

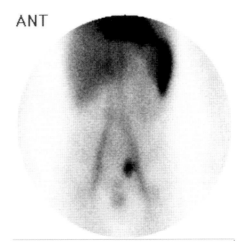

ANT

FIGURE 15.18 Positive ^{99}Tc-labeled red cell scan in a patient with active bleeding. Bleeding was first seen at 4.5 minutes.

Angiography

Mesenteric angiography may diagnose small bowel bleeding in one of two ways: by demonstration of extravasation of contrast, if the rate of blood loss is greater than 0.5 mL/min (Figure 15.19); or by the finding of an early filling and

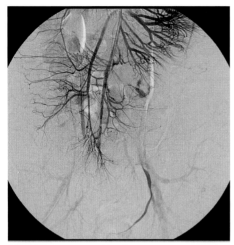

FIGURE 15.19 Active bleeding seen at angiography in an 18-year-old man with Ehlers–Danlos syndrome. The lesion was successfully embolized with coils (see Figure 15.24). Subsequent capsule endoscopy was normal. (Courtesy of Dr. Richard Waugh).

persistent vein typical of an AVM even when not bleeding. In highly selected patients the yield of angiography may be 40–50% in obscure GI bleeding.[46-48] It is usually reserved for patients in whom bleeding is very rapid, producing hemodynamic instability. If a bleeding point is found, then therapy is possible by infusing agents such as vasopressin or octreotide or by embolization of any feeding vessel.

Push enteroscopy

The development of push enteroscopy was a significant step forward in the ability to diagnose small bowel disease, in particular in patients with obscure GI bleeding.[1,49-51] The longer Sonde enteroscope had been available for some time, but was limited by its lack of maneuverability, the inability to treat any lesions found, and the time taken for the procedure.[52] It is estimated that the push enteroscope reaches up to 160 cm beyond the ligament of Treitz, although the reported depth of insertion varies considerably.[1,53,54] An overtube is often used to maximize the depth of insertion, although with experience this is not necessary.

The diagnostic yield of push enteroscopy has varied from 38% to 75% in published studies. The most common lesions found in the small intestine of patients with obscure GI bleeding are angioectasias, in 8–45%. Other vascular abnormalities such as blue rubber bleb nevus syndrome are found less commonly. The likelihood of finding a cause for the bleeding is generally similar whether push enteroscopy is performed for overt or occult bleeding,[12,55] although not all workers agree.[56] In my own experience to date of 347 patients undergoing push enteroscopy for obscure GI bleeding, a small bowel site was found in 101 (29%). Fifty of 139 (36%) with overt bleeding had a small bowel abnormality, as did 51 of 208 (25%) with anemia. Of the abnormal findings, 89% were vascular lesions, with all but 2 either single or multiple angioectasias. The other 2 patients had blue rubber bleb nevus syndrome. Lesions within reach

of conventional upper GI endoscopy were found in 17% of patients. This has been a common finding in other studies of push enteroscopy as well.[50,53,54,56,57]

Push enteroscopy is generally well tolerated but requires sedation and attendance at an endoscopy facility. Complications are uncommon but there is a risk of mucosal tearing or perforation, particularly with the use of an overtube.

Surgical endoscopy

Intraoperative enteroscopy is regarded as the gold standard for investigation of small bowel disease, including obscure GI bleeding. Until the advent of capsule endoscopy it was the only means of examining the entire length of the small intestine. With this technique, a bleeding source has been found in 55–75% of patients with obscure GI bleeding.[56,58,59] However, the need for a laparotomy and its associated risk and morbidity have generally made this procedure reserved for those with life-threatening or recurrent severe bleeding.

Capsule endoscopy

Capsule endoscopy allows for the first time a simple and safe method for examining all of the small intestinal mucosa. It has quickly become the diagnostic procedure of choice in patients with obscure GI bleeding, which is its main indication.[42,60-65] A likely or possible cause of blood loss has been found in 52–97% of patients in reported studies, generally within a range of 55–75% (Table 15.2). The majority of lesions detected are vascular abnormalities, between approximately 30% and 50% overall, but representing around 40–80% of lesions found. Small bowel ulcers and tumors are found much less frequently.

Angioectasias are the most common vascular abnormality. They can be isolated but often are multiple and found at any site along the small intestine. Other lesions such as Dieulafoy lesions, blue rubber blebs, and small bowel varices are found occasionally. Active bleeding from any of these abnormalities can be seen easily, aided by the suspected blood indicator (SBI). It is not always possible to identify the actual bleeding point if bleeding is profuse. If it is, an angioectasia or Dieulafoy lesion is the most likely underlying pathology (Figure 15.20).

Angioectasias are not always symptomatic and can be found as an incidental finding. For this reason, even if angioectasias are identified at capsule endoscopy, other abnormalities should still be carefully sought (Figure 15.21).

Simethicone has been reported to minimize bubbles in the lumen.[75] Oral purgatives can be used to empty the small intestine prior to capsule endoscopy, although their benefit in terms of reducing luminal contents has yet to be confirmed. Prokinetics such as metoclopramide increase the likelihood of the capsule passing along the entire small intestine and reaching the colon.[76] Whether these techniques lead to an improved diagnostic yield is still being evaluated.

The timing of capsule endoscopy in patients with obscure GI bleeding is also important. The diagnostic yield is highest

Table 15.2 Frequency of small bowel vascular and other lesions in patients with obscure GI bleeding undergoing capsule endoscopy

Number of patients	Number with positive diagnosis (%)	Small bowel vascular abnormalities Number (% yield)	Small bowel vascular abnormalities % of lesions found	Ulceration Number (%)	Tumor Number (%)	Other Number (%)	Reference
32	21 (66%)	17 (53%)	81%	2 (6%)	2 (6%)	7 (22%)	Ell et al, 2002[62]
20	11 (55%)	9 (45%)	81%	1 (5%)	1 (5%)	0	Lewis & Swain, 2002[61]
20	15 (75%)	8 (40%)	53%	n/a	n/a	n/a	Scapa et al, 2002[a60]
47	32 (68%)	21 (45%)	66%	1 (2%)	4 (9%)	6 (13%)	Chong et al, 2003[a65]
33	25 (76%)	15 (45%)	60%	7 (21%)	1	2	Hartmann et al, 2003[66]
50	34 (68%)	24 (48%)	71%	5 (10%)	2 (4%)	3 (6%)	Mylonaki et al, 2003[64]
58	40 (69%)	30 (52%)	75%	8 (14%)	2 (3%)	0	Saurin et al, 2003[31]
21	12 (57%)	3 (14%)	25%	0	1 (5%)	8 (38%)	Van Gossum et al, 2003[32]
20	14 (70%)	11 (55%)	79%	2 (10%)	0	0	Adler et al, 2004[67]
78	45 (58%)	26 (33%)	58%	11 (24%)	0	8 (18%)	Fireman et al, 2004[a68]
15	8 (53%)	2 (13%)	25%	3 (20%)	2 (13%)	1 (7%)	Magnano et al, 2004[69]
42	31 (74%)	21 (50%)	68%	7 (17%)	2 (5%)	1 (2%)	Mata et al, 2004[70]
100	62 (62%)	41 (41%)	66%	13 (13%)	2 (2%)	6 (6%)	Pennazio et al, 2004[39]
92	60 (65%)	47 (51%)	78%	3 (3%)	6 (7%)	4 (4%)	Selby, 2004[40]
12	10 (83%)	5 (42%)	50%	1 (8%)	3 (25%)	1 (8%)	Sriram, 2004[a71]
64	40 (63%)	18 (28%)	45%	18 (28%)	23 (36%)	0	Bresci et al, 2005[72]
108	56 (52%)	46 (43%)[b]	82%	n/a	n/a	n/a	Kalantzis et al, 2005[a73]
70	68 (97%)	26 (36%)	38%	17 (28%)	2 (3%)	0	Napierkowski et al, 2005[a74]

[a] Data extracted from study of a larger number of patients with suspected small bowel disease.
[b] "Specific" angioectasias only. Other vascular abnormalities not listed.
n/a = data not available from the published results.

in patients with ongoing overt bleeding.[39,40,73,77] Pennazio found a lesion in 21 of 23 (92.3%) patients in this group.[39] Eighteen of these abnormalities were vascular in nature: 13 angioectasias, Dieulafoy lesions in 2, jejunal varices in 2, and mucosal bleeding in 1. Similarly, in their comparison with intraoperative enteroscopy, Hartmann et al found a small bowel abnormality in all 11 patients with ongoing

bleeding, again mostly angioectasias.[68] The likelihood of finding a lesion at capsule endoscopy performed in patients while in hospital for management of their bleeding is also high, 9 of 10 in one series, including all 8 with ongoing bleeding.[40] The diagnostic yield in another study was 91% in a group in whom capsule endoscopy was performed within 15 days of their obscure GI bleed, but only 34% in a

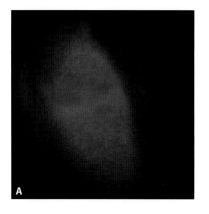
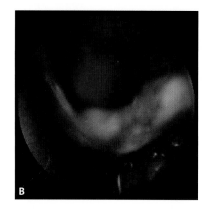

FIGURE 15.20 (a) Incidental large angioectasia in the mid small intestine in a patient with obscure GI bleeding. This was not bleeding. However, further down the small bowel there was a mucosal tumour that was bleeding (b). (Courtesy of Dr Henry Debinski.)

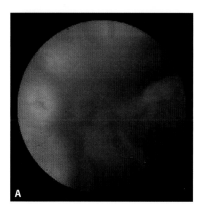
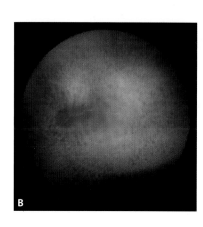

FIGURE 15.21 A 71-year-old woman with melena. (a) Active bleeding was seen in the initial images at capsule endoscopy. Capsule transit was very slow, and 2 hours later the bleeding angioectasia was visible (b).

group in whom it was performed after this.[72] This evidence supports early capsule endoscopy in patients with overt obscure GI bleeding, particularly if it is continuing.

In patients with previous overt bleeding and occult bleeding the diagnostic yield of capsule endoscopy is lower. Pennazio et al found a cause of bleeding in only 12.9% of patients whose capsule endoscopy had been performed 10 days to one year after their overt bleed.[39] In contrast, Hartmann et al found a cause in 67% of patients in this group, the same as that in the occult group.[77] A third study also found no difference in the frequency of a positive finding between patients with previous overt or occult obscure bleeding. Other demographic and clinical features were also unable to predict the finding of a small bowel vascular lesion or other abnormality by capsule endoscopy.[40]

There are now a number of studies comparing capsule endoscopy with other diagnostic techniques for the investigation of small bowel disease, in particular in patients with obscure GI bleeding. Clinical experience indicates that small bowel contrast radiology, either follow-through or enteroclysis, rarely detects vascular lesions. In most of the studies comparing capsule endoscopy with push enteroscopy, normal small bowel radiology was a requirement of entry (Table 15.3).[61,63,70] Nevertheless, the diagnostic yield in these studies was still high. In a series of consecutive patients undergoing capsule endoscopy for obscure bleeding, small bowel follow-through was reported as normal in all 88 patients in whom it had been performed, yet a vascular abnormality was found in 51%.[40] Direct comparisons of

capsule endoscopy with these radiological procedures have involved only small numbers of patients. In the first of these, 22 patients underwent barium follow-through or capsule endoscopy, 13 for obscure GI bleeding.[42] None of the 8 vascular abnormalities (all angioectasias) was detected radiologically. Hara et al examined 40 patients with small bowel follow-through (36) or enteroclysis (4), mostly for obscure GI bleeding.[43] Capsule endoscopy found a lesion in 22 (55%) but only one of the radiological examinations was abnormal, showing ileal ulcers. None of the angioectasias was identified on x-ray. Contrast-enhanced CT was able to identify masses in 3 patients but none of the vascular lesions. In a comparison with CT enteroclysis, Voderholzer et al made a diagnosis in 4 of 8 patients with obscure GI bleeding using capsule endoscopy (2 angioectasias) but in only one with CT (a suspected jejunal angioma).[78] The new technique of magnetic resonance enteroclysis has yet to be fully evaluated but, like the other radiological methods, will likely be of more value in diagnosing inflammatory bowel disease than vascular lesions.[79] These studies confirm the clear superiority of capsule endoscopy over radiology not just for the diagnosis of small bowel vascular lesions but for all small bowel pathology.

In patients with obscure GI bleeding, capsule endoscopy will find approximately twice as many lesions overall as push enteroscopy (Table 15.3). This diagnostic superiority of capsule endoscopy is also maintained when only the finding of a vascular abnormality is considered. Analysis of the Given Imaging clinical database of 345 patients with

Table 15.3 Studies comparing capsule endoscopy (VCE) with push enteroscopy (PE) in patients with obscure gastrointestinal bleeding. Overall diagnostic yield and comparative frequency of vascular lesions

Number	Overall yield (%)		Small bowel vascular lesions (%)		Reference
	VCE	PE	VCE	PE	
20	11 (55%)	6 (30%)	9 (45%)	6 (30%)	*Lewis & Swain, 2002[61]
32	21 (66%)	9 (28%)	17 (53%)	7 (22%)	Ell et al, 2002[62]
20	14 (70%)	9 45%)	12 (60%)	7 (35%)	*Selby & Shackell, 2002[63]
33	25 (76%)	7 (21%)	15 (45%)	5 (5%)	Hartmann et al, 2003[66]
50	34 (68%)	16 (32%)	24 (48%)	15 (30%)	Mylonaki et al, 2003[64]
58	40 (69%)	22 (38%)	30 (52%)	17 (29%)	Saurin et al, 2003[31]
21	12 (57%)	15 (71%)	4 (19%)	4 (19%)	Van Gossum et al, 2003[32]
20	14 (70%)	5 (25%)	11 (55%)	3 (15%)	Adler et al, 2004[67]
42	31 (74%)	8 (19%)	21 (50%)	7 (17%)	*Mata et al, 2004[70]

* In these three studies small bowel follow-through was normal in all 54 patients in whom it was performed prior to capsule endoscopy.

obscure GI bleeding who had small bowel vascular lesions has confirmed the advantage of capsule endoscopy over push enteroscopy. The lesions were found only by capsule endoscopy in 66.4%, by both capsule endoscopy and push enteroscopy in 26.7%, and by push enteroscopy alone in only 7%.[80]

While the above studies have demonstrated a significant advantage of capsule endoscopy over standard diagnostic modalities, does it stand up to the gold standard of intraoperative enteroscopy? In a landmark study, Hartmann et al performed intraoperative enteroscopy in 47 patients with obscure GI bleeding within one week of capsule endoscopy.[77] In 11 of these the bleeding was ongoing overt, in 24 it was previously overt, and in 12 it was occult. Upper GI endoscopy, colonoscopy, and push enteroscopy were all non-diagnostic prior to capsule endoscopy. A source of bleeding was found in 74% of patients, including all of those with ongoing overt bleeding, and 67% of the other groups. Angioectasias were the most common lesion found, in 22 patients (46.8%). In patients where these angioectasias were multiple, more were seen at intraoperative enteroscopy. Active bleeding from an unidentifiable underlying site was seen in a further 2 but this was not seen at intraoperative enteroscopy. Less common lesions including ulcers, erosions, varices, and bleeding diverticulum were seen equally with both procedures. This study showed capsule endoscopy to have a sensitivity of 95%, specificity 75%, positive predictive value 95%, and negative predictive value 86%.

Double balloon enteroscopy (DBE) is a new technique which allows more extensive endoscopic examination of the small intestine, using either an oral (antegrade) or an anal (retrograde) approach.[81,82] It utilizes a 200 cm enteroscope and an overtube, both of which have a balloon at their tip. This "push-and-pull" method permits complete small bowel visualization in 45–86% of patients in whom it is attempted, although this is not always necessary.[81,83,84] It can be performed under conscious sedation, although it takes approximately 75 minutes for each approach. A cause of obscure GI bleeding has been found in 54% and 66% of patients in the two largest studies to date.[83,84] Angioectasias are again amongst the most common findings. These can then be treated endoscopically when found, using argon plasma coagulation or other modalities. Although there have not been any direct comparisons to date between DBE and capsule endoscopy for the diagnosis of vascular abnormalities of the small bowel, the reports to date have shown a comparative diagnostic yield.[83-85] DBE is likely to replace intraoperative enteroscopy for most patients with bleeding vascular abnormalities of the small intestine as its availability becomes more widespread.

There is limited experience with capsule endoscopy in the pediatric age group but the early data indicate that it is as useful in children as it is in adults.[86] In 3 of 4 children with obscure GI bleeding in one series a possible vascular abnormality was found: blue rubber bleb nevus syndrome in 1 and venous ectasia in 2.[87]

Management

In general, vascular abnormalities of the small bowel are readily amenable to therapy. The method used depends on the nature and number of the lesions, the site along the small intestine, the rate of bleeding, and the presence of any underlying disease. Options include endoscopic treatment, angiography, surgery or medical therapy.

Endoscopic therapy

Angioectasias can be treated endoscopically by any of the techniques used on vascular lesions elsewhere in the GI tract. Access to the lesion may be by push enteroscopy, if the lesion is in the duodenum or proximal jejunum, or by double balloon enteroscopy using either the antegrade or retrograde route. Ileal lesions near the ileocecal valve may also be accessible with a colonoscope. The most commonly employed methods are heater probe, bipolar coagulation or argon plasma coagulation (Figures 15.22, 15.23).[12,88,89] Injection sclerotherapy and neodymium:yttrium:aluminium garnet (Nd:YAG) laser therapy have largely been superseded by other techniques.[90] Difficulties arise if there are multiple angioectasias. If one is actively bleeding, then deciding which is the significant lesion is simple. However, most angioectasias are not bleeding at either capsule endoscopy or enteroscopy and therefore the definite source of blood loss cannot be identified with certainty. In this situation, all visible lesions need to be ablated and the likelihood of further bleeding is high.

Endoscopic therapy of small bowel angioectasias has been shown to improve patient outcome, with cessation of further bleeding or reduction in the need for transfusion. Askin and Lewis cauterized 55 patients with bleeding from small bowel angioectasias and compared the outcome at 1 year with a group of patients who did not have their angioectasias cauterized.[88] There was a major difference in subsequent transfusion requirement between the two groups, with a significant fall in those who underwent endoscopic therapy. Similar results have been described using heater probe ablation.[12,89]

Treatment of Dieulafoy lesions within reach of an endoscope or enteroscope is usually successful by injection of adrenalin, thermocoagulation, band ligation or haemoclipping.[24] However, most experience to date has been with gastroduodenal lesions. Many of the small bowel Dieulafoy lesions have required surgery.[25] If they are identified at angiography, then embolization of the feeding vessel is possible.

Interventional radiology

In patients with rapid, uncontrolled bleeding from small bowel vascular lesions and in whom enteroscopy is not possible or who are not fit for surgery, an attempt can be made to stop the hemorrhage either by infusion of agents, such as vasopressin or octreotide, or by embolization of the source vessel with particles or coils (Figure 15.24).[91] Although the numbers in reported series are small, this form of therapy can be very successful. It relies on the demonstration of active bleeding or a definite vascular malformation. Use of vasopressin is associated with a risk of cardiovascular events including arrhythmias, myocardial infarction, and distal arterial thrombosis.[92] It has now largely been replaced by octreotide, which has a better safety profile. Embolization is associated with a risk of ischemia and infarction of the devascularized bowel segment or production of a fistula. Such complications are said to be less frequent when embolizing small bowel than colonic lesions.[91]

The treatment options in patients with small bowel varices include surgical resection, embolization or transjugular intrahepatic portosystemic shunt (TIPS).[28,30,33]

Surgery

Until the advent of push enteroscopy and capsule endoscopy, intraoperative enteroscopy was the last option for patients with clinically significant obscure GI bleeding where the diagnosis was unclear on preoperative investigations. Enteroscopy is complete in approximately 90% of patients and a source of bleeding is found in 55–75%. Any vascular

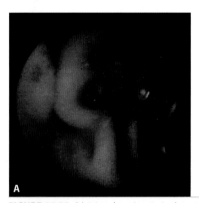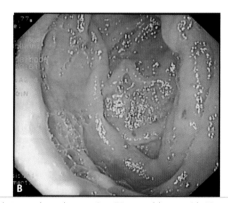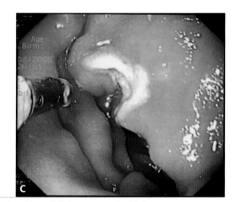

FIGURE 15.22 (a) Jejunal angioectasia detected at capsule endoscopy in a 71-year-old man with 18 months of iron deficiency anemia. (b) At enteroscopy, two small angioectasias were seen. These were ablated by heater probe thermocoagulation (c).

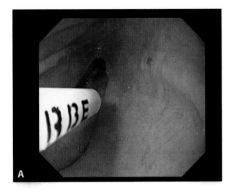 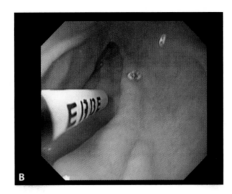

FIGURE 15.23 Hereditary hemorrhagic telangiectasia. Two lesions visible in the jejunum, (a) before and (b) after argon plasma coagulation at double balloon enteroscopy. (Courtesy of Dr. Arthur Kaffes).

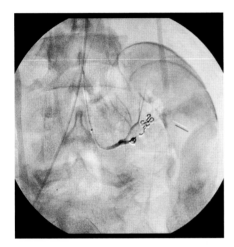

FIGURE 15.24 The same patient as in Figure 15.19. Coils have been placed into the feeding vessel with cessation of bleeding. (Courtesy of Dr. Richard Waugh).

lesions can be treated appropriately.[58,59,93–95] The best results occur in patients with isolated vascular lesions. However, up to 30% of patients re-bleed after surgery for obscure GI bleeding, most commonly because there are multiple angioectasias; the same problems exist with enteroscopy.[93,96] For this reason, every attempt should be made to identify an active bleeding source prior to surgery. Surgery is associated with significant morbidity, including the risk of postoperative ileus.

Fortunately, the introduction of double balloon enteroscopy means that surgery for vascular abnormalities will mostly be reserved for patients with ongoing rapid bleeding in whom endoscopic or radiological therapy has failed.

Medical therapy

A variety of medical treatments have been tried in patients with persistent bleeding from small bowel angioectasias, particularly associated with syndromes such as HHT. Medical therapy is mainly used when the abnormalities are multiple and distributed widely along the small intestine, when endoscopic and/or surgical treatment has failed to stop the bleeding, and when simple treatment with iron fails to control anemia.[97] It can also be given when significant co-

morbidity prevents other forms of intervention. Hormonal therapy with estrogen, either alone or in combination with a progestogen, is the most commonly used form of treatment. Anecdotal success has been described in patients with chronic renal failure, HHT or von Willebrand disease.[1,8,98,99] A placebo-controlled crossover trial in 10 patients with bleeding vascular malformations demonstrated a significant fall in transfusion requirements with 6 months of ethynylestradiol 0.05 mg and norethisterone 1 mg.[100] However, a later study of 72 similar patients failed to confirm this benefit using 1–2 years of lower dose ethynylestradiol (0.01 mg) and norethisterone 2 mg.[101] It therefore seems likely that the higher dose of estrogen is needed.[102] Hormonal therapy may also be more effective in HHT than in patients with acquired angioectasias.[101] Such treatment is not without risk: deep venous thrombosis, uterine bleeding, gynecomastia, and cardiac failure are amongst possible side effects, although their frequency has been low in clinical trials.

Other forms of treatment tried include subcutaneous octreotide,[103,104] somatostatin,[105] danazol,[106] and aminocaproic acid.[107] However, the number of patients in these reports is small and no large clinical trials have been performed.

Outcome following capsule endoscopy

Capsule endoscopy has not only increased the diagnostic yield in patients with obscure GI bleeding, but this benefit transfers to improved patient outcome, particularly because of the identification and treatment of vascular abnormalities. In the first study to show this, Pennazio et al followed 91 of their 100 patients with obscure GI bleeding after capsule endoscopy for a mean of 18 months.[39] All 23 patients with ongoing overt bleeding underwent either endoscopic, surgical or medical treatment. No further bleeding occurred in 20, including 11 of 13 with angioectasias, both patients with Dieulafoy lesions, 1 with active mucosal bleeding, and 1 of 2 with jejunal varices. In the patients with previous obscure bleeding, an AVM continued to bleed, as did a treated Dieulafoy lesion. In their group with occult bleeding, the anemia resolved in 6 of 10 patients with angioectasias, although only one underwent endoscopic treatment. In a smaller study, Moreno et al treated 67% of patients with obscure GI bleeding in whom a cause was found.[108] Six of 9 had resolution of their anemia.

A diagnosis at capsule endoscopy also leads to fewer subsequent investigations and offers significant cost savings.

There are still unanswered questions relating to capsule endoscopy in the investigation of patients with obscure GI bleeding. Particularly important is the issue of a negative study despite a high index of suspicion of ongoing bleeding and the ruling out of a tumor or a significant inflammatory lesion. Is this a false negative or a true negative examination? Has capsule endoscopy missed a Dieulafoy lesion or small angioectasia? Should the patient undergo repeat endoscopy and/or colonoscopy, push enteroscopy, double balloon enteroscopy or another capsule endoscopy? Should empirical hormone therapy be used? Only experience and further studies with sufficient duration of followup will address these issues. The number of patients who have undergone repeat capsule endoscopy for obscure GI bleeding to date is small, but in one series of 13 patients with recurrent bleeding, vascular abnormalities were seen in several patients after an initial non-diagnostic study.[109] In another report, AVMs were found in 2 of 10 patients with persistent iron deficiency anemia who had had an initial negative capsule endoscopy.[110]

Conclusion

The development of capsule endoscopy has demonstrated that small bowel vascular abnormalities are the most common cause of obscure GI bleeding. The diagnostic yield is significantly greater than with any of the previously available techniques apart from intraoperative enteroscopy. Once found, these lesions are readily amenable to therapy, whether endoscopic, surgical or medical. The choice of treatment will depend on the abnormality found and the clinical situation. Patient outcome has been improved by capsule endoscopy and significant savings made, especially in those with bleeding vascular lesions. Management of patients with specific bleeding syndromes such as HHT and blue rubber bleb nevus syndrome will also be aided significantly by capsule endoscopy.

References

1. Zuckerman G, Prakash C, Askin M, et al. AGA technical review on the evaluation and management of occult and obscure gastrointestinal bleeding. Gastroenterology 2000;118:201–21.

2. Lewis B. Small intestinal bleeding. Gastroenterol Clin N Am 1994;23:67–91.

3. Rockey DC. Occult gastrointestinal bleeding. N Engl J Med 1999;341:38–46.

4. Bayrak-Toydemir P, Mao R, Lewin S, et al. Hereditary hemorrhagic telangiectasia: an overview of diagnosis and management in the molecular era for clinicians. Genet Med 2004;6:175–91.

5. Longacre AV, Gross CP, Gallitelli M, et al. Diagnosis and management of gastrointestinal bleeding in patients with hereditary hemorrhagic telangiectasia. Am J Gastroenterol 2003;98:59–65.

6. Ingrosso M, Sabba C, Pisani A, et al. Evidence of small-bowel involvement in hereditary hemorrhagic telangiectasia: a capsule-endoscopic study. Endoscopy 2004;36:1074–9.

7. Kjeldsen AD, Kjeldsen J. Gastrointestinal bleeding in patients with hereditary hemorrhagic telangiectasia. Am J Gastroenterol 2000;95:415–8.

8. Proctor DD, Henderson KJ, Dziura JD, et al. Enteroscopic evaluation of the gastrointestinal tract in symptomatic patients with hereditary hemorrhagic telangiectasia. J Clin Gastroenterol 2005;39:115–9.

9. Oranje AP. Blue rubber bleb nevus syndrome. Pediatr Dermatol 1986;3:304–10.

10. Moodley M, Ramdial P. Blue rubber bleb nevus syndrome: case report and review of the literature. Pediatrics 1993;92:160–2.

11. Ertem D, Acar Y, Kotiloglu E, et al. Blue rubber bleb nevus syndrome. Pediatrics 2001;107:418–20.

12. Shackel NA, Bowen DG, Selby WS. Video push enteroscopy in the investigation of small bowel disease: defining clinical indications and outcomes. Aust NZ J Med 1998;28:198–203.

13. Fish L, Fireman Z, Kopelman Y, et al. Blue rubber bleb nevus syndrome: small-bowel lesions diagnosed by capsule endoscopy. Endoscopy 2004;36:836.

14. Fishman SJ, Smithers CJ, Folkman J, et al. Blue rubber bleb nevus syndrome: surgical eradication of gastrointestinal bleeding. Ann Surg 2005;241:523–8.

15. Small intestine. In: Morson BC, Dawson IMP, Day DW, et al, eds. Morson & Dawson's Gastrointestinal pathology. Blackwell Scientific Publications, Oxford, 1990, pp. 334–50.

16. Veyradier A, Balian A, Wolf M, et al. Abnormal von Willebrand factor in bleeding angiodysplasias of the digestive tract. Gastroenterology 2001;120:346–53.

17. Foutch PG. Angiodysplasia of the gastrointestinal tract. Am J Gastroenterol 1993;88:807–18.

18. Vincentelli A, Susen S, Le Tourneau T, et al. Acquired von Willebrand syndrome in aortic stenosis. N Engl J Med 2003;349:343–9.

19. Navab F, Masters P, Subramani R, et al. Angiodysplasia in patients with renal insufficiency. Am J Gastroenterol 1989;84:1297–301.

20. Fressinaud E, Meyer D. International survey of patients with von Willebrand disease and angiodysplasia. Thromb Haemost 1993;70:546.

21. Shindler DM. Aortic stenosis and gastrointestinal bleeding. Arch Intern Med 2004;164:103–4.

22. Bhutani MS, Gupta SC, Markert RJ, et al. A prospective controlled evaluation of endoscopic detection of angiodysplasia and its association with aortic valve disease. Gastrointest Endosc 1995;42:398–402.

23. Warkentin TE, Moore JC, Morgan DG. Gastrointestinal angiodysplasia and aortic stenosis. N Engl J Med 2002;347:858–9.

24. Schmulewitz N, Baillie J. Dieulafoy lesions: a review of 6 years of experience at a tertiary referral center. Am J Gastroenterol 2001;96:1688–94.

25. Blecker D, Bansal M, Zimmerman RL, et al. Dieulafoy's lesion of the small bowel causing massive gastrointestinal bleeding: two case reports and literature review. Am J Gastroenterol 2001;96:902–5.

26. Norton ID, Petersen BT, Sorbi D, et al. Management and long-term prognosis of Dieulafoy lesion. Gastrointest Endosc 1999;50:762–7.

27. Ueno N, Tada S, Nakamura T, et al. Bleeding jejunal Dieulafoy lesion. Gastrointest Endosc 2002;55:558.

28. Tang SJ, Zanati S, Dubcenco E, et al. Diagnosis of small-bowel varices by capsule endoscopy. Gastrointest Endosc 2004;60:129–35.

29. Lopez MJ, Cooley JS, Petros JG, et al. Complete intraoperative small-bowel endoscopy in the evaluation of occult gastrointestinal bleeding using the sonde enteroscope. Arch Surg 1996;131:272–7.

30. Tang SJ, Jutabha R, Jensen DM. Push enteroscopy for recurrent gastrointestinal hemorrhage due to jejunal anastomotic varices: a case report and review of the literature. Endoscopy 2002;34:735–7.

31. Saurin JC, Delvaux M, Gaudin JL, et al. Diagnostic value of endoscopic capsule in patients with obscure digestive bleeding: blinded comparison with video push-enteroscopy. Endoscopy 2003;35:576–84.

32. Van Gossum A, Hittelet A, Schmit A, et al. A prospective comparative study of push and wireless-capsule enteroscopy in patients with obscure digestive bleeding. Acta Gastroenterol Belg 2003;66:199–205.

33. Joo YE, Kim HS, Choi SK, et al. Massive gastrointestinal bleeding from jejunal varices. J Gastroenterol 2000;35:775–8.

34. Peters J, Reilly P, Merine D, et al. Vascular insufficiency. In: Yamada T, Alpers D, Owyang C, et al, eds. Textbook of gastroenterology. JB Lippincott, Philadephia, 1991, pp. 2188–217.

35. Clouse RE. Vascular ectasias, tumors and malformations. In: Yamada T, Alpers D, Owyang C, et al, eds. Textbook of gastroenterology. JB Lippincott, Philadephia, 1991, pp. 2180–2.

36. Non-epithelial tumours. In: Morson BC, Dawson IMP, Day DW, eds. Morson & Dawson's Gastrointestinal pathology. Blackwell Scientific Publications, Oxford, 1990, pp. 382–3.

37. Kim YS, Chun HJ, Jeen YT, et al. Small bowel capillary hemangioma. Gastrointest Endosc 2004;60:599.

38. Khurana V, Dala R, Barkin JS. Small bowel cavernous hemangioma. Gastrointest Endosc 2004;60:96.

39. Pennazio M, Santucci R, Rondonotti E, et al. Outcome of patients with obscure gastrointestinal bleeding after capsule endoscopy: report of 100 consecutive cases. Gastroenterology 2004;126:643–53.

40. Selby W. Can clinical features predict the likelihood of finding abnormalities when using capsule endoscopy in patients with GI bleeding of obscure origin? Gastrointest Endosc 2004;59:782–7.

41. Moch A, Herlinger H, Kochman ML, et al. Enteroclysis in the evaluation of obscure gastrointestinal bleeding. Am J Roentgenol 1994;163:1381–4.

42. Costamagna G, Shah SK, Riccioni ME, et al. A prospective trial comparing small bowel radiographs and video capsule endoscopy for suspected small bowel disease. Gastroenterology 2002;123:999–1005.

43. Hara AK, Leighton JA, Sharma VK, et al. Small bowel: preliminary comparison of capsule endoscopy with barium study and CT. Radiology 2004;230:260–5.

44. Smith R, Copely DJ, Bolen FH. 99mTc RBC scintigraphy: correlation of gastrointestinal bleeding rates with scintigraphic findings. Am J Roentgenol 1987;148:869–74.

45. Zuckerman GR, Prakash C. Acute lower intestinal bleeding: part I: clinical presentation and diagnosis. Gastrointest Endosc 1998;48:606–17.

46. Boley SJ, Sprayregen S, Sammartano RJ, et al. The pathophysiologic basis for the angiographic signs of vascular ectasias of the colon. Radiology 1977;125:615–21.

47. Fiorito JJ, Brandt LJ, Kozicky O, et al. The diagnostic yield of superior mesenteric angiography: correlation with the pattern of gastrointestinal bleeding. Am J Gastroenterol 1989;84:878–81.

48. Lau WY, Ngan H, Chu KW, et al. Repeat selective visceral angiography in patients with gastrointestinal bleeding of obscure origin. Br J Surg 1989;76:226–9.

49. Lewis BS, Waye JD. Small bowel enteroscopy in 1988: pros and cons. Am J Gastroenterol 1988;83:799–802.

50. Harris A, Dabezies MA, Catalano MF, et al. Early experience with a video push enteroscope. Gastrointest Endosc 1994;40:62–4.

51. Barkin JS, Chong J, Reiner DK. First-generation video enteroscope: fourth-generation push-type small bowel enteroscopy utilizing an overtube. Gastrointest Endosc 1994;40:743–7.

52. Gostout CJ. Sonde enteroscopy. Technique, depth of insertion, and yield of lesions. Gastrointest Endosc Clin N Am 1996;6:777–92.

53. Chong J, Tagle M, Barkin JS, et al. Small bowel push-type fiberoptic enteroscopy for patients with occult gastrointestinal bleeding or suspected small bowel pathology. Am J Gastroenterol 1994;89:2143–6.

54. Barkin JS, Lewis BS, Reiner DK, et al. Diagnostic and therapeutic jejunoscopy with a new, longer enteroscope. Gastrointest Endosc 1992;38:55–8.

55. Chak A, Koehler MK, Sundaram SN, et al. Diagnostic and therapeutic impact of push enteroscopy: analysis of factors associated with positive findings. Gastrointest Endosc 1998;47:18–22.

56. Zaman A, Katon RM. Push enteroscopy for obscure gastrointestinal bleeding yields a high incidence of proximal lesions within reach of a standard endoscope. Gastrointest Endosc 1998;47:372–6.

57. Schmit A, Gay F, Adler M, et al. Diagnostic efficacy of push-enteroscopy and long-term follow-up of patients with small bowel angiodysplasias. Dig Dis Sci 1996;41:2348–52.

58. Cave DR, Cooley JS. Intraoperative enteroscopy. Indications and techniques. Gastrointest Endosc Clin N Am 1996;6:793–802.

59. Flickinger EG, Stanforth AC, Sinar DR, et al. Intraoperative video panendoscopy for diagnosing sites of chronic intestinal bleeding. Am J Surg 1989;157:137–44.

60. Scapa E, Jacob H, Lewkowicz S, et al. Initial experience of wireless-capsule endoscopy for evaluating occult gastrointestinal bleeding and suspected small bowel pathology. Am J Gastroenterol 2002;97:2776–9.

61. Lewis BS, Swain P. Capsule endoscopy in the evaluation of patients with suspected small intestinal bleeding: Results of a pilot study. Gastrointest Endosc 2002;56:349–53.

62. Ell C, Remke S, May A, et al. The first prospective controlled trial comparing wireless capsule endoscopy with push enteroscopy in chronic gastrointestinal bleeding. Endoscopy 2002;34:685–9.

63. Selby W, Shackell N. A prospective comparison between the M2A capsule and push enteroscopy for the investigation of obscure gastrointestinal bleeding. A final report. J Gastroenterol Hepatol 2002;17:A137.

64. Mylonaki M, Fritscher-Ravens A, Swain P. Wireless capsule endoscopy: a comparison with push enteroscopy in patients with gastroscopy and colonoscopy negative gastrointestinal bleeding. Gut 2003;52:1122–6.

65. Chong AKK, Taylor ACF, Miller AM, et al. Initial experience with capsule endoscopy at a major referral hospital. Med J Aust 2003;178:537–40.

66. Hartmann D, Schilling D, Bolz G, et al. Capsule endoscopy versus push enteroscopy in patients with occult gastrointestinal bleeding. Z Gastroenterol 2003;41:377–82.

67. Adler D, Knipschield M, Gostout C. A prospective comparison of capsule endoscopy and push enteroscopy in patients with GI bleeding of obscure origin. Gastrointest Endosc 2004;59:492–8.

68. Fireman Z, Eliakim R, Adler S, et al. Capsule endoscopy in real life: a four-centre experience of 160 consecutive patients in Israel. Eur J Gastroenterol Hepatol 2004;16:927–31.

69. Magnano A, Privitera A, Calogero G, et al. The role of capsule endoscopy in the work-up of obscure gastrointestinal bleeding. Eur J Gastroenterol Hepatol 2004;16:403–6.

70. Mata A, Bordas JM, Feu F, et al. Wireless capsule endoscopy in patients with obscure gastrointestinal bleeding: a comparative study with push enteroscopy. Aliment Pharmacol Ther 2004;20:189–94.

71. Sriram PV. Wireless capsule endoscopy: Experience in a tropical country. J Gastroenterol Hepatol 2004;19:63–7.

72. Bresci G, Parisi G, Bertoni M, et al. The role of video capsule endoscopy for evaluating obscure gastrointestinal bleeding: usefulness of early use. J Gastroenterol 2005;40:256–9.

73. Kalantzis N, Papanikolaou IS, Giannakoulopoulou E, et al. Capsule endoscopy; the cumulative experience from its use in 193 patients with suspected small bowel disease. Hepatogastroenterology 2005;52:414–9.

74. Napierkowski JJ, Maydonovitch CL, Belle LS, et al. Wireless capsule endoscopy in a community gastroenterology practice. J Clin Gastroenterol 2005;39:36–41.

75. Albert J, Gobel CM, Lesske J, et al. Simethicone for small bowel preparation for capsule endoscopy: A systematic, single-blinded, controlled study. Gastrointest Endosc 2004;59:487–91.

76. Selby W. Complete small-bowel transit in patients undergoing capsule endoscopy: determining factors and improvement with metoclopramide. Gastrointest Endosc 2005;61:80–5.

77. Hartmann D, Schmidt H, Bolz G, et al. A prospective two-center study comparing wireless capsule endoscopy with intraoperative enteroscopy in patients with obscure GI bleeding. Gastrointest Endosc 2005;61:826–832.

78. Voderholzer WA, Ortner M, Rogalla P, et al. Diagnostic yield of wireless capsule enteroscopy in comparison with computed tomography enteroclysis. Endoscopy 2003;35:1009–14.

79. Schreyer AG, Golder S, Seitz J, et al. New diagnostic avenues in inflammatory bowel diseases. Capsule endoscopy, magnetic resonance imaging and virtual enteroscopy. Dig Dis 2003;21:129–37.

80. Friedman S. Comparison of capsule endoscopy to other modalities in small bowel. Gastrointest Endosc Clin N Am 2004;14:51–60.

81. Yamamoto H, Sekine Y, Sato Y, et al. Total enteroscopy with a nonsurgical steerable double-balloon method. Gastrointest Endosc 2001;53:216–20.

82. Gerson LB. Double-balloon enteroscopy: the new gold standard for small-bowel imaging? Gastrointest Endosc 2005;62:71–5.

83. Yamamoto H, Kita H, Sunada K, et al. Clinical outcomes of double-balloon endoscopy for the diagnosis and treatment of small-intestinal diseases. Clin Gastroenterol Hepatol 2004;2:1010–6.

84. May A, Nachbar L, Ell C. Double-balloon enteroscopy (push-and-pull enteroscopy) of the small bowel: feasibility and diagnostic and therapeutic yield in patients with suspected small bowel disease. Gastrointest Endosc 2005;62:62–70.

85. Matsumoto T, Esaki M, Moriyama T, et al. Comparison of capsule endoscopy and enteroscopy with the double-balloon method in patients with obscure bleeding and polyposis. Endoscopy 2005;37:827–32.

86. Seidman EG, Sant'Anna AM, Dirks MH. Potential applications of wireless capsule endoscopy in the pediatric age group. Gastrointest Endosc Clin N Am 2004;14:207–17.

87. Guilhon de Araujo Sant'Anna AM, Dubois J, Miron MC, et al. Wireless capsule endoscopy for obscure small-bowel disorders: final results of the first pediatric controlled trial. Clin Gastroenterol Hepatol 2005;3:264–70.

88. Askin MP, Lewis BS. Push enteroscopic cauterization: long-term follow-up of 83 patients with bleeding small intestinal angiodysplasia. Gastrointest Endosc 1996;43:580–3.

89. Morris AJ, Mokhashi M, Straiton M, et al. Push enteroscopy and heater probe therapy for small bowel bleeding. Gastrointest Endosc 1996;44:394–7.

90. Sargeant IR, Loizou LA, Rampton D, et al. Laser ablation of upper gastrointestinal vascular ectasias: long term results. Gut 1993;34:470–5.

91. Rosen RJ, Sanchez G. Angiographic diagnosis and management of gastrointestinal hemorrhage. Current concepts. Radiol Clin N Am 1994;32:951–67.

92. Gomes AS, Lois JF, McCoy RD. Angiographic treatment of gastrointestinal hemorrhage: comparison of vasopressin infusion and embolization. Am J Roentgenol 1986;146:1031–7.

93. Desa LA, Ohri SK, Hutton KA, et al. Role of intraoperative enteroscopy in obscure gastrointestinal bleeding of small bowel origin. Br J Surg 1991;78:192–5.

94. Lewis BS, Wenger JS, Waye JD. Small bowel enteroscopy and intraoperative enteroscopy for obscure gastrointestinal bleeding. Am J Gastroenterol 1991;86:171–4.

95. Ress AM, Benacci JC, Sarr MG. Efficacy of intraoperative enteroscopy in diagnosis and prevention of recurrent, occult gastrointestinal bleeding. Am J Surg 1992;163:94–8.

96. Szold A, Katz LB, Lewis BS. Surgical approach to occult gastrointestinal bleeding. Am J Surg 1992;163:90–2.

97. Barkin JS, Ross BS. Medical therapy for chronic gastrointestinal bleeding of obscure origin. Am J Gastroenterol 1998;93:1250–4.

98. Bronner MH, Pate MB, Cunningham JT, et al. Estrogen-progesterone therapy for bleeding gastrointestinal telangiectasias in chronic renal failure. An uncontrolled trial. Ann Intern Med 1986;105:371–4.

99. Van Cutsem E, Piessevaux H. Pharmacologic therapy of arteriovenous malformations. Gastrointest Endosc Clin N Am 1996;6:819–32.

100. Van Cutsem E, Rutgeerts P, Vantrappen G. Treatment of bleeding gastrointestinal vascular malformations with oestrogen-progesterone. Lancet 1990;335:953–5.

101. Junquera F, Feu F, Papo M, et al. A multicenter, randomized, clinical trial of hormonal therapy in the prevention of rebleeding from gastrointestinal angiodysplasia. Gastroenterology 2001;121:1073–9.

102. Madanick RD, Barkin JS. Hormonal therapy in angiodysplasia: should we completely abandon its use? Gastroenterology 2002;123:2156–7.

103. Orsi P, Guatti-Zuliani C, Okolicsanyi L. Long-acting octreotide is effective in controlling rebleeding angiodysplasia of the gastrointestinal tract. Dig Liver Dis 2001;33:330–4.

104. Rossini FP, Arrigoni A, Pennazio M. Octreotide in the treatment of bleeding due to angiodysplasia of the small intestine. Am J Gastroenterol 1993;88:1424–7.

105. Andersen MR, Aaseby J. Somatostatin in the treatment of gastrointestinal bleeding caused by angiodysplasia. Scand J Gastroenterol 1996;31:1037–9.

106. Haq AU, Glass J, Netchvolodoff CV, et al. Hereditary hemorrhagic telangiectasia and danazol. Ann Intern Med 1988;109:171.

107. Saba HI, Morelli GA, Logrono LA. Brief report: treatment of bleeding in hereditary hemorrhagic telangiectasia with aminocaproic acid. N Engl J Med 1994;330:1789–90.

108. Moreno C, Arvanitakis M, Deviere J, et al. Capsule endoscopy examination of patients with obscure gastrointestinal bleeding: evaluation of clinical impact. Acta Gastroenterol Belg 2005;68:10–14.

109. Jones BH, Fleischer DE, Sharma VK, et al. Yield of repeat wireless video capsule endoscopy in patients with obscure gastrointestinal bleeding. Am J Gastroenterol 2005;100:1058–64.

110. Bar-Meir S, Eliakim R, Nadler M, et al. Second capsule endoscopy for patients with severe iron deficiency anemia. Gastrointest Endosc 2004;60:711–13.

CHAPTER **16**

Benign and Malignant Tumors of the Small Bowel

Blair S Lewis

KEY POINTS

1. The incidence of cancer of the small bowel is relatively low: approximately 5000 cases are diagnosed in the United States annually with approximately 1000 deaths.

2. Small bowel tumors are typically overlooked. Due to the inaccessibility of the small bowel to conventional diagnostic modalities, the diagnosis and localization of small bowel tumors remains a clinical challenge.

3. Until recently, the diagnostic modalities for investigating small intestinal pathology have been suboptimal. Thus, historically, small bowel tumors carry a poor prognosis. Early consideration of this diagnosis along with newer modalities to evaluate the small bowel may improve this disease's prognosis.

4. Small bowel tumors are a significant cause of obscure gastrointestinal bleeding. These lesions should be particularly considered in the younger patient. Video capsule endoscopy is the highest yield diagnostic test for these lesions.

Introduction

The small intestine is considered to be an uncommon place for neoplasms. Most physicians when speaking of illness of the small bowel are concerned with vascular lesions or inflammatory illnesses such as Crohn's or celiac disease. Small bowel tumors account for only 5% of all gastrointestinal (GI) tract tumors. The majority of these lesions are benign. Classically, the diagnosis of a small bowel malignancy is often delayed and thus the prognosis in patients with malignant tumors is quite poor. In 1980, Herbsman et al reported that survival of more than 6 months for adenocarcinoma of the small bowel was rare.[1] In 2006, it is expected that 5420 new cases will be reported along with 1070 deaths.[2] It has been shown that early diagnosis improves survival. Of 71 patients treated for obscure GI bleeding, Szold et al reported 19 patients with tumors detected early by enteroscopy.[3] In this series, 13 patients were long-term survivors and 6 died of metastatic disease. In a retrospective review of 144 patients with primary cancer of the small intestine, the overall 5-year survival was 57% and the median survival was 52 months.[4] Not surprisingly, survival was best for early stage tumors and those that could be completely resected.

The failure to diagnose tumors early is due to two major factors. The first reason is that physicians fail to consider tumors as a source of patients' symptoms. Tumors typically present with vague early symptoms and there is an absence of physical findings. Anemia is present in 88% of patients. Since bleeding is often the sole symptom when a tumor initially presents, the diagnosis is overlooked. Gross bleeding is the presenting complaint in 25–53% of patients with small bowel tumors. They are the second most common cause of small intestinal hemorrhage, after vascular lesions[5,6] and account for 5–10% of all cases of small intestinal hemorrhage.[7,8] These patients are generally younger than patients with angioectasias of the small bowel, with an average age of 51 compared to 69.[9] In 1987, Thompson et al reported 37 patients with obscure GI bleeding.[10] Fifteen patients were younger than 50 years of age, and all but one had a small bowel tumor identified as the culprit lesion. This finding led the author to advocate early surgery in young patients with obscure bleeding. Berner et al reported a series also suggesting that small bowel tumors must be searched for in younger patients.[11] The average age of patients with a tumor was 51 years. Angioectasias, although present in all age groups, were more common in elderly patients. In addition, young patients with small bowel tumors tend to require fewer transfusions, presumably because they tolerate the anemia. Therefore, it can be suggested that tumors be searched for in younger patients with obscure bleeding, even if the effect on the patient's quality of life seems mild. Lewis reported gross bleeding as the presentation in 62% of 13 patients with small bowel tumors, while 38% presented with occult blood in the stool.[9] According to Lewis, the type of bleeding, whether frank blood loss or occult blood in the stool, is not an effective means of differentiating bleeding secondary to angioectasia from that caused by a small bowel tumor.[9] Patients often go on to develop symptoms as the disease progresses. The most frequent symptoms are abdominal pain, weight loss, nausea, vomiting, bleeding, jaundice, and anorexia.[12] Patients present with pain 16% of the time and with intussusception 12% of the time. While benign lesions are more likely to cause pain with small bowel obstruction and intussusception, malignant lesions tend to cause pain syndromes that are less specific for small bowel pathology. Unfortunately, by the time they are diagnosed, most small bowel malignancies have advanced beyond the early stage of neoplasm.

The second reason that tumors of the small bowel are not diagnosed early is that, until recently, the diagnostic modalities for investigating small intestinal pathology have been sub-optimal. Due to the inaccessibility of the small bowel to conventional diagnostic modalities, the diagnosis and localization of small bowel tumors has been a clinical challenge. A small bowel series has long been considered the mainstay in the evaluation of the small intestine. However, data show a relatively low yield of positive findings for patients with occult bleeding or iron deficiency. It is estimated that only approximately 5% of small bowel follow-through exams will detect an intestinal bleeding site. Rabe et al reported a yield of 5.6% in a series of 215 small bowel series performed for obscure bleeding.[13] Fried et al made no diagnosis in 28 exams.[13] Gordon et al made diagnoses in 3 of 46 patients (6.5%) with iron deficiency anemia who underwent small bowel follow-through exams.[15] These included one with a jejunal ulcer and two with an abnormal terminal ileum. Rockey and Cello evaluated 29 patients with iron deficiency anemia and negative esophagogastroduodenoscopies (EGD) and colonoscopies using enteroclysis in 26 and small bowel series in 3. No lesions were identified.[16] Noninvasive barium studies have a particularly low yield for diagnosing the source of obscure gastrointestinal bleeding. Although better than small bowel series, enteroclysis is reported to have a 10–20% yield.[17] Bleeding scans and angiography, although superior to barium studies, require active bleeding at the time of testing. While computed tomography (CT) may be useful in diagnosing extraluminal and metastatic spread of small bowel malignancies, its role in detecting small intraluminal and mucosal lesions has been limited, with a diagnostic yield as low as 20%.[18] Endoscopic evaluation of the small intestine has been demonstrated to be the best means at present for the early diagnosis of tumors of the small bowel, which are discussed below.

Stromal tumors

Gastrointestinal stromal cell tumors (GISTs) can be located throughout the small bowel. These tumors are believed to arise from the intestinal pacemaker cells that are found in the smooth muscle layer of the intestine. Pathologically they can be diagnosed by immunohistochemical staining for the c-kit protein. This is considered to be a sensitive marker for GISTs. GISTs are the most common tumors that bleed. Bleeding may be brisk and occurs in these submucosal tumors when there is central tumor necrosis and subsequent ulceration of the overlying mucosa (Figure 16.1). Due to their vascularity, ^{99m}Tc pertechnetate scanning may be positive in GISTs; angiography has been reported to show a tumor blush in 86% of lesions. There is no sex predilection and these lesions are most frequently seen in the fifth to seventh decade. Gradual but more chronic blood loss is usually associated with other small bowel tumors including carcinoid, adenocarcinoma, and lymphomas. GISTs can vary in size and the endoscopic appearance does not predict the extent of the extramucosal component.

Adenomas and adenocarcinoma

Adenomatous polyps and adenocarcinoma are most frequently found within the proximal bowel with 90% of lesions located within the duodenum and the first 20 cm of the jejunum. Tubular, tubulovillous, and villous adenomas are all seen in the small bowel (Figure 16.2). These lesions are generally identified within reach of push enteroscopy. Endoscopic biopsy is recommended and polypectomy is readily accomplished even with flat lesions. One helpful guideline to therapy in the small bowel is to consider it

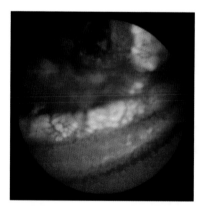

FIGURE 16.1 A stromal cell tumor with central ulceration and necrosis.

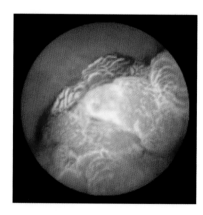

FIGURE 16.2 A tubular adenoma of the small bowel.

similar to therapies delivered in the cecum. Both organs are thin walled and perforate more easily than other areas of the gastrointestinal tract. Adenomas of the small bowel are associated with familial polyposis and Gardner's syndrome. Up to 90% of patients with these diseases will have adenomas of the duodenum.[19] Periampullary adenomas and adenocarcinomas are most typical in Gardner's syndrome. Most authors suggest surveillance of these patients with a combination of push enteroscopy and duodenoscopy using a side-viewing endoscope.[19] Small intestinal adenocarcinoma is also more common in patients with small intestinal Crohn's disease as well as in patients with celiac disease (Figure 16.3).

Adenocarcinoma of the small bowel is often circumferential and quite exophytic. It has an apple core appearance similar to cancers in the colon. If a cancer is seen within the duodenum, the differential should also include invading pancreatic cancer. Due to the liquid nature of food within the small bowel, cancers are typically quite advanced prior to the development of obstructive symptoms. This late diagnosis contributes to the relatively poor outcomes in these patients, with 5-year survivals less than 25%.

Non-neoplastic polyps

Hyperplastic and hamartomatous polyps can occur within the small bowel. These tend to be pedunculated, in marked contrast to adenomatous polyps within the small bowel, which tend to be sessile (Figure 16.4). These polyps can occur

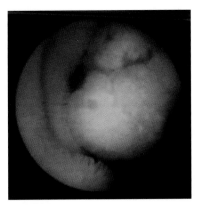

FIGURE 16.3 An adenocarcinoma of the small bowel.

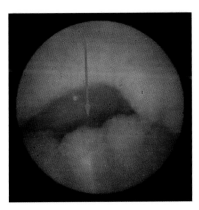

FIGURE 16.4 The edge of a pedunculated hamartoma polyp.

de novo or can be associated with a polyposis syndrome such as Peutz–Jeghers. Endoscopic polypectomy of these pedunculated lesions is readily accomplished.

Lipomas of the small bowel are also seen. Typically these polyps are yellow in color, submucosal, and quite soft and pliable on manipulation with the biopsy forceps (Figure 16.5). When the tip of the forceps is pushed into the body of a lipomatous polyp, the lipoma is easily "indented" — the so-called "pillow sign." Lipomas are usually asymptomatic unless they grow to a large size. Lipomas are the most common cause of intussusception among adults, they may ulcerate and cause bleeding, and large lipomas also have the potential to cause intestinal obstruction. Endoscopic polypectomy is not performed in these patients unless the lesion is symptomatic, due to the high risk of perforation or snare entrapment within the fatty tissue.

Carcinoid

Carcinoid tumors are submucosal neoplasms consisting of cells that stain for neural markers such as synaptophysin and chromogranin A. While not true carcinomas, they may metastasize and cause the carcinoid syndrome. Next to the appendix, the small intestine is the most common location for carcinoid tumors, and they tend to be located distally in the small bowel, with the ileum the most common location.

Size of the lesion is an important predictor of metastatic potential; lesions less than 1 cm are uncommonly associated with metastatic disease. Carcinoid tumors appear as small submucosal nodules that are often umbilicated (Figure 20.6). As these tumors grow in size, ulceration may occur with the potential for bleeding.

Lymphoma

Primary lymphoma of the small bowel is generally a discrete tumor in the United States and "developed" countries, and tends to involve the distal jejunum or ileum (Figure 20.7). Primary lymphoma of the small bowel is uncommon and may be associated with celiac disease or human immunodeficiency virus (HIV) infection. Celiac disease is associated

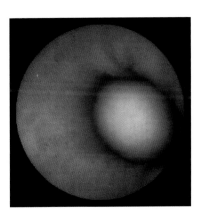

FIGURE 16.5 A lipoma of the small bowel.

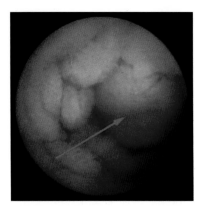

FIGURE 16.6 An umbilicated carcinoid of the ileum.

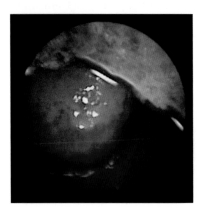

FIGURE 16.7 An ulcerated lymphoma.

with T-cell lymphomas, while HIV-associated lymphomas are generally B-cell lymphomas which virtually always present in extranodal sites and involve the gastrointestinal tract in approximately 25% or more of cases. Most primary small bowel lymphomas not associated with celiac disease are B-cell lymphomas and have been given the name mucosa-associated lymphoid tissue (MALT) lymphomas.

In developing countries, a diffuse primary small intestinal lymphoma labeled immunoproliferative small intestinal disease (IPSID) occurs. This disease is also known by other terms such as Mediterranean lymphoma or alpha-chain disease. It is characterized by an intense infiltration of the lamina propria with lymphocytes and plasma cells and an extensive follicular lymphoid hyperplasia. Over a number of years, frank lymphoma can develop. Infection is felt to play an important role in the development of IPSID and the disease is reversible if treated with antibiotics (tetracycline) in its early stages.

Lymphomas can have several different appearances. A classification of these appearances has been created and includes a nodular pattern, an infiltrative pattern, and an ulcerating pattern.[20] Halphen et al, in a review of 120 patients with primary small bowel lymphoma, found the infiltrative pattern, in which the mucosa is firm and motionless, to be most indicative of lymphoma.[21] The other patterns may be mimicked by celiac disease and radiation enteritis among others. While only limited, discrete regions of the small intestine are generally involved in primary small intestinal lymphoma, the involved area will be extensive in IPSID.

Metastatic disease

Metastatic disease can also migrate to the small bowel. Melanoma, breast cancer, and lung cancer are the most common to metastasize to the small intestine.[22] They may present clinically with bleeding (from ulceration), intussusception, or, rarely, obstruction. Metastatic melanoma can often be suspected by its pigmented nature (Figure 16.8). Pigmentation is not necessary, however, and amelanotic melanoma may be seen. Often, the typical bulls-eye appearance seen in the stomach is not observed in the small bowel. Other tumors that metastasize to the small bowel include colon cancer, renal cell cancer, osteogenic sarcoma, Meckel cell carcinoma of the skin, and germ cell cancers. As mentioned above, pancreatic cancer can directly invade the duodenum and present with bleeding or obstruction.

Endoscopic diagnosis

The use of endoscopy in the diagnosis of small bowel tumors is relatively new. In 1980, Martin et al reported on the diagnosis of 25 intestinal tumors.[23] Upper endoscopy and colonoscopy were performed in all patients, but did not help to make the final diagnosis. Enteroscopy was not utilized. This report included 9 sarcomas of the intestine, 7 adenocarcinomas, 5 leiomyomas, 1 lymphoma, 2 hamartomas, and 1 adenomatous polyp. Barium studies made the diagnosis in 56% of patients with positive findings on small bowel series in 13 and a diagnostic enteroclysis in 1. Still 44% of the tumors were missed by barium studies and the diagnosis was finally made by angiography in 6 and exploratory laparotomy in 5.

It was not until 1982 that the first report of the use of enteroscopy in the diagnosis of a small bowel tumor was made. Shinya and McSherry reported on the initial use of both Sonde and push enteroscopy and described finding a duodenal adenocarcinoma and a jejunal hemangiolymphangioma.[24] The role of enteroscopy in the diagnosis of small bowel tumors has developed since that time. Often, small bowel tumors were diagnosed by other means and were confirmed by enteroscopy. Parker and Agayoff reported finding a large neurofibroma within the proximal jejunum.[25] Hashmi et al reported a 22-year-old woman presenting with

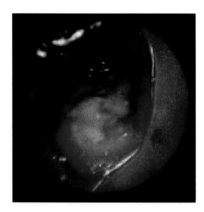

FIGURE 16.8 An ulcerated metastatic implant of melanoma.

melena.[26] The jejunal leiomyoma was diagnosed initially by angiography and was subsequently confirmed by push enteroscopy and enteroclysis. Shigematsu et al reported 3 patients with lymphangiomas of the small bowel diagnosed on small bowel series and subsequently confirmed on push enteroscopy.[26] Watatani et al reported, in 1989, a 73-year-old woman with nausea and vomiting in whom a small bowel series showed a distal duodenal lesion.[27] Push enteroscopy not only confirmed this lesion, but a biopsy was performed that revealed this to be an adenocarcinoma.

At the same time, enteroscopy was being employed in the evaluation of patients with unexplained gastrointestinal bleeding. It is through this indication that enteroscopy diagnosed small bowel tumors without any prior diagnostic examination. Foutch reported finding a jejunal leiomyoma in a 65-year-old man with unexplained gastrointestinal bleeding.[29] The patient's previous evaluations including angiography and small bowel series were non-diagnostic and the lesion was found using push enteroscopy. Hall et al reported finding an adenocarcinoma of the third portion of the duodenum in a patient with celiac disease.[30] An upper GI series and abdominal CT scan had been normal. Lewis et al reported finding 13 small bowel tumors with a combination of push and Sonde enteroscopy during evaluation of 258 patients with obscure gastrointestinal bleeding.[9] Tumors discovered included 4 lymphomas, 3 adenocarcinomas, 2 leiomyomas, 2 lipomas, 1 leiomyosarcoma, and 1 carcinoid. All patients had non-diagnostic barium studies including 6 negative enteroclysis in 4 patients. Seven patients had negative angiographic studies. Push enteroscopy discovered 5 of the lesions while Sonde enteroscopy discovered 8 of the tumors.

Push enteroscopy is quite effective in identifying small bowel tumors and other causes of intestinal bleeding. There have been several series examining the value of push enteroscopy. Reported yields of push enteroscopy in patients with obscure gastrointestinal bleeding have varied from 13% to 38%.[29,31,32] Messer reported finding the bleeding site in 20 of 52 patients (38%) with obscure bleeding.[11] Tumors made up 55% of findings. The small bowel tumors included leiomyomas in 4, adenocarcinoma in 4, lipoma in 1, lymphangioma in 1, and melanoma in 1. Foutch also reported a yield of 38% in his report of push enteroscopic examinations in 39 patients with unexplained bleeding.[29] Tumors were found to be the cause of bleeding in 3 patients, accounting for 15% of the overall findings. These included a leiomyoma, a metastatic lung cancer lesion, and a large lipoma. These lesions had been missed by previous barium studies.

Push enteroscopy can also be therapeutic, and polypectomy of small intestinal adenomas or inflammatory polyps can be accomplished. Surveillance of patients with a polyposis syndrome can also be performed with push enteroscopy, allowing biopsy and polypectomy of larger lesions. Iida et al reported on using push enteroscopy to examine 10 patients with polyposis syndromes, finding jejunal adenomas in 90%.[19]

Push enteroscopy can also be used in the performance of enteroclysis, which in turn may help diagnose an intestinal tumor. Nasojejunal tubes have been placed using push enteroscopy and a Seldinger technique.[33] The push enteroscope is placed into the jejunum initially and then a guidewire is advanced through the endoscope's biopsy channel. Finally the endoscope is removed leaving the guidewire in place, over which a tube for the performance of enteroclysis is advanced.[31,34,35] Cohen reported on using this technique to combine push enteroscopy and enteroclysis in 4 patients.[34] Three had normal examinations, but a fourth had a metastatic melanoma found on the push examination that was associated with other metastases documented on the enteroclysis.

Double balloon enteroscopy is a new form of push enteroscopy developed to allow even deeper small bowel intubation. The procedure is designed to pleat the small bowel onto an overtube much in the same way that the small bowel is pleated onto an enteroscope by a surgeon while performing intraoperative enteroscopy. The procedure involves using an overtube preloaded onto an enteroscope and both the overtube and enteroscope have balloons at their tips. When inserted and the balloons inflated, the assembly can be withdrawn causing the pleating effect. May et al reported using this new technology in 137 patients.[36] Twenty-seven tumors were diagnosed including GISTs, hamartomas, and primary adenocarcinomas.

Intraoperative enteroscopy also plays a role in the management of small bowel tumors. Although one would think that, at exploration, tumors of the small intestine would be visible or at least palpable to the surgeon, often small tumors and polyps can be missed. Bracke et al reported using intraoperative enteroscopy to localize a jejunal hamartoma in a 67-year-old man who presented with bleeding.[37] The lesion was diagnosed preoperatively by enteroclysis but could not be felt at exploration. Webb reported using intraoperative enteroscopy to identify small bowel polyps in patients with familial polyposis.[38] Takehara et al reported using the same techniques in an 18-year-old woman with Peutz–Jeghers syndrome.[39] Endoscopic polypectomy was performed intra-operatively in this patient as well. Mathus-Vliegan and Tytgat have also reported intraoperative endoscopic small bowel polypectomies in patients with Peutz–Jeghers syndrome.[40]

Wireless capsule endoscopy is a relatively new tool for investigating the small bowel.[41] It is already recognized as the state-of-the-art method to examine the small bowel and it is clear that capsule endoscopy permits the early diagnosis of tumors when all other modalities fail. The first series of small bowel tumors diagnosed by capsule endoscopy reported a 3.8% rate of primary tumors.[42] This study included 130 patients. In describing the series of 5 small bowel tumors, de Mascarenhas-Saraiva and da Silva Araujo Lopes concluded that the accuracy of capsule endoscopy in diagnosing the tumors seemed to be superior to that of other methods. Several case reports have also attested to the diagnostic ability of capsule endoscopy in detecting tumors.[42–46] Cobrin et al reported that the prevalence of small bowel tumors may be higher than predicted in the pre-capsule era.[47] Their data suggest that 9% of obscure gastrointestinal bleeding is due to small bowel tumors. The calculated number of capsule studies needed to diagnose a small bowel tumor in the setting of obscure gastrointestinal bleeding was 12. A pooled analysis of 24 studies included a total of 530 patients, 310 of whom had obscure gastrointestinal bleeding.[48] The patients had undergone an average of 7.4 diagnostic tests prior to being diagnosed. Eighty-six of the 1349 pathologies identified at capsule endoscopy (6.4%) were intestinal neoplasms. Another pooled analysis, strictly of patients with tumors diagnosed by capsule endoscopy, was reported by Schwartz and Barkin.[49] Eighty-nine tumors were reported including 87 small bowel tumors, 1 cecal cancer, and 1 gastric tumor. These patients had undergone an average of 4.6 negative examinations prior to the diagnosis being made by capsule endoscopy. These evaluations included 40 small bowel series, 24 CT scans, 26 push enteroscopies, 16 enteroclyses, and 6 angiographies. Malignant tumors constituted 61% of the tumors identified. Capsule endoscopy has also been used to evaluate patients with polyposis syndromes including familial polyposis and Peutz–Jeghers syndrome.[50-52] Again, capsule endoscopy appears to be superior to small bowel series and MR enterography in the detection of these lesions.

Endoscopic appearances of tumors

The endoscopic appearance of a small bowel mass can be deceiving to the endoscopist. The variety of pathologies seen within the small bowel cannot be matched by the colon or the stomach. Thus the well-trained endoscopist may still be able to say only that a tumor was present and not know the underlying pathology. Many small bowel tumors are submucosal, also adding to the difficulty of visual diagnosis and even diagnosis by endoscopic biopsy. Submucosal tumors include leiomyomas, carcinoids, lipomas, and metastatic disease. With the small space of the small bowel and the large nature of a tumor, the typical changes suggestive of a submucosal process may be missed. Typically the endoscopist looks for visible mucosa and a vascular pattern across the tumor to confirm its submucosal nature. Bridging folds may also help in this regard. In the small bowel, the mucosa may be pulled so tightly over the mass that it becomes transparent, masking the standard changes. GISTs can vary in size and the endoscopic appearance does not predict the size of the extramucosal component. Occasionally central ulceration or umbilication may be seen. Lymphomas can have several different appearances. A classification of these appearances has been created and includes a nodular pattern, an infiltrative pattern, and an ulcerating pattern.[20] Halphen et al, in a review of 120 patients with primary small bowel lymphoma, found the infiltrative pattern, in which the mucosa is firm and motionless, to be most indicative of lymphoma.[21] The other patterns may be mimicked by celiac disease and radiation enteritis among others. Adenocarcinoma is circumferential and often quite exophytic appearing like the endoscopic appearance of colon cancer. Metastatic melanoma can often be suspected by its pigmented nature. Carcinoid appears as small submucosal nodules.

Summary

As the field of endoscopy has continued to develop, technical advances allow the visualization of the entire small bowel in a noninvasive form. Capsule endoscopy has revolutionized the evaluation of the small bowel and permits the early diagnosis of small bowel tumors. In turn, patient management is improved, limiting testing, directing surgery, and hopefully saving lives.

References

1. Herbsman H, Wetstein L, Rosen Y, et al. Tumors of the small intestine. Curr Probl Surg 1980;17:121.

2. American Cancer Society; New York, 2006 Cancer Facts and Figures 2005, p. 4.

3. Szold A, Katz LB, Lewis BS. Surgical approach to occult gastrointestinal bleeding. Am J Surg 1992;163:90-2.

4. North JH, Pack MS. Malignant tumors of the small intestine: a review of 144 cases. Am Surg 2000;66:46-51.

5. Rossini F, Risio M, Pennazio M. Small bowel tumors and polyposis syndromes. Gastrointest Endosc Clin North Am 1999;9:93-114.

6. Conn M. Tumors of the small intestine. In: DiMarino A, Benjamin S, eds. Gastrointestinal disease: an endoscopic approach. Blackwell Science, Malden, Mass., 1997, pp. 551-66.

7. Martin L, Max M, Richardson J, Peterson G. Small bowel tumors: continuing challenge. South Med J 1980;73:981-5.

8. Ashley S, Wells S. Tumors of the small intestine. Semin Oncol 1988;15:116-28.

9. Lewis B, Kornbluth A, Waye J. Small bowel tumors: the yield of enteroscopy. Gut 1991;32:763-5.

10. Thompson JN, Salem RR, Hemingway AP, et al. Specialist investigation of obscure gastrointestinal bleeding. Gut 1987; 28:47-51.

11. Berner JS, Mauer K, Lewis BS. Push and sonde enteroscopy for the diagnosis of obscure gastrointestinal bleeding. Am J Gastroenterol 1994;89:2139-42.

12. Torres M, Matta E, Chinea B, et al. Malignant tumors of the small intestine. J Clin Gastroenterol 2003;37:372-80.

13. Rabe F, Becker G, Begozzi M, et al. Efficacy study of the small-bowel examination. Radiology 1981;140:47-50.

14. Fried A, Poulos A, Hatfield D. The effectiveness of the incidental small-bowel series. Radiology 1981;140:45-6.

15. Gordon SR, Smith RE, Power GC. The role of endoscopy in the evaluation of iron deficiency anemia in patients over the age of 50. Am J Gastroenterol 1994;89:1963-7.

16. Rockey DC, Cello JP. Evaluation of the gastrointestinal tract in patients with iron-deficiency anemia. N Engl J Med 1993;329:1691-5.

17. Lewis B, Goldfarb N. Review article: the advent of capsule endoscopy — a not-so-futuristic approach to obscure gastrointestinal bleeding. Aliment Pharmacol Ther 2003; 17:1085-96.

18. Hara AK, Leighton JA, Sharma VK, Fleisher DE. Small bowel: preliminary comparison of capsule endoscopy with barium study and CT. Radiology 2004;230:260-5.

19. Iida M, Matsui T, Itoh H, et al. The value of push-type jejunal endoscopy in familial adenomatosis coli/Gardner's syndrome. Am J Gastroenterol 1990;85:1346–8.

20. Barakat M. Endoscopic features of primary small bowel lymphoma: a proposed endoscopic classification. Gut 1982; 23:36–41.

21. Halphen M, Najjar T, Jaafoura H, et al. Diagnostic value of upper intestinal fiber endoscopy in primary small intestinal lymphoma. Cancer 1986;58:2140–5.

22. Kadakia S, Parker A, Canalses L. Metastatic tumors to the upper gastrointestinal tract: endoscopic experience. Am J Gastroenterol 1992;87:1418–23.

23. Martin L, Max M, Richardson J, Peterson G. Small bowel tumors: continuing challenge. South Med J 1980;73:981–5.

24. Shinya H, McSherry C. Endoscopy of the small bowel. Surg Clin North Am 1982;62:821–4.

25. Parker H, Agayoff J. Enteroscopy and small bowel biopsy utilizing a peroral colonoscope. Gastrointest Endosc 1983; 29:139–40.

26. Hashmi M, Sorokin J, Levine S. Jejunal leiomyoma: an endoscopic diagnosis. Gastrointest Endosc 1985;31:81–3.

27. Shigematsu A, Iida M, Hatanaka M, et al. Endoscopic diagnosis of lymphangioma of the small intestine. Am J Gastroenterol 1988;83:1289–93.

28. Watatani M, Yasuda N, Imamoto H, et al. Primary small intestinal adenocarcinoma diagnosed by endoscopic examination prior to operation. Gastroenterol Jpn 1989; 24:402–6.

29. Foutch GP, Sawyer R, Sanowski R. Push-enteroscopy for diagnosis of patients with gastrointestinal bleeding of obscure origin. Gastrointest Endosc 1990;36:337–41.

30. Hall M, Cooper B, Rooney N, Thompson H. Coeliac disease and malignancy of the duodenum. Gut 1991;32:90–2.

31. Foutch P, Sanowski R, Kelly S. Enteroscopy for detection of small bowel tumors. Am J. Gastroenterol 1985;80:887–90.

32. Messer J, Romeu J, Waye J, Dave P. The value of proximal jejunoscopy in unexplained gastrointestinal bleeding. Gastrointest Endosc 1984;30:151.

33. Lewis B, Mauer K, Bush A. The rapid placement of jejunal feeding tubes; the Seldinger technique applied to the gut. Gastrointest Endosc 1990;36:739–40.

34. Cohen M, Barkin J. Enteroscopy and enteroclysis: the combined procedure. Am J Gastroenterol 1989;84:1413–5.

35. McGovern R, Barkin J. Enteroscopy and enteroclysis: an improved method for combined procedure. Gastrointest Radiol 1990;15:327–8.

36. May A, Nachbar L, Ell C. Double-balloon enteroscopy of the small bowel: feasibility and diagnostic and therapeutic yield in patients with suspected small bowel disease. Gastrointest Endosc 2005;62:62–70.

37. Bracke P, Degryse H, Goovaerts G, et al. Polypoid hamartoma of the jejunum. Gastrointest Radiol 1991;16:113–4.

38. Webb W. Intra-operative endoscopy of the total gastrointestinal tract in familial polyposis syndrome. Gastrointest Endosc 1979;25:167.

39. Takehara H, Okada A, Nishi M, et al. Intra-operative total enteroscopy for the management of Peutz-Jegher's syndrome. Acta Paediatr Jpn 1992;34:569–72.

40. Mathus-Vliegen E, Tytgat G. Intraoperative endoscopy: technique, indications and results. Gastrointest Endosc 1986;32:381–4.

41. O'Loughlin C, Barkin JS. Wireless capsule endoscopy: summary. Gastrointest Endosc Clin N Am 2004;14:229–37.

42. de Mascarenhas-Saraiva MNG, da Silva Araujo Lopes LM. Small-bowel tumors diagnosed by capsule endoscopy: report of five cases. Endoscopy 2003;35:865–8.

43. Kimchi NA, Broide E, Zehavi S, Halevy A, Scapa E. Capsule endoscopy diagnosis of celiac disease and ileal tumors in a patient with melena of obscure origin. Isr Med Assoc J 2005;7:412–3.

44. Kruger S, Noack F, Blochle C, Feller AC. Primary malignant melanoma of the small bowel: a case report and review of the literature. Tumori 2005;91:73–6.

45. Coates SW Jr, DeMarco DC. Metastatic carcinoid tumor discovered by capsule endoscopy and not detected by esophagogastroduodenoscopy. Dig Dis Sci 2004;49:639–41.

46. Forner A, Mata A, Puig M, et al. Ileal carcinoid tumor as a cause of massive lower-GI bleeding: the role of capsule endoscopy. Gastrointest Endosc 2004;60:483–5.

47. Cobrin G, Pittman R, Lewis B. Increased diagnostic yield of small bowel tumors with capsule endoscopy. Cancer 2006;107:22–7.

48. Eisen G, Lewis BS, Friedman S. A pooled analysis to evaluate results of capsule endoscopy trials. Endoscopy 2005;37:960–5.

49. Schwartz G, Barkin J. Small bowel tumors. Gastrointest Endosc Clin N Am 2006;16:267–75.

50. Soares J, Lopes L, Vilas Boas G, Pinho C. Wireless capsule endoscopy for evaluation of phenotypic expression of small-bowel polyps in patients with Peutz-Jeghers syndrome and in symptomatic first-degree relatives. Endoscopy 2004; 36:1060–6.

51. Caspari R, von Falkenhausen M, Krautmacher C, Schild H, Heller J, Sauerbruch T. Comparison of capsule endoscopy and magnetic resonance imaging for the detection of polyps of the small intestine in patients with familial adenomatous polyposis or with Peutz-Jeghers' syndrome. Endoscopy 2004;36:1054–9.

52. De Palma GD, Rega M, Ciamarra P, Di Girolamo E, Patrone F, Mastantuono L, Simeoli I. Small-bowel polyps in Peutz-Jeghers syndrome: diagnosis by wireless capsule endoscopy. Endoscopy 2004;36:1039.

CHAPTER **17**

Malabsorption

Peter H R Green and Moshe Rubin

KEY POINTS

1. Capsule endoscopy has a role in the diagnosis of celiac disease and in the evaluation of patients with symptoms despite a gluten-free diet.

2. Mucosal diseases will be discovered incidentally during capsule endoscopy.

3. Persons performing capsule endoscopy need to be aware of the variety of abnormalities that occur in small intestinal mucosal diseases.

Introduction

The role of capsule endoscopy in evaluation of diseases of the small intestine that can cause malabsorption has received little attention. In this chapter on malabsorption, we will focus on celiac disease, which is common, even in developing countries. We will also discuss other small intestinal mucosal diseases that may cause symptoms attributed to malabsorption of nutrients.

Celiac disease

Celiac disease is a gluten sensitive enteropathy that occurs in genetically predisposed individuals.[1] Those with celiac disease develop an immunological reaction to gluten, the main storage protein of wheat, and similar proteins in rye and barley.[2] Gliadin is the most studied component of gluten. Recently, the mechanism of the immunological response has been further explained by the recognition of a toxic fragment of gliadin, a 33 amino acid component (33 mer) that is resistant to digestion.[3] The immune reaction in the lamina propria is triggered when this 33 mer is deamidated by tissue transglutaminase and binds to either DQ2 or DQ8 molecules on antigen presenting cells. An inflammatory process is then initiated by gliadin restricted CD4+ T-cells that results in villous atrophy.[1]

Villous atrophy and intraepithelial lymphocytosis are the histologic hallmarks of the disease.[4] The intraepithelial lymphocytosis is, however, considered to be the result of different mechanisms, involving the innate immune system.[5]

While celiac disease was formerly considered to be a pediatric malabsorption syndrome, it is now recognized primarily as an adult disease[6] that more closely resembles a multisystem disorder.[7] The clinical presentation among adults has changed from a diarrhea predominant disorder to presentations that can involve any organ system.[8] Patients may be overweight or even obese at presentation.[6] Patients frequently present with dyspeptic symptoms or esophageal reflux,[8-10] irritable bowel syndrome,[11] iron deficiency, or neurological disorders.[12]

While the diagnosis is usually straightforward, it may be difficult in some. The gold standard of diagnosis is the duodenal biopsy. People come to biopsy either because of symptoms, positive serologic tests or the recognition of mucosal abnormalities at endoscopy. The serologic tests include antigliadin, endomysial, and tissue transglutaminase antibodies. The recent National Institutes of Health (NIH) consensus development conference on celiac disease recommended that tissue transglutaminase or endomysial antibodies (EMA) should serve as the serologic tests used in the diagnosis of celiac disease. The low specificity of the antigliadin antibodies reduces their usefulness.[13,14]

Celiac disease is estimated to occur in about 1% of the population.[13] It occurs on every continent and is increasingly recognized in developing countries.[15] The disease is considered to be markedly under-diagnosed, at least in the United States. As an example of the high rate of under-diagnosis, it appears that duodenal biopsy is performed infrequently at upper gastrointestinal endoscopy, even when clinically indicated. Analysis of the Clinical Outcomes Research Initiative (CORI) database, maintained by the American Society for Gastrointestinal Endoscopy (ASGE), revealed that duodenal biopsy was performed in only 7% of cases when iron deficiency was the indication for esophagogastroduodenoscopy (EGD), 6% for weight loss, and 19% for those with diarrhea.[16] Biopsy of the duodenum to diagnose or exclude the presence of celiac disease would be appropriate in all these settings.

Endoscopic findings in celiac disease

Characteristic endoscopic findings have been described in the duodenum in patients with celiac disease. These are described on visualization of the inflated descending duodenum and include reduced duodenal folds,[17] scalloping of folds,[18] mucosal fissures, crevices or grooves,[19,20] mosaic pattern, and visible submucosal vessels.[21]

Several studies reveal the sensitivity of these signs in the detection of celiac disease to range from 50% to 94%.[22–25] Reduced folds was the most sensitive sign in two studies[22,25] and scalloping or mosaic pattern in one.[23] The greatest number of studies are toward the lower value, closer to 50%, mainly due to their absence when lesser degrees of villous atrophy are present.[20,23,24,26]

These endoscopic signs, however, have high specificity for celiac disease, 95–100%.[24,25] They are encountered in other disease processes, though rarely. Case reports and case series have documented several other causes of these mucosal abnormalities (mainly scalloping) including tropical sprue,[27,28] giardiasis, eosinophilic enteritis, and HIV related diseases,[27] Crohn's disease,[29] and amyloidosis.[30]

Generally, the terminology developed at endoscopy has also been applied to the findings at capsule endoscopy, though there has been no systematic review of the applicability of this terminology to the abnormalities seen at capsule endoscopy in patients with celiac disease. The mucosa in celiac disease at capsule endoscopy may appear scalloped (Figure 17.1). The mosaic appearance of the mucosa is also apparent (Figure 17.2). The capsule also provides a magnified view of the mucosa, allowing visualization of villi; in celiac disease the mucosa may be atrophic and villi not seen (Figure 17.3). Capsule endoscopy is, however, different to regular endoscopy, for the bowel is not distended. Capsule endoscopy is a more physiological endoscopy. We have identified a previously undescribed sign in people with celiac disease, that of layering or stacking of folds (Figure 17.4).

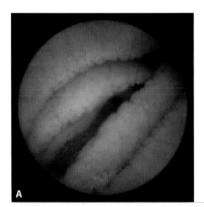
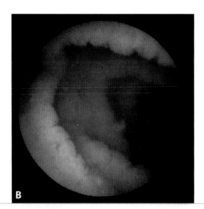
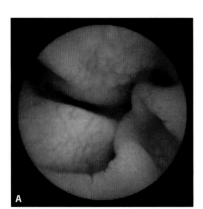

FIGURE 17.1 Scalloping of mucosal folds.

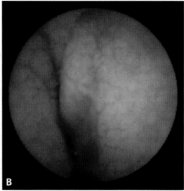

FIGURE 17.2 Mosaic appearance to the mucosa.

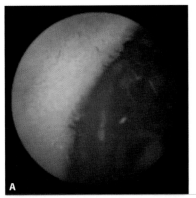
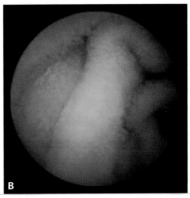
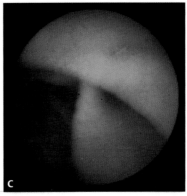

FIGURE 17.3 (a) Normal villi. (b) Patchy areas of villous atrophy. (c) Absent villi; an erosion is visualized as well.

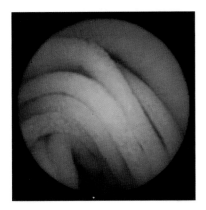

FIGURE 17.4 Layering of folds.

Role of capsule endoscopy in celiac disease

There are limited published studies that include case reports and case series on the role of capsule endoscopy in patients with celiac disease. In addition a consensus paper on the role of capsule endoscopy in celiac disease was presented recently at the 3rd International Conference on Capsule Endoscopy, 2005.[31]

The areas that need to be addressed include the role of capsule endoscopy in the diagnosis of celiac disease, in the assessment of new or persistent symptoms in those who already have the diagnosis of celiac disease, and in surveillance for malignancy.

Role of capsule endoscopy in the diagnosis of celiac disease.

Due to the specificity of the visual endoscopic markers of celiac disease, capsule endoscopy may replace EGD and biopsy in selected patients with positive endomysial or tissue transglutaminase IgA antibodies who were unwilling or unable to undergo EGD. Only those with more severe degrees of villous atrophy will be detected by this technique, because lesser degrees of villous atrophy may not be detected. The patients with partial villous atrophy frequently have a normal upper endoscopy[23] and may well have a normal capsule endoscopy, though this has not been studied.

The high specificity of the mucosal abnormalities in patients with celiac disease was confirmed by Petroniene

et al in 10 patients with celiac disease evaluated by capsule endoscopy. The sensitivity and specificity for recognizing villous atrophy was 70% and 100% respectively.[32]

Recognition of the mucosal changes of celiac disease as an incidental finding at endoscopy in patients undergoing endoscopy for a variety of conditions including abdominal pain, dyspepsia, and gastroesophageal reflux has become a major mode of diagnosis of patients with celiac disease.[8,33] There is no doubt that the diagnosis of celiac disease will be established in some patients who undergo capsule endoscopy for a variety of symptoms and in whom it was not considered prior to the procedure. This was demonstrated in a case report of a patient who underwent capsule endoscopy to evaluate gastrointestinal bleeding.[34]

Role of capsule endoscopy in patients with complicated celiac disease

There are data supporting the role of capsule endoscopy in patients with complicated celiac disease. These include single case reports of patients with celiac disease in whom capsule endoscopy demonstrated intussusception, ulcerative ileo-jejunitis, and enteropathy-associated lymphoma.[35–37] In addition, we have studied 47 patients with known celiac disease who had already undergone a large series of investigations to evaluate abdominal pain, bleeding, refractory iron deficiency, or previous small intestinal cancer or adenomas. In this cohort of patients with complicated celiac disease, unexpected findings detected at capsule endoscopy included jejunal or ileal ulceration in 45% (n = 21) (Figure 17.5), cancer (1) (Figure 17.6), polyps (1), stricture (1), submucosal mass (1), ulcerated nodular mucosa suspicious for lymphoma (2), and intussusception (1).[38]

In view of the concern for the development of complications of long-standing celiac disease such as lymphoma,[39,40] ulcerative jejunitis,[41] and adenocarcinoma,[42] those patients who develop "alarm" symptoms while on a gluten-free diet often undergo extensive radiological and even surgical evaluation. We consider that capsule endoscopy should be performed early when symptoms such as pain, fever, weight loss or evidence of bleeding occur in patients who are adherent to a gluten-free diet. One problem is that the lesions identified at capsule endoscopy beyond the range of conventional endoscopy may need to be biopsied. The

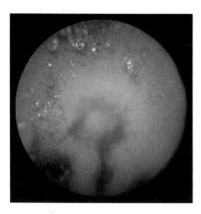

FIGURE 17.5 Jejunal ulceration in a patient with celiac disease and abdominal pain.

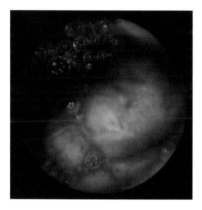

FIGURE 17.6 Jejunal adenocarcinoma not visualized by enteroclysis in a patient with celiac disease and who has occult blood in his stool.

recent availability of double balloon enteroscopy, which allows biopsy of lesions in the more distal small bowel, will help address this problem.[43]

Role of capsule endoscopy in surveillance for malignancy

Celiac disease is associated with an increased risk of intestinal lymphoma,[44,45] typically of a T-cell type,[40,46] as well as small intestinal adenocarcinoma that probably arises from adenomas.[42,47,48] The risk of malignancy is reduced by adherence to a gluten-free diet.[49] In addition, recent population-based studies have demonstrated that the risk of malignancy may not be as great as previously considered in studies based on patients attending hospital clinics or centers.[50–53]

It is unclear who should undergo surveillance capsule endoscopy. We would suggest that candidates include elderly patients recently diagnosed with celiac disease. In addition, those diagnosed in childhood who are re-diagnosed as adults may be at increased risk of adenocarcinoma.[42]

Conclusion

Celiac disease is common and frequently not considered as part of the differential diagnosis of a variety of different symptoms. It is therefore imperative that physicians performing capsule endoscopy, and those charged with reviewing the images, be aware of the variety of appearances of the mucosa in those with celiac disease. In addition, studies are

needed to determine the role of capsule endoscopy in the diagnosis and management of those with celiac disease.

Other causes of malabsorption

Malabsorption of nutrients can arise from intraluminal causes of maldigestion, diseases of the mucosa, and problems with lymphatic obstruction. The role of capsule endoscopy in patients with malabsorption syndromes other than celiac has not been systematically addressed. However, it is clear that some patients will be encountered who have malabsorption and are undergoing capsule endoscopy. Overall it appears that capsule endoscopy has a low yield in the evaluation of patients with chronic diarrhea.[54]

Of the intraluminal causes of malabsorption, patients with strictures may present with bacterial overgrowth. While there have been no studies addressing bacterial overgrowth, strictures may well be found at capsule endoscopy as an unexpected finding.[55] In addition parasites may be recognized, especially in tropical countries.[56,57]

Small bowel mucosal disease can result from infection, inflammatory conditions, and infiltrative diseases. Opportunistic infections in HIV disease can cause characteristic changes in the mucosa recognized at endoscopy[58] and may be recognized at capsule endoscopy.[59]

Tropical sprue is a presumed infectious disease that occurs primarily in people who live in or visit endemic areas, including the Caribbean, South and Southeast Asia. Mucosal damage including villous atrophy, villous blunting, crypt hyperplasia, and inflammation occurs to a variable degree resulting in malabsorption. Endoscopically the mucosa can resemble that seen in celiac disease.[27] The use of capsule endoscopy in this disease remains to be studied.

Tuberculosis of the small intestine may be encountered at capsule endoscopy, especially in developing countries.[60]

Whipple's disease, caused by *Tropheryma whippelii*, is a rare, multisystem infectious disease that may affect the small bowel. Symptoms include pain, bleeding, diarrhea, weight loss, and weakness. Fritscher-Ravens et al reported a patient with Whipple's disease who had diffuse mucosal involvement throughout the small intestine with focal jejunal bleeding.[61] Gay et al studied a patient with Whipple's disease before and after treatment with antibiotics.[62] They reported

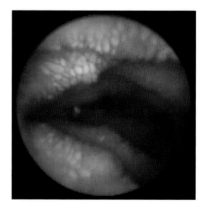

FIGURE 17.7 Intestinal lymphangiectasia.

finding delayed transit and diffusely edematous, ulcerated, and friable mucosa in both the jejunum and ileum. These abnormalities all resolved after treatment.

Intestinal lymphangiectasia will be recognized in patients with obstructed mesenteric lymphatics or those undergoing capsule endoscopy with protein-losing enteropathy. There are case reports, in abstract form, of intestinal lymphangiectasia recognized at capsule endoscopy.[63,64] In our experience it is very useful to give these patients a fatty meal the night before the capsule study (Figure 17.7).

Conclusions

Capsule endoscopy lends itself to the evaluation of the variety of diseases that can cause malabsorption. Of these, celiac disease is the most important because it is common, occurs worldwide, and may be difficult to diagnose or result in complications including ulceration, intussusception, and malignancy. Other causes of malabsorption are uncommon but may be encountered by those performing capsule endoscopy. However, we will discover much about the small intestine as we begin to identify and map the various abnormalities of the small intestine with this new tool.

References

1. Alaedini A, Green PH. Narrative review: celiac disease: understanding a complex autoimmune disorder. Ann Intern Med 2005;142:289–98.

2. Green PH, Jabri B. Coeliac disease. Lancet 2003;362:383–91.

3. Shan L, Molberg O, Parrot I, et al. Structural basis for gluten intolerance in celiac sprue. Science 2002;297:2275–9.

4. Marsh MN. Gluten, major histocompatibility complex, and the small intestine. A molecular and immunobiologic approach to the spectrum of gluten sensitivity ('celiac sprue'). Gastroenterology 1992;102:330–54.

5. Meresse B, Chen Z, Ciszewski C, et al. Coordinated induction by IL15 of a TCR-independent NKG2D signaling pathway converts CTL into lymphokine-activated killer cells in celiac disease. Immunity 2004;21:357–66.

6. Murray JA, Van Dyke C, Plevak MF, Dierkhising RA, Zinsmeister AR, Melton LJ 3rd. Trends in the identification and clinical features of celiac disease in a North American community, 1950–2001. Clin Gastroenterol Hepatol 2003;1:19–27.

7. Green PH. The many faces of celiac disease: Clinical presentation of celiac disease in the adult population. Gastroenterology 2005;128:S74–8.

8. Lo W, Sano K, Lebwohl B, Diamond B, Green PH. Changing presentation of adult celiac disease. Dig Dis Sci 2003;48:395–8.

9. Iovino P, Ciacci C, Sabbatini F, Acioli DM, D'Argenio G, Mazzacca G. Esophageal impairment in adult celiac disease with steatorrhea. Am J Gastroenterol 1998;93:1243–9.

10. Cuomo A, Romano M, Rocco A, Budillon G, Del Vecchio Blanco C, Nardone G. Reflux oesophagitis in adult coeliac disease: beneficial effect of a gluten free diet. Gut 2003; 52:514–7.

11. Sanders DS, Carter MJ, Hurlstone DP, Pearce A, Ward AM, McAlindon ME, Lobo AJ. Association of adult coeliac disease with irritable bowel syndrome: a case-control study in patients fulfilling ROME II criteria referred to secondary care. Lancet 2001;358:1504–8.

12. Chin RL, Sander HW, Brannagan TH, Green PH, Hays AP, Alaedini A, Latov N. Celiac neuropathy. Neurology 2003; 60:1581–5.

13. Statement. NIH Consensus Development Conference on Celiac Disease http://www.consensus.nih.gov/cons/118/ 118cdc_intro.htm. Bethesda, Washington, DC, 2004.

14. Rostom A, Dube C, Cranney A, et al. The diagnostic accuracy of serologic tests for celiac disease: A systematic review. Gastroenterology 2005;128:S38–46.

15. Malekzadeh R, Sachdev A, Fahid Ali A. Coeliac disease in developing countries: Middle East, India and North Africa. Best Pract Res Clin Gastroenterol 2005;19:351–8.

16. Harewood GC, Holub JL, Lieberman DA. Variation in small bowel biopsy performance among diverse endoscopy settings: results from a national endoscopic database. Am J Gastroenterol 2004;99:1790–4.

17. Brocchi E, Corazza GR, Caletti G, Treggiari EA, Barbara L, Gasbarrini G. Endoscopic demonstration of loss of duodenal folds in the diagnosis of celiac disease. N Engl J Med 1988;319:741–4.

18. Jabbari M, Wild G, Goresky CA, Daly DS, Lough JO, Cleland DP, Kinnear DG. Scalloped valvulae conniventes: an endoscopic marker of celiac sprue. Gastroenterology 1988;95:1518–22.

19. Siegel LM, Stevens PD, Lightdale CJ, Green PH, Goodman S, Garcia-Carrasquillo RJ, Rotterdam H. Combined magnification endoscopy with chromoendoscopy in the evaluation of patients with suspected malabsorption. Gastrointest Endosc 1997;46:226–30.

20. Smith AD, Graham I, Rose JD. A prospective endoscopic study of scalloped folds and grooves in the mucosa of the duodenum as signs of villous atrophy. Gastrointest Endosc 1998;47:461–5.

21. Niveloni S, Fiorini A, Dezi R, et al. Usefulness of videoduodenoscopy and vital dye staining as indicators of mucosal atrophy of celiac disease: assessment of interobserver agreement. Gastrointest Endosc 1998; 47:223–9.

22. Maurino E, Bai JC. Endoscopic markers of celiac disease. Am J Gastroenterol 2002;97:760–1.

23. Dickey W, Hughes D. Disappointing sensitivity of endoscopic markers for villous atrophy in a high-risk population: implications for celiac disease diagnosis during routine endoscopy. Am J Gastroenterol 2001;96:2126–8.

24. Bardella MT, Minoli G, Radaelli F, Quatrini M, Bianchi PA, Conte D. Reevaluation of duodenal endoscopic markers in the diagnosis of celiac disease. Gastrointest Endosc 2000;51:714–6.

25. Oxentenko AS, Grisolano SW, Murray JA, Burgart LJ, Dierkhising RA, Alexander JA. The insensitivity of endoscopic markers in celiac disease. Am J Gastroenterol 2002;97:933–8.

26. Tursi A, Brandimarte G, Giorgetti GM, Gigliobianco A. Endoscopic features of celiac disease in adults and their correlation with age, histological damage, and clinical form of the disease. Endoscopy 2002;34:787–92.

27. Shah VH, Rotterdam H, Kotler DP, Fasano A, Green PH. All that scallops is not celiac disease. Gastrointest Endosc 2000;51:717–20.

28. Tawil SC, Brandt LJ, Bernstein LH. Scalloping of the valvulae conniventes and mosaic mucosa in tropical sprue. Gastrointest Endosc 1991;37:365–6.

29. Culliford A, Markowitz D, Rotterdam H, Green PH. Scalloping of duodenal mucosa in Crohn's disease. Inflamm Bowel Dis 2004;10:270–3.

30. Michael H, Brandt LJ, Tanaka KE, Berkowitz D, Cardillo M, Weidenheim K. Congo-red negative colonic amyloid with scalloping of the valvulae conniventes. Gastrointest Endosc 2001;53:653–5.

31. Cellier C, Green, PH, Collin P, Murray J. ICCE consensus for celiac disease. Endoscopy 2005;37(10):1055–9.

32. Petroniene R, Dubcenco E, Baker JP, et al. Given capsule endoscopy in celiac disease: evaluation of diagnostic accuracy and interobserver agreement. Am J Gastroenterol 2005;100:685–94.

33. Green PH, Shane E, Rotterdam H, Forde KA, Grossbard L. Significance of unsuspected celiac disease detected at endoscopy. Gastrointest Endosc 2000;51:60–5.

34. Kimchi NA, Broide E, Zehavi S, Halevy A, Scapa E. Capsule endoscopy diagnosis of celiac disease and ileal tumors in a patient with melena of obscure origin. Isr Med Assoc J 2005;7:412–3.

35. Willingham FF, Opekun AR, Graham DY. Endoscopic demonstration of transient small bowel intussusception in a patient with adult celiac disease. Gastrointest Endosc 2003;57:626–7.

36. Apostolopoulos P, Alexandrakis G, Giannakoulopoulou E, Kalantzis C, Papanikolaou IS, Markoglou C, Kalantzis N. M2A wireless capsule endoscopy for diagnosing ulcerative jejunoileitis complicating celiac disease. Endoscopy 2004;36:247.

37. Joyce AM, Burns DL, Marcello PW, Tronic B, Scholz FJ. Capsule endoscopy findings in celiac disease associated enteropathy-type intestinal T-cell lymphoma. Endoscopy 2005;37:594–6.

38. Culliford A, Daly J, Diamond B, Rubin M, Green PH. The value of wireless capsule endoscopy in patients with complicated celiac disease. Gastrointest Endosc 2005;62:55–61.

39. Green PH, Fleischauer AT, Bhagat G, Goyal R, Jabri B, Neugut AI. Risk of malignancy in patients with celiac disease. Am J Med 2003;115:191–5.

40. Cellier C, Delabesse E, Helmer C, et al. Refractory sprue, coeliac disease, and enteropathy-associated T-cell lymphoma. French Coeliac Disease Study Group. Lancet 2000;356:203–8.

41. Green JA, Barkin JS, Gregg PA, Kohen K. Ulcerative jejunitis in refractory celiac disease: enteroscopic visualization. Gastrointest Endosc 1993;39:584–5.

42. Rampertab SD, Forde KA, Green PH. Small bowel neoplasia in coeliac disease. Gut 2003;52:1211–4.

43. Yamamoto H, Kita H, Sunada K, et al. Clinical outcomes of double-balloon endoscopy for the diagnosis and treatment of small-intestinal diseases. Clin Gastroenterol Hepatol 2004;2:1010–6.

44. Selby WS, Gallagher ND. Malignancy in a 19-year experience of adult celiac disease. Dig Dis Sci 1979;24:684–8.

45. Awrich AE, Irish CE, Vetto RM, Fletcher WS. A twenty-five year experience with primary malignant tumors of the small intestine. Surg Gynecol Obstet 1980;151:9–14.

46. Spencer J, MacDonald TT, Diss TC, Walker-Smith JA, Ciclitira PJ, Isaacson PG. Changes in intraepithelial lymphocyte subpopulations in coeliac disease and enteropathy associated T cell lymphoma (malignant histiocytosis of the intestine). Gut 1989;30:339–46.

47. Holmes GK, Dunn GI, Cockel R, Brookes VS. Adenocarcinoma of the upper small bowel complicating coeliac disease. Gut 1980;21:1010–6.

48. Nielsen SN, Wold LE. Adenocarcinoma of jejunum in association with nontropical sprue. Arch Pathol Lab Med 1986;110:822–4.

49. Holmes GK, Prior P, Lane MR, Pope D, Allan RN. Malignancy in coeliac disease — effect of a gluten free diet. Gut 1989;30:333–8.

50. Card TR, West J, Holmes GK. Risk of malignancy in diagnosed coeliac disease: a 24-year prospective, population-based, cohort study. Aliment Pharmacol Ther 2004;20:769–75.

51. West J, Logan RF, Smith CJ, Hubbard RB, Card TR. Malignancy and mortality in people with coeliac disease: population based cohort study. BMJ 2004;329:716–9.

52. Catassi C, Bearzi I, Holmes GK. Association of celiac disease and intestinal lymphomas and other cancers. Gastroenterology 2005;128:S79–86.

53. Farre C, Domingo-Domenech E, Font R, et al. Celiac disease and lymphoma risk: a multicentric case-control study in Spain. Dig Dis Sci 2004;49:408–12.

54. Kalantzis N, Papanikolaou IS, Giannakoulopoulou E, et al. Capsule endoscopy; the cumulative experience from its use in 193 patients with suspected small bowel disease. Hepatogastroenterology 2005;52:414–9.

55. Romero Vazquez J, Caunedo Alvarez A, Rodriguez-Tellez M, Sanchez Yague A, Pellicer Bautista F, Herrerias Gutierrez JM. [Previously unknown stricture due to radiation therapy diagnosed by capsule endoscopy.]. Rev Esp Enferm Dig 2005;97:449–54.

56. Sriram PV, Rao GV, Reddy DN. Wireless capsule endoscopy: experience in a tropical country. J Gastroenterol Hepatol 2004;19:63–7.

57. Soares J, Lopes L, Villas-Boas G, Pinho C. Ascariasis observed by wireless-capsule endoscopy. Endoscopy 2003;35:194.

58. Poorman JC, Katon RM. Small bowel involvement by Mycobacterium avium complex in a patient with AIDS: endoscopic, histologic, and radiographic similarities to Whipple's disease. Gastrointest Endosc 1994;40:753–9.

59. Cello JP. Capsule endoscopy features of human immunodeficiency virus and geographical diseases. Gastrointest Endosc Clin N Am 2004;14:169–77.

60. Reddy DN, Sriram PV, Rao GV, Reddy DB. Capsule endoscopy appearances of small-bowel tuberculosis. Endoscopy 2003;35:99.

61. Fritscher-Ravens A, Swain CP, von Herbay A. Refractory Whipple's disease with anaemia: first lessons from capsule endoscopy. Endoscopy 2004;36:659–62.

62. Gay G, Roche JF, Delvaux M. Capsule endoscopy, transit times, and Whipple's disease. Endoscopy 2005;37:272–3.

63. Tatar EL, Siddiqui H, Shen EH, Pitchumoni C. Lymphangiectasias found on Pillcam, are they clinically significant? In: International Conference on Capsule Endoscopy, Florida, 2005.

64. Peretti N, Sant'Anna1 AMGA, Dirks MH, Seidman EG. Capsule endoscopy detects lymphangiectasia missed by other means. In: International Conference on Capsule Endoscopy, Florida, 2005.

CHAPTER **18**

Small Bowel Transplantation and Graft Versus Host Disease

Roberto de Franchis • Emanuele Rondonotti • Federica Villa • Clementina Signorelli • Carla Abbiati, and Gizela Beccari

KEY POINTS

1. At the present time the post surgical management of small bowel transplantation requires aggressive immunosuppressant therapy and strict surveillance of the graft performed by repeated trans-stomal endoscopies.

2. VCE appears to be a promising tool for the surveillance of the graft over time, since it allows a painless exploration of the entire transplanted small bowel.

3. The diagnosis of intestinal GVHD is very difficult because of the lack of specific symptoms and the presence of confounding variables.

4. At present, the gold standard for the diagnosis of GVHD is simultaneous upper and lower endoscopy with mucosal biopsies, but VCE has been found to be more sensitive and better tolerated than traditional endoscopy.

Capsule endoscopy in small bowel transplantation

Introduction

The general term "intestinal/multivisceral transplantation" refers to a heterogeneous group of transplants involving the whole small bowel (jejunum plus ileum), transplanted "en bloc," simultaneously with or without one or more segments of the upper or lower gastrointestinal tract. This may include a "visceral component" such as stomach, duodenum, or colon with or without one or more solid abdominal organs such as liver, pancreas, and sometimes kidney/s.[1]

Experimental animal models for small bowel transplantation were initiated 20–30 years ago.[2,3] The initial clinical experience yielded high morbidity and mortality rates because of the frequency of technical, immunological, and infectious complications.[4–6] It is only since the advent of more refined harvesting, preservation procedures, improved surgical techniques, more effective immunosuppression, and more sophisticated intra- and postoperative monitoring and treatment protocols that intestinal and multivisceral transplantation has become a clinical reality. However, the optimal management of small bowel transplantation remains controversial.[1]

In 2002 the U.S. Health Care Financing Administration considered intestinal, liver–intestinal, and multivisceral transplantation as the standard of care for patients with irreversible failure of the intestine and failed total parenteral nutrition.[7]

According to the International Intestinal Transplantation Registry,[8] between April 1985 and 31 May 2003, 61 transplantation centers worldwide performed 989 small bowel transplantations in 923 patients of which 433 were small bowel alone, 386 were combined small bowel and liver, and 170 were multiorgan.

Indications for small bowel–multivisceral transplantation

Small bowel transplantation is performed in patients with irreversible intestinal failure. The diagnosis of irreversible intestinal failure should be made only after optimal utilization of the currently available medical and surgical therapeutic modalities to enhance gut adaptation.[9] At the present time, irreversibility of this condition is an essential prerequisite for transplantation. Intestinal failure is most commonly due to congenital or post-surgical short gut syndrome as a consequence of intestinal atresia, midgut volvulus, gastroschisis, abdominal trauma, necrotizing enterocolitis, Crohn's disease, mesenteric vascular thrombosis, and/or surgical adhesions. Children represent almost 50% of small bowel recipients for short bowel syndrome. The major cause of death in children requiring parenteral nutrition for short bowel syndrome is hepatic failure due to cholestasis and recurrent sepsis.[10]

Other indications include motility disorders such as hollow visceral myopathy and/or neuropathy (total intestinal aganglionosis), small bowel neoplasms (mesenteric desmoid tumor, diffuse gastrointestinal polyposis, Gardner's syndrome, and other large benign unresectable masses), microvillous inclusion disease, selective autoimmune enteropathy, and radiation enteritis (Table 18.1).[6,9,11,12]

For patients with intestinal failure, total parenteral nutrition is the mainstay of medical therapy, showing 1- and 4-year survival rates of 94% and 80% respectively.[13,14] Patients are considered as candidates for small bowel transplantation when they can no longer be supported by total parenteral nutrition because of complications of their disease or of total parenteral nutrition. The latter include impending liver failure, loss of central venous access, multiple line infections, and frequent episodes of severe dehydration despite intravenous fluid replacement.[9]

Some patients develop total parenteral nutrition associated liver disease. The pathogenesis is not fully understood. It may be reversible in the early phase, but may progress to irreversible cirrhosis and liver failure.[15] Irreversibility of liver disease is likely when signs of portal hypertension develop, there is reduced liver synthetic function, or severe bridging fibrosis–cirrhosis is present on liver histology.[11]

The loss of venous access is a frequent indication for small bowel transplantation. These patients should be referred for surgery before exhausting all reliable venous access, because good venous access is needed for several months after transplantation in order to administer fluids, immunosuppression, and antibiotics.

Factors such as the presence of an indwelling catheter, translocation of enteral organisms, and loss of gut-associated lymphoid tissue (GALT) are considered responsible for recurrent infective episodes seen in patients with intestinal failure. If these are mild, patients are not candidates for intestinal transplantation. However, patients with severe complications such as brain abscess, infective endocarditis, and multiorgan failure should be considered for transplantation. Similarly, patients with multidrug-resistant organisms (i.e. vancomycin-resistant *Enterococcus faecium*) that colonize their mucocutaneous surfaces should be evaluated for small bowel transplantation.[11]

Patients with complications of total parenteral nutrition are often terminally ill and these complications have contributed to the poor survival rate after these procedures. As experience increases and results improve, patients are now being considered for transplantation earlier in the course of the disease.[6]

For each patient selected for small bowel transplantation, the cause of intestinal failure and extent of the primary disease determine the algorithm of the evaluation process. The functional status of the native liver, as assessed from the results of biochemistry, imaging studies, and histology,[9] is the critical determinant of the type of intestinal graft needed.

Post-surgical management: immunosuppressive therapies and possible complications

Clinical and experimental evidence clearly demonstrates high immunogenicity of the intestinal graft[16,17]; the large amount of lymphatic tissue and the expression of Class II major histocompatibility antigens (MHC) on the gut surface make the small bowel highly vulnerable to rejection and serve as a source for aggressive, and often lethal, graft versus host reactions.

Much remains to be learned about the immunology of intestinal allograft rejection but experimental models suggest that rejection is caused by IL2 and IFN-γ secretion, by Th1 lymphocyte activity and by activated Th2 lymphocytes that secrete IL4, IL10, and IL13; the interrelationship between these lymphocyte populations will determine whether or not the graft is rejected or tolerated.[18]

In the early 1990s, small bowel transplantation became a clinical reality owing to substantial progress in harvesting and preservation procedures, surgical techniques, and the development of new immunosuppressant drugs, particularly tacrolimus, which replaced cyclosporine. This latter change yielded a marked increase in 1-year graft survival (from 17% to 65%).[6,12] The addition of mycophenolate mofetil, which inhibits lymphocyte proliferation,[19] and the addition of bone marrow from the donor to induce tolerance to the graft and to permit drug-free graft acceptance over the long term, may improve results still further.[20] On the basis of this evidence, the most commonly used immunomodulatory regimen now consists of a combination of tacrolimus, mycophenolate mofetil, and steroids.

Acute rejection is treated with high doses of steroids and an increased dose of tacrolimus. Statistically, most cases

Table 18.1 Specific indications for small bowel transplantation: the Cumulative World Experience (CWE)[12]

Indication	Number of patients (%)

Short bowel syndrome
    Crohn's disease
    Mesenteric artery thrombosis
    Necrotizing enterocolitis
    Intussusception
	114 (62%)

Malabsorption syndrome
    Gastric ectasia
    Intestinal atresia
	23 (12%)

Motility disorder
    Intestinal pseudo-obstruction
    Hirschsprung's disease
	15 (8%)

Neoplastic disease
    Endocrine tumors
    Familial polyposis coli
    Desmoid tumors
	23 (12%)

Primary and secondary transplant failure	10 (6%)
Total	185 (100%)

of acute intestinal allograft rejection occur within the first 3 months of transplantation. Nonetheless, severe acute rejection resulting in allograft loss can occur 1 year or more after transplantation.[21] Most rejection episodes are mild and do not progress to graft loss. However, when there is no response to therapy, monoclonal antibodies to lymphocytes are given.

Despite the introduction of these drugs, the incidence of acute allograft rejection remains high and is the reason for graft removal in 56% of recipients worldwide.[8] Thus interest in alternative/supplemental therapeutic agents (monoclonal antibodies, azathioprine, sirolimus, cyclophosphamide) and new strategies (transplant of bone marrow with new preconditioning regimens) continues.

The immunosuppression regimens needed to avoid allograft rejection or graft versus host reaction often induce severe adverse events: tacrolimus may cause headache, tremor, numbness around the mouth, diarrhea, hyperkalemia, hyperglycemia, and renal failure; mycophenolate mofetil often induces gastritis, diarrhea, and, in high dosages, bone marrow suppression, but the most common, and potentially lethal, are opportunistic infections. Thus specific post-surgical management protocols for the treatment and prophylaxis of infection, similar to those used for solid organ recipients, have been developed. In addition, selective gut decontamination is used for 1–2 weeks postoperatively and during moderate to severe rejection episodes. Chronic viral and protozoal prophylaxis with ganciclovir for cytomegalovirus and Epstein–Barr virus and trimethoprim plus sulfamethoxazole for *Pneumocystis carinii* are routine. The realization of the importance of infectious complications in rejection, previously demonstrated with liver transplantation, is even more applicable with the intestine, because a disrupted mucosal barrier quickly creates a lethal environment. The paradoxical therapeutic philosophy of treating infection-relatable rejection with prompt increase in immunosuppression, in addition to systemic and local antibiotic therapy, is of the utmost importance in preventing or stopping bacterial translocation among intestinal transplant recipients.[9,22]

Nevertheless, despite developments in immunosuppression and prophylaxis protocols, opportunistic infections and graft rejection remain the main complications of small bowel transplantation, and early diagnosis of postoperative complications, although sometimes difficult to achieve, is a major determinant of successful small bowel transplantation (Table 18.2).[12] Postoperative monitoring is aimed at detecting the onset of post-transplant complications as early as possible, as well as at assessing the intestinal graft's anatomic and functional integrity.

Monitoring of graft conditions and complications

Invasive methods

At the present time, endoscopy of the transplanted graft is an essential tool in the postoperative assessment of intestinal transplant recipients, because clinical signs and symptoms of intestinal graft rejection are nonspecific.[23–26] In general, trans-stomal surveillance enteroscopies are

Table 18.2 Complications of small bowel transplantation[12]

Complication	No of patients (%)
Sepsis	34 (40%)
Multiorgan failure	24 (28%)
Graft thrombosis	3 (4%)
Neurological problems	1 (1%)
Rejection	4 (5%)
Bleeding	4 (5%)
Lymphoma	9 (11%)
Other/unknown	5 (6%)
Total	84 (100%)

performed twice a week for the first month after small bowel transplantation, once a week for the next 2 months, monthly for the next 3 months, and every 3–6 months thereafter. Typical endoscopic features of acute graft rejection include edema, erythema, friability, erosions, and granularity of the mucosa.[23] These findings are often patchy or segmental, and in about one third of patients with graft rejection the mucosa, visualized by trans-stomal enteroscopy, is normal.[1,23] Biopsies are routinely taken during trans-stomal enteroscopy for pathologic examination and detection of common infectious agents. Early histological features of acute rejection include shortened and blunted villi, lymphocytic infiltrates in the lamina propria, cryptitis and crypt apoptosis, exfoliation of the mucosal surface, and ulcerations.[11,27]

Recently, the use of zoom video-endoscopes was proposed to provide a more accurate evaluation of the mucosal lining. Examination of the villous micro-texture on zoom video-endoscopy provides assessment of height, blunting, and erythema of the villi similar to the microscopic examination of the endoscopic biopsy.[28,29] However, because endoscopy only allows partial exploration of the transplanted graft and causes discomfort in these frail patients, novel noninvasive markers and endoscopic methodologies have been studied.

Noninvasive methods

Serum intestinal fatty acid binding protein is an enterocyte-specific protein that is detectable in serum after intestinal injury, but it has not been found to be useful in clinical intestinal allograft rejection.[30] A relationship between serum citrulline levels and intestinal function has been reported in patients with short gut syndrome. This observation can be extended to the phenomenon of rejection in small bowel allograft.[11,31]

In 2001, a video capsule was developed (Given Imaging, Yoqneam, Israel) that allowed a complete and minimally invasive examination of the small bowel. The device has been proven to be safe and well tolerated. It takes two images per second at a 1:8 magnification, which allows visualization of the individual villi in the normal small bowel (Figure 18.1).

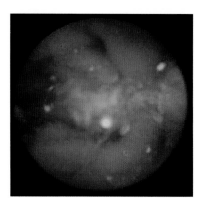

FIGURE 18.1 Capsule enteroscopy: normal terminal ileum.

Role of capsule enteroscopy in monitoring graft conditions

There are only two reports on the monitoring of small bowel transplanted patients using video capsule endoscopy (VCE).[32,33] In the first case report, the patient underwent transplantation for post-surgical short bowel due to a superior mesenteric artery embolus.[32] Biopsies of the upper jejunum showed no signs of rejection. To visualize the entire graft, a video capsule endoscopy was performed 9 weeks after transplantation. The dominant finding was blunting of villi in the middle part of the jejunum. The ileum appeared nearly normal morphologically, except for slight hyperemia in the middle portion and dilated lymphatic vessels in the distal portion. There was no overt evidence of rejection. The authors concluded that the use of capsule endoscopy facilitated the noninvasive visualization of bowel segments that could not be reached endoscopically.

In the second report,[33] capsule endoscopy was used to evaluate patients at different time intervals after transplantation, and capsule endoscopy findings were compared with those obtained from trans-stomal traditional endoscopy. Four patients received isolated small bowel transplants and one received a multivisceral transplant.[1] In all patients, the transplanted small bowel was connected proximally to the stomach with an end-to-side anastomosis and distally to the rectum with an ileo-rectal anastomosis. All patients had a protective ileostomy and were on immunosuppressive, antibiotic, and antimycotic drugs. After transplantation, all patients underwent repeated trans-stomal retrograde ileoscopy with biopsy, using a magnifying endoscope. Capsule endoscopy was performed at 20 days

up to 6 months after transplantation, 0–13 days after the previous ileoscopy. During ileoscopy all patients complained of bloating and some discomfort. The capsule was swallowed easily and passed naturally in all patients without adverse events. In one patient the capsule remained in the stomach throughout the recording time; this was probably due to a lack of motor coordination between the stomach and the jejunal graft. In the others good quality images of the small bowel were obtained. At routine trans-stomal endoscopy the appearance of the ileal mucosa was normal in all patients (Figure 18.2), both with the standard view (Figure 18.2a) and with magnification (Figure 18.2b). Ileal histology showed mild inflammatory infiltration and edema in the lamina propria in all cases. On capsule endoscopy the appearance of the mucosa in the ileal segments reached by retrograde ileoscopy was normal. However, mucosal changes were observed in more proximal segments in 3 of the 4 patients in whom capsule endoscopy yielded small bowel images. These changes included diffusely blunted, ridge-shaped or convoluted villi and isolated hyperemic spots in a patient examined 20 days after transplantation (Figures 18.3, 18.4), small areas with blunted villi and isolated petechiae (Figure 18.5) in a patient examined at 6 weeks, and diffuse blunted edematous villi with isolated small erosions in a patient examined at 2 months. In the fourth patient, studied 6 months after small bowel transplantation, normal well-shaped long villi were observed. Capsule enteroscopy was better tolerated than retrograde ileoscopy in all patients. Mucosal changes were identified in 3/4 patients in proximal segments beyond the reach of retrograde ileoscopy, demonstrating a possible advantage of capsule enteroscopy, which allows the examination of the entire transplanted graft compared with conventional retrograde ileoscopy.

The significance of these mucosal changes is not yet clear. The time interval between transplantation and capsule enteroscopy varied between patients, ranging between 20 days and 6 months. It is of note that the severity of the mucosal changes was greater in the patient examined at 20 days than in those examined at 6 weeks and 2 months, while the patient examined at 6 months had a normal mucosa. This may represent the normal evolution of the graft over time.

Clearly, more research is needed to interpret the findings of capsule endoscopy in relation to conventional endoscopy and biopsy. Once this information is available, capsule

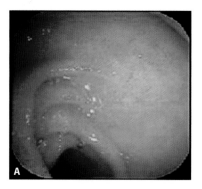

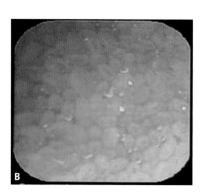

FIGURE 18.2 Retrograde trans-stomal ileoscopy: normal terminal ileum. (a) Normal view. (b) 100× magnification.

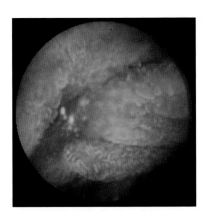

FIGURE 18.3 Capsule enteroscopy: ridge-shaped and convoluted villi in a patient examined 20 days after transplantation.

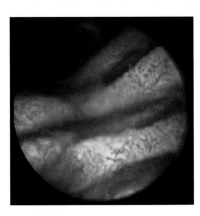

FIGURE 18.4 Capsule enteroscopy: blunted and ridge-shaped whitish villi and isolated hyperemic spot in a patient examined 20 days after transplantation.

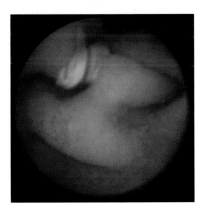

FIGURE 18.5 Capsule enteroscopy: blunted villi and isolated petechiae in a patient examined at 6 weeks after transplantation.

endoscopy could become the first step in the endoscopic monitoring of patients after small bowel transplantation since it is well tolerated and allows a complete examination of the transplanted bowel. Standard ileoscopy with biopsy could be reserved for further assessment in patients in whom mucosal lesions are identified by capsule enteroscopy and when histology is mandatory to confirm the presence and degree of rejection.

Use of capsule endoscopy in intestinal graft versus host disease

Introduction

Allogenic hematopoietic stem cell transplantation (HCT) can be used for treating a variety of hematological malignancies, solid tumors, and non-malignant stem cell disorders. However, a common complication of this treatment is graft versus host disease (GVHD); this condition is the major complication of HCT and represents the primary cause of morbidity and mortality.[34] It is calculated that approximately half of the patients who develop clinically significant GVHD die of the disease or of therapy-related complications.[35] GVHD occurs when the donor-derived T-lymphocytes recognize host cells as foreign and initiate an immune response.[36]

Human leukocyte antigen (HLA) differences between the hematopoietic stem cell donor and transplant recipient is the factor most frequently involved in the development and amplification of GVHD. In mismatched grafts, the incidence of GVHD is about 70–80%, while in patients with identical HLA typing it ranges from 40% to 60%.[34]

Several factors may be implicated in the development of graft versus host reaction; however, three conditions[37] have been identified that are necessary for GVHD to develop:

1. The graft must contain immunologically competent cells.
2. The host must possess important transplantation alloantigens that are lacking in the donor graft, so that the host appears as foreign to the graft and is, therefore, capable of stimulating it antigenically.
3. The host itself must be incapable of mounting an effective immunological reaction against the graft, at least for a time sufficient for the latter to manifest its immunological capabilities; that is, it must have the "security of tenure."

Graft versus host disease may be acute or chronic; each has a different presentation and pathogenesis. By definition, acute GVHD develops within 100 days following allogenic transplantation and involves different tissues, such as the epithelial cells of the skin, the mucosa of the gastrointestinal tract, and the bile ducts. Chronic GVHD occurs after 100 days post transplantation and the clinical manifestations of this syndrome are arthralgia, arthritis, and serositis. Additionally, a rare hyperacute form exists, occurring in the first week post transplantation, with fever, hepatitis, enteritis, erythroderma, skin desquamation, and vascular leakage.[36]

Acute GVHD: mechanisms and manifestations

The GVHD syndrome is a consequence of damage to host tissues by activated donor-derived T-lymphocytes in response to major histocompatibility antigen (MHC) disparities. The T-cells do not recognize the antigens alone, but in combination with the MHC of the antigen-presenting cells (APC), that are usually self. The mechanisms that cause acute GVHD can be divided into the three components[38]: cellular damage induced in pre-conditioning, induction and expansion of donor T-lymphocytes, and direct and indirect cytotoxicity to host cells.

In phase 1, GVHD starts during the pre-conditioning regimen, when the immunological systems are suppressed by total body irradiation or high-dose chemotherapy to prevent graft rejection. This can cause substantial damage in host tissues and induce dysregulated secretion of many cytokines such as TNF-α, IL1, IL6, granulocyte and macrophage colony stimulating factor,[36] and up-regulation of cytokines and adhesion molecules,[38] with resultant injury to the gastrointestinal tract, liver, and skin.

In phase 2, the donor-derived T-lymphocytes recognize and reach foreign host antigens presented by antigen-presenting cells in conjunction with the major histo-compatibility complex. After that, the donor T-cells clonally expand and differentiate into Th1 lymphocytes that secrete IFN-γ and IL2. The vascular endothelium is the first contact area with new alloantigens, and serves as a substrate to which donor T-cells may adhere. This allows activation of the latter, in conjunction with adhesion molecules such as E-selectin and the integrin family, ICAM-1, PECAM-1, and VCAM-1.[36]

In phase 3, host cells are injured both directly by activated T-cells and by secondary mechanisms. Th1 cells induce activation of cytotoxic T-cells that stimulate the secretion of many important cytokines. These play a fundamental role in the pathogenesis of GVHD because they activate other T-cells, allowing the expansion of NK cells and NK-like cells,[36] which cause additional tissue damage.

The clinical manifestations of acute GVHD include skin changes with a macropapular rash, extensive exanthema, bulla formation or desquamation. In the liver there may be injury to biliary canaliculi with cholestatic jaundice. In the lymph nodes there may be a reduction of germinal centers and peripheral blood counts may be reduced. Changes in the gastrointestinal tract are described below.

Chronic GVHD

Chronic GVHD (CGVHD) occurs more than 100 days after transplantation with an incidence of about 33%. It frequently occurs after acute GVHD and, for this reason, it has often been considered as a late phase of acute GVHD. It has been shown that, in the development of CGVHD, thymic atrophy with loss of epithelial thymic secretory functions and depletion of lymphocytes plays an important role in the development of alloreactivity.

The clinical manifestations of CGVHD are similar to those of acute GVHD: there are skin lesions such as erythema, rapid desquamation, and development of lichen planus, alterations of liver function, and ophthalmic symptoms such as keratoconjunctivitis sicca; gastrointestinal involvement is uncommon but dysphagia, abdominal pain, and weight loss may occur.

Intestinal GVHD: pathogenesis and manifestations

The most common manifestations of intestinal involvement during GVHD are nausea, severe secretory diarrhea with alteration of plasma electrolytes, abdominal cramps and pain, intestinal bleeding, and paralytic ileus. These manifestations are common and serious problems after stem cell transplantation. The intestinal mucosa contains many lymphocytes located in the Peyer's patches and in the lamina propria. This group of lymphocytes represents

the so-called "gut-associated lymphoid tissue" (GALT) that provides a biological defense against foreign antigens. Any alteration in this system involving tissue injury may produce an inflammatory response that leads to the secretion and activation of many cytokines, which may initiate GVHD.[38]

Several reports[39,40] have shown that the microbial environment, including the normal flora, may also influence the development of GVHD, acting as a trigger, perhaps by sharing antigenic epitopes with gut epithelial cells or by activating latent virus-inducing antigens on the cell surface.

Studies have shown that, during the pre-conditioning phase, even the bacterial endotoxin/lipopolysaccharide (LPS) of normal flora can be injurious. In this phase, the permeability of the gut is increased by chemotherapy and whole body irradiation. Endotoxins and LPS pass the intestinal barrier and reach the systemic circulation where they stimulate the production of TNF-α, IL1, and IL12 from lymphocytes, which in turn stimulate the activation of granulocytes and macrophages.

These inflammatory mediators may directly damage the mucosa. Mouse studies have suggested that TNF-α and IFN-γ can mediate injury of the intestinal epithelium. Histologically, from the stomach to the rectum, single cell necrosis, destruction of the intestinal crypts, and, in the most severe forms, complete loss of the epithelium, may occur (Figure 18.6).[41]

Intestinal GVHD: use of traditional methods for diagnosis

Endoscopy

The diagnosis of intestinal GVHD in patients with bone marrow transplantation is very difficult because of the lack of specific symptoms and the presence of confounding variables. The differential diagnosis includes gastrointestinal toxicity associated with the pre-transplant conditioning regimen, medications, and enteric infections such as cytomegalovirus or herpes simplex virus.[42,43] The current gold standard for the diagnosis of GVHD is simultaneous upper and lower endoscopy with histological examination of mucosal biopsies. The endoscopic findings vary enormously, from a normal appearance to severe inflammation with erythema, ulceration, and exudates.[42] Endoscopic findings can be graded according to a validated scale (Table 18.3).[44]

Table 18.3 Endoscopic scale for grading GVHD[44]

Endoscopic grade	Findings
0	Normal mucosa
1	Loss of vascular marking and/or mild focal erythema
2	Moderate edema and/or erythema
3	Edema, erosions, and/or bleeding
4	Ulceration, exudates, and bleeding

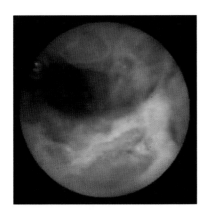

FIGURE 18.6 Capsule enteroscopy: diffuse jejunal ulceration in a patient with GVHD.

Histologic changes of GVHD (both acute and chronic) include apoptosis of the crypt epithelial cells, drop-out and disappearance of crypts, and a patchy lymphocytic infiltration.[43] The importance of mucosal biopsy is emphasized by studies showing that between 30% and 80% of recipients of allogenic transplant with gastrointestinal symptoms have histological GVHD despite minimally abnormal findings on endoscopy.[43] Although recent studies show a strong correlation between endoscopic findings and both acute and chronic GVHD,[42] the current opinion is that macroscopic findings may be useful to raise the early suspicion of gastrointestinal GVHD, but a histologic evaluation of the gastrointestinal mucosa is needed to confirm the diagnosis and to evaluate the severity of the condition.[42] The reported degree of concordance of histological findings between upper and lower endoscopy ranges from 66% to 96%. Some investigators suggest that since GVHD involves the whole gut, either upper or lower endoscopy, and even simple rectal or gastric biopsies may be sufficient for diagnosis.[43,44] However, the diagnosis, extent, and severity of GVHD are best assessed by bidirectional endoscopy and biopsy.[45]

Radiology

If the patient is critically ill, and endoscopy would be hazardous and evaluation of the small bowel involvement is important, conventional radiology such as computed tomography (CT), plain abdominal radiography or barium studies can be used.[46,47] A variety of small bowel abnormalities can be seen on barium studies in patients with GVHD. These may include edema of mucosal folds of the ileum and jejunum, effacement of folds towards the ileum, thickening of the bowel wall, intestinal pneumatosis, spasm, and stenoses with pre-stenotic dilatation or air–fluid levels.[46] The most common findings on CT are discontinuous small bowel wall thickening and engorgement of the vasa recta adjacent to the bowel segments in a high proportion of the patients.[47] Radiology can also identify the involvement of the colon and of the upper gastrointestinal tract, which may show thickening of the esophagus or loss of haustration, thumbprinting, spasm, and ulceration in the colon.[46,47] In general, endoscopy is regarded as the gold standard for the diagnosis of GVHD. Radiology should be used when

endoscopy is unsafe or as a complementary exam to define the extension and the severity of the disease.

Transabdominal ultrasonography

Transabdominal ultrasonography is a new method of evaluation of the bowel in GVHD. This is a noninvasive procedure that might be used for early diagnosis and for monitoring the response to therapy. Sonographic patterns are variable and nonspecific: the most common findings are dilatation of colon (predominantly in the ascending colon) and bowel wall thickening, most frequently in the ileocecal region.[48,49] Although the gold standard for the diagnosis of GVHD is endoscopy, transabdominal sonography might be used as a noninvasive tool to identify GVHD before the appearance of clinical symptoms and to define the extension and severity of the disease.[48,49]

Intestinal GVHD: use of video capsule endoscopy

At present, there is only one study on the use of capsule endoscopy in GVHD.[50] The major indication for the investigation of these patients was the persistence of profuse diarrhea. In this study, 10 consecutive patients with suspected acute GVHD were evaluated by esophagogastroduodenoscopy with gastric and duodenal biopsies and VCE. Capsule images were scored according to a standard classification[44] and compared with the endoscopic and histologic findings. Importantly, 5 patients had a normal VCE, which ruled out GVHD, suggesting an alternative cause of the patients' diarrhea. VCE was found to be more sensitive than traditional upper endoscopy in the diagnosis of gastrointestinal GVHD and allowed mapping of often patchy intestinal lesions along the entire length of the small bowel[50] (Figure 18.6). VCE was well tolerated. This procedure had a high negative predictive value for GVHD in this study, suggesting that it may be suitable for screening purposes. The authors concluded that this procedure could be used both in patients with suspected GVHD and also in the followup of patients with known GVHD to monitor response to treatment and avoid excessive immunosuppression.

References

1. Scotti-Foglieni T, Tinozzi SD, Abu-Elmagd K, Starzl TE. Enteroscopy of the transplanted small bowel. In: Rossini FP, Gay G, eds. Atlas of enteroscopy. Springer, Milan, 1998, pp. 151–69.

2. Lillehei RC, Groot B, Miller FA. The physiological response of the small bowel of the dog to ischemia, including prolonged preservation of the small bowel with the successful replacement and survival. Ann Surg 1959;150:543–60.

3. Monchik GJ, Russel PS. Transplantation of the small bowel in the rat: technical and immunological considerations. Surgery 1971;70:693–702.

4. Alican F, Hardy JD, Cayirily M, et al. Intestinal transplantation: laboratory experience and report of a clinical case. Am Surg 1971;121:150–1.

5. Fortner JG, Sichuk G, Litwin SD, et al. Immunological response to an intestinal allograft with HLA identical donor-recipient. Transplantation 1972;14:531–2.

6. Niv Y, Mor E, Tzakis AG. Small bowel transplantation — a clinical review. Am J Gastroenterol 1999;94:3126–30.

7. Abu-Elmagd K, Bond G, Reyes J, Fung J. Intestinal transplantation: a coming of age. Adv Surg 2002;36:65–101.

8. International Intestinal Transplantation Registry site, 1997; http://www.intestinaltransplant.org/registry.htm; http://www.intestinaltransplant.org/ITR_Reports/Report_2003/ITR%202003%20Final%20Summary%20Slides_files/frame.htm

9. Abu-Elmaged K, Bond G. Gut failure and abdominal visceral transplantation. Proc Nutr Soc 2003;62;727–37.

10. Ricour C, Gorski AM, Goulet O, et al. Home parenteral nutrition in children; eight years of experience with 112 patients. Hum Nutr Clin Nutr 1990;9:65–71.

11. Mittal NK, Tzakis A, Kato T, Thompson JF. Current status of small bowel transplantation in children: update 2003. Pediatr Clin North Am 2003;50:1419–33.

12. Grant D. Current results of intestinal transplantation: International Transplant Registry. Lancet 1996;347:1801–3.

13. Howard L, Malone M. Current status of home parenteral nutrition in the United States. Transplant Proc 1996;28:2691–5.

14. Howard L, Hassan N. Home parenteral nutrition 25 years later. Gastrointest Clin North Am 1998;27:481–512.

15. Sondheimer JM, Asturias E, Cadnapaphornchai M. Infection and cholestasis in neonates with intestinal resection and long term parenteral nutrition. J Pediatr Gastroenterol Nutr 1998;27:131–37.

16. Nishida S, Levi D, Kato T, et al. Ninety-five cases of intestinal transplantation at the University of Miami. J Gastrointest Surg 2002;6:233–9.

17. Zhang Z, Zhu L, Quan D, et al. Pattern of liver, kidney, heart and intestine allograft rejection in different mouse strain combinations. Transplantation 1996;62:1267–72.

18. Turka LA. Immune mediators in transplant rejection and tolerance. Transpl Imunol 1997;13:5–7.

19. European MMF Cooperative Study Group. Placebo-controlled study of mycophenolate mofetil combined with cyclosporine and corticosteroids for prevention of acute rejection. Lancet 1995;345:1321–5.

20. Kartzas T, Khan F, Tzakis AG. Clinical intestinal transplantation. Experience in Miami. Transpl Proc 1997;29:1787–9.

21. Sudan DL, Kaufman SS, Shaw BW, et al. Isolated intestinal transplantation for intestinal failure. Am J Gastroenterol 2000;95:1506–15.

22. Abu-Elmagd K, Todo S, Tzakis A, et al. Three years clinical experience with intestinal transplantation. J Am Coll Surg 1994;179:385–400.

23. Sigurdsson L, Reyes J, Putnam PE, et al. Endoscopies in pediatric small intestinal transplant recipient: five year experience. Am J Gastroenterol 1998;93:207–11.

24. Grover R, Lear PA, Ingham Clark CL, Pockley AG, Wood RFM. Method for diagnosing rejection in small bowel transplantation. Br J Surg 1993;80:1024–26.

25. Garau P, Orenstein SR, Neigut DA, Putnam PE, Reyes J, Tzakis AG, Kocoshis SA. Role of endoscopy following small intestinal transplantation in children. Transpl Proc 1994;26:136–7.

26. Hassanein T, Schade RR, Soldevilla-Pico C, et al. Endoscopy is essential for early detection of rejection in small bowel transplantation recipients. Transpl Proc 1994;26:1414–5.

27. Lee RG, Nakamura K, Athanassios CT, et al. Pathology of human intestinal transplantation. Gastroenterology 1996;110:1820–34.

28. Kato T, O'Brien CB, Nishida S, et al. The first case report of the use of a zoom videoendoscope for evaluation of small bowel graft mucosa in a human after intestinal transplantation. Gastrointest Endosc 1999;50:257–61.

29. Kato T, O'Brien CB, Berho M, et al. Improved rejection surveillance in intestinal transplant recipient with frequent use of zoom video endoscopy. Transpl Proc 2000;32:1200.

30. Kaufman SS, Lyden ER, Marks WH, et al. Lack of utility of intestinal fatty acid binding protein levels in predicting intestinal allograft rejection. Transplantation 2001;71:1058–60.

31. Pappas PA, Saudubray JM Tzakis AG, et al. Serum citrulline and rejection in small bowel transplantation: a preliminary report. Transplantation 2001;72:1212–6.

32. Beckurts KT, Stippel D, Scleimer K, Benz C, Dienes HP, Holscher AH. First case of isolated small bowel transplantation at the University of Cologne: rejection free course under quadruple immunosuppression and endoluminal monitoring with video-capsule. Transpl Proc 2004;36:340–2.

33. de Franchis R, Rondonotti E, Abbiati C, Beccari G, Merighi A, Pinna A, Villa E. Capsule endoscopy in small bowel transplantation. Dig Liver Dis 2003;35:728–31.

34. Anasetti C. Advances in the prevention of graft versus host disease after hematopoietic cell transplantation. Transplantation 2004;77:79–83.

35. Terdiman JP, Linker AC, Ries CA, Damon LE, Rugo HS, Ostroff JW. The role of endoscopic evaluation in patients with suspected intestinal graft versus host disease after allogeneic bone marrow transplantation. Endoscopy 1996;28:680–5.

36. Goker H, Haznedaroglu IC, Chao NJ. Acute graft vs host disease: Pathobiology and management. Exp Hematol 2001;29:259–77.

37. Billingham RE. The biology of graft vs host reactions. In: The Harvey Lectures. Academy Press, New York, 1966;62:21–78.

38. Takatsuka H, Iwasaki T, Okamoto T, Kakishita E. Intestinal graft versus host disease. Drugs 2003;63:1–15.

39. Clift RA, Buckner CD, Appelbaum FR, et al. Allogenic marrow transplantation in patients with acute myeloid leukaemia in first remission: randomized trial of two irradiation regimens. Blood 1990;76:1867–71.

40. Rindgen O. Viral infection and graft versus host disease. In: Burakoff SJ, Deeg HJ, Ferrara J, Atkinson K, eds. Graft versus host disease. Marcel Dekker, New York, 1990, p. 467.

41. Roy J, Platt JL, Weisdorf J. The immunopathology of upper gastrointestinal acute graft versus host disease. Transplantation 1993;55:572–7.

42. Cruz-Corea M, Poonawala A, Abraham SC, Zahurak M, Vogelsang G, Kalloo AN, Lee LA. Endoscopic findings predict the histologic diagnosis in gastrointestinal graft-versus-host disease. Endoscopy 2002;34;808–13.

43. Ponec RJ, Hackman RC, McDonald GB. Endoscopic and histologic diagnosis of intestinal graft-versus-host disease after marrow transplantation. Gastrointest Endosc 1998;49:612–21.

44. Brand RE, Tarantolo MR, Bishop ZS, et al. The correlation of endoscopic grading to clinical and pathologic staging of acute gastrointestinal graft-versus-host disease. Blood 1998;49(suppl.1):45.

45. Roy J, Snover D, Weisdorf S, et al. Simultaneous upper and lower biopsy in the diagnosis of intestinal graft-versus-host disease. Transplantation 1991;51:642–6.

46. Schuttevaer HM, Kroon HM, Chandie Shaw P. Graft-versus-host disease of gastrointestinal tract. Diagn Imaging Clin Med 1986;55:254–61.

47. Kalantari BN, Mortele KJ, Cantisani V, et al. CT features with pathologic correlation of acute gastrointestinal graft-versus-host disease after bone marrow transplantation in adults. AJR Am J Roentgenol 2003;181:1621–5.

48. Klein SA, Martin H, Schreiber-Dietrich D, Hermann S, Caspary WF, Hoelzer D, Dietrich F. A new approach to evaluating intestinal graft-versus-host disease by transabdominal sonography and colour doppler imaging. Br J Haematol 2001;155:929–34.

49. Gorg C, Wollenberg B, Beyer J, Stolte MS, Neubauer A. High resolution ultrasonography in gastrointestinal graft-versus-host disease. Ann Hematol 2005;84:33–9.

50. Yakoub-Agha IY, Maunoury V, Wacrenier A, et al. Impact of small bowel exploration using video capsule endoscopy in the management of acute gastrointestinal graft versus host disease. Transplantation 2004;78:1697–701.

Section FOUR

Non-Small Bowel Indications

CHAPTER **19**

Capsule Endoscopy in the Stomach and Colon

Virender K Sharma

KEY POINTS

1. The small bowel capsule may reveal significant findings in the stomach and colon.

2. In the stomach the most common findings are peptic ulcers, porta; hypertensive gastropathy, GAVE and occasionally tumors.

3. Findings in the colon are generally limited by the poor quality of the bowel preparation.

4. The suspected blood indicator may detect areas of colonic bleeding.

5. Colonic findings on small bowel capsule endoscopy include diverticulosis, AVM's, inflammatory bowel disease, polyps and tumors.

Introduction

Wireless video capsule endoscopy (VCE) is a novel endoscopic technology that enables direct visualization of the entire small intestine mucosa.[1] The advent of capsule endoscopy has led to improved diagnostic yield in small bowel diseases such as obscure gastrointestinal (GI) bleeding, Crohn's disease, celiac disease, and small bowel tumors.[2] The capsule endoscope naturally passes through the complete GI tract and is expelled in the stool. However, due to limitations in capsule endoscopy technology, evaluation of the GI tract other than small bowel has been limited. Rapid transit of the small bowel capsule through the esophagus limits its ability to capture adequate esophageal images. The large gastric lumen results in poor illumination and incomplete visualization of the gastric mucosa and hence an inadequate examination of the stomach. Presence of stool in an unprepared colon masks colonic findings. In addition the patients evaluated using small bowel capsule endoscopy have undergone prior upper and lower GI endoscopy, excluding patients with pathology in these regions, further limiting our knowledge regarding the accuracy of the capsule to detect pathology in stomach and colon. Despite this, gastric or colonic pathology may be found in up to 14% of patients undergoing capsule endoscopy for obscure GI bleeding.[3]

Improvements in future capsule technology such as esophageal and colonic capsule endoscopy will allow us to better evaluate the portions of the GI tract that are currently not evaluable using the current small bowel capsule endoscope. The current chapter deals with endoscopic findings in the stomach and colon visualized on small bowel capsule endoscopy.

Gastric findings on small bowel capsule endoscopy

The capsule endoscope remains in the stomach for an adequate amount of time to obtain a large number of images at the frame rate of two images per second. However, the large gastric lumen, lack of gastric distension, and large surface area result in poor visualization, limiting the accuracy of capsule endoscopy in diagnosing gastric findings. However, capsule endoscopy can detect gastric findings that are diffuse or those in the antrum and pyloric region where the gastric lumen tapers down, resulting in adequate illumination and visualization. Gastric lesions missed at prior endoscopy may be seen on capsule endoscopy and should prompt repeat esophagogastroduodenoscopy (EGD).[4]

Acid peptic disease

Acid peptic disease due to *Helicobacter pylori* infection or non-steroidal anti-inflammatory drugs (NSAIDs) manifests as erosions and/or ulcerations, both of which can cause obscure GI bleeding. In addition NSAID use can result in injury to both small bowel and stomach and hence gastric findings due to NSAID injury can be seen in patients undergoing small bowel capsule endoscopy for evaluation of NSAID enteropathy (see Chapter 14).

Diagnosis

Acid peptic injury to the stomach is easily diagnosed on traditional endoscopy. However, the lesions can be transient and may have healed at the time of endoscopy. Although not very sensitive in picking out focal gastric findings, the capsule can detect erosions and ulcerations (Figure 19.1), especially in the gastric antrum where good visualization is possible.

Treatment

Treatment of acid peptic injury to the stomach includes treatment of the causative agent, i.e. antibiotic treatment for *H. pylori* infection, or stopping NSAIDs and antisecretory therapy with proton pump inhibitors or H_2-receptor antagonists to promote healing.

Portal hypertensive gastropathy

Portal hypertensive gastropathy (congestive gastropathy) results from an increase in portal venous pressure and hepatic sinusoidal resistance and a decrease in hepatic blood flow in patients with chronic liver disease and liver cirrhosis.[5] Portal hypertensive gastropathy, although mostly asymptomatic, may result in iron deficiency anemia from chronic blood loss or rarely overt gastrointestinal bleeding. The bleeding occurs from spontaneous rupture of the ectatic blood vessels due to increased portal pressure.

Diagnosis

Portal hypertensive gastropathy characteristically appears as a fine white reticular pattern separating areas of pinkish mucosa on endoscopy, giving the gastric mucosa a "snakeskin," "reticular," or "cobblestone" appearance (Figure 19.2). Mucosal changes are predominantly seen in the fundus and body; however, in more severe cases they can be diffuse and involve the antrum. In a patient with chronic liver disease, the diagnosis is made on endoscopy. Pathologic examination reveals edema with capillary and venous dilatation in the submucosa extending into the mucosa.[6]

Portal hypertensive gastropathy changes are diffuse and can be easily detected on capsule endoscopy (Figure

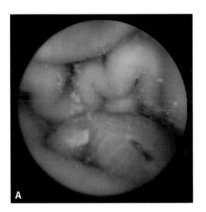
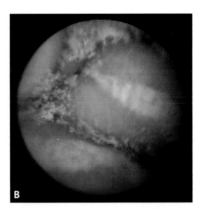

FIGURE 19.1 NSAID gastropathy. (a) Erosions seen on capsule endoscopy. (b) Linear ulcerations in the body.

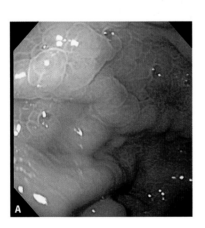
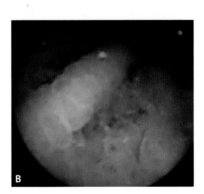

FIGURE 19.2 Portal hypertensive gastropathy — characteristic appearance of fine white reticular pattern separating areas of pinkish mucosa on endoscopy, also called "snakeskin," "reticular" or "cobblestone" appearance. (a) Endoscopic view. (b) Capsule endoscopy.

19.2b). Eisen et al used esophageal capsule endoscopy to evaluate patients with chronic liver disease. They reported a sensitivity of 100% and specificity of 77% compared to upper endoscopy for the detection of portal hypertensive gastropathy.[7]

Treatment

Decreasing portal pressure using beta-blocker medications (propranolol, atenolol), transjugular intrahepatic portosystemic shunts (TIPS), portosystemic shunt surgery, and liver transplantation are the mainstays of long-term treatment of bleeding from portal hypertensive gastropathy. Acute hemostasis using endoscopic therapy for focal bleeding lesions and medications that decrease splanchnic pressure such as vasopressin, somatostatin or octreotide have been used, but their efficacy for this indication has not been studied in controlled trials.[6]

Gastric antral vascular ectasia (GAVE) or watermelon stomach

Gastric antral vascular ectasia is a rare cause of obscure GI bleeding that on endoscopy appears as linear streaks of red mucosa radiating from the pylorus to the antrum, giving it the typical appearance and name of watermelon stomach. GAVE can sometimes be confused with portal hypertensive gastropathy, and both conditions can occur in patients with cirrhosis. In addition, GAVE can be seen in patients without portal hypertension and liver disease. Despite its typical endoscopic appearance GAVE is one of the more common lesions in patients with obscure GI bleeding. GAVE is often confused with antral gastropathy, which can also have a streaky erythematous appearance and hence GAVE can be missed on upper endoscopy. Since the histologic changes are predominantly in the submucosa, superficial mucosal biopsies may be normal. Deeper biopsies containing submucosal tissue reveal ectatic blood vessels with spindle cell proliferation and fibrohyalinosis. A punctate form of GAVE has also been described and appears to be more common in patients with liver disease and cirrhosis.[8]

GAVE can present both as iron deficiency anemia from chronic blood loss or overt GI bleeding. As in portal hyper-

tensive gastropathy, the bleeding in GAVE also occurs from spontaneous rupture of ectatic blood vessels.

Diagnosis

The diagnosis is based upon the classic endoscopic appearance; it may be confirmed with endoscopic biopsy, endoscopic ultrasound, tagged red blood cell scan, or CT scan. GAVE is one of the gastric lesions commonly seen on capsule endoscopy (Figure 19.3) in patients with obscure GI bleeding.

Treatment

Medical management with oral or parenteral iron therapy is the mainstay of treatment in patients with GAVE, with endoscopic therapy reserved for severe bleeding requiring transfusion. Since bleeding from GAVE is mostly chronic, blood transfusions may be required in cases not responding to parenteral iron therapy. Endoscopic thermal therapies with heater probe, gold probe, argon plasma coagulator or laser therapy may decrease transfusion requirements in patients with severe bleeding, however they are rarely able to completely obliterate GAVE.[9] Portal decompression with TIPS or portovenous shunting does not reduce bleeding, underscoring the uncertain relationship of GAVE to portal hypertension. Hormonal therapy has been tried in these patients; however, evidence of its effectiveness is lacking. In severe cases that do not respond to endoscopic therapy, antrectomy can be performed and is curative in severe cases of GAVE. We have had good success with antral band ligation in patients with severe GAVE, resulting in reduction in the number of endoscopies and transfusion requirement and improvement in the endoscopic appearance of GAVE.[10]

Gastric tumors

Gastric tumors are easily detected on traditional endoscopy, and patients with known gastric tumors ordinarily would not undergo capsule endoscopy, hence our knowledge of accuracy of capsule endoscopy in detecting gastric tumors is limited. Gastric tumors (Figure 19.4) can be seen in patients undergoing capsule endoscopy for evaluation of small bowel involvement in polyposis syndromes (e.g. familial adenomatous polyposis).[11]

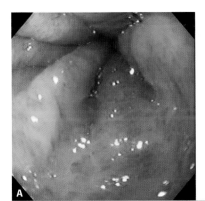 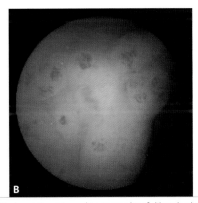 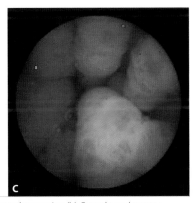

FIGURE 19.3 Gastric antral vascular ectasia (GAVE). (a) Endoscopic view — linear streaks of dilated submucosal vascular ectasias. (b) Capsule endoscopy — punctate form of GAVE. (c) Capsule endoscopy — more typical linear streaks of submucosal vascular ectasias.

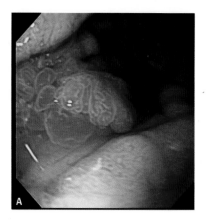
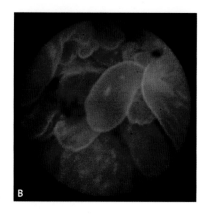

FIGURE 19.4 Giant hyperplastic gastric polyp in a patient with familial polyposis. (a) Endoscopic view. (b) Capsule endoscopy.

Colonic findings on small bowel capsule endoscopy

Colonic imaging with the small bowel capsule is limited due to poor preparation and slow colonic transit. Presence of stool in the unprepared colon limits endoscopic visualization. Also, due to poor transit the capsule mainly stays in the right colon and does not obtain complete colonic images. In patients undergoing small bowel capsule endoscopy, evaluation of the colonic segment of the study in an unprepared colon is not routinely performed. However, certain colonic pathologies can be seen on capsule endoscopy that can help in diagnosing the etiology of patients' complaints.

The suspected blood indicator (SBI) is a computer algorithm that detects various shades of red and hence red lesions such as active bleeding, arteriovenous malformations, and erythema due to inflammation. SBI can detect colonic findings in an unprepared colon, and the colonic segment where SBI is positive should be evaluated for possible pathology.[12] In a prepared colon, colonic findings, especially in the right colon, can be visualized on small bowel capsule endoscopy.

Diverticulosis

Herniation of the colonic mucosa through the muscular layer of the colonic wall results in diverticulum formation. The herniation results from increased intraluminal pressures and weakness in the wall created by the colonic arteries, vasa recti, entering the colon. As the diverticulum herniates, the vasa recti become draped over the diverticular orifice. Over time, the vasa recti, lined only by the colonic mucosa, weaken resulting in eccentric thickening of the intima and thinning of the media. These changes result in segmental weakness of the artery and eventually to rupture into the lumen causing an arterial bleed that presents as painless bright red blood per rectum. Although the bleeding is usually painless, patients can have mild crampy abdominal discomfort due to colonic spasm from intraluminal blood. Diverticular bleeding is usually intermittent and self-limiting.[13]

Diagnosis

Diverticulosis can be easily diagnosed on colonoscopy, barium radiography or abdominal CT. Bleeding from diverticulosis usually resolves by the time the patient undergoes an endoscopy and active bleeding is rarely seen. The patient's clinical presentation, presence of colonic diverticulosis, and absence of any other lesion responsible for bleeding help diagnose diverticular bleeding. The rebleeding rate approaches 25% after the initial bleeding episode. Capsule endoscopy can visualize diverticulosis (Figure 19.5) and in the event of active bleeding at the time of capsule endoscopy the SBI can suggest diverticulosis as the colonic source of bleeding.

Treatment

Most diverticular bleeds are self-limited and managed supportively. Active diverticular bleeding can be treated using endoscopic thermal therapy, endoscopic injection therapy with epinephrine, argon plasma coagulation or endoscopic clip application. Unstable patients can be treated with angiographic embolization while surgical resection of the diseased segment of colon is limited to patients with persistent or recurrent diverticular bleeding.[13]

Arteriovenous malformations

Arteriovenous malformations (AVMs) or angiodysplasias are dilated tortuous submucosal vessels composed of

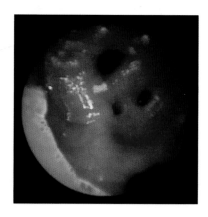

FIGURE 19.5 Diverticulosis. Capsule endoscopy showing multiple colonic diverticula. The suspected blood indicator revealed bleeding limited to the colon, suggesting colonic diverticulosis as the source of the patient's bleeding.

endothelial lining without a smooth muscle component to the wall. Colonic AVMs are an uncommon source of bleeding in younger patients; however, the incidence and the risk of bleeding increase with age due to degeneration of the vessel walls. Thus, AVMs may account for up to a quarter of the cases of lower GI bleeding in patients over the age of 65 years. Most of the bleeding AVMs are in the right side of the colon. Bleeding from AVMs tends to be slow, episodic, and self-limited. The presentation can be as obscure occult or overt bleeding, and recurrent or persistent bleeding is common unless AVMs are treated endoscopically, surgically or radiologically.[14]

Diagnosis

The typical appearance of a spider-like vascular lesion (Figure 19.6) in the right colon is diagnostic on endoscopy. However, due to alterations in the splanchnic pressures with sedative medication, these lesions can be less apparent on colonoscopy. The SBI can alert to the presence of AVMs in the colon in a patient undergoing capsule endoscopy for obscure GI bleeding.

Treatment

Patients with obscure occult bleeding can be managed with oral or parenteral iron therapy. Endoscopic thermal therapy with bipolar probe, heater probes or argon plasma coagulation and endoscopic clip placement can all achieve obliteration of AVMs and definitive hemostasis in patients with active bleeding.[15] Surgery is limited to patients with diffuse segmental disease or disease not responding to endoscopic treatment.

Inflammatory bowel disease

Inflammatory bowel disease refers to both Crohn's disease and ulcerative colitis. Patients with Crohn's disease can have cecal involvement with erosion and ulceration that may be visible on capsule endoscopy. Hematochezia is a less common initial presentation of Crohn's disease involving the ileocecal region; iron deficiency anemia due to chronic blood loss is more typically seen.

Diagnosis

Endoscopy with histologic confirmation on biopsies has been the mainstay for diagnosing inflammatory bowel disease. At endoscopy, the anatomic distribution of disease and type of ulcer lesion can differentiate between Crohn's disease and ulcerative colitis.[16] Barium radiography, CT enterography, and colography are helpful in the diagnosis of these conditions. Colonic findings of inflammatory bowel disease can be visible on capsule endoscopy as edema, erythema, erosions or frank ulcerations (Figure 19.7).

Treatment

Treatment of inflammatory bowel disease includes 5-ASA agents, systemic and topical steroids, immunosuppressive

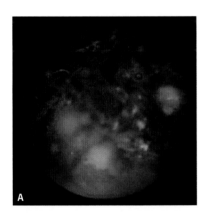
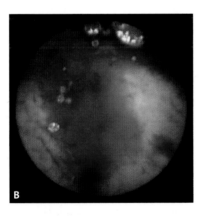

FIGURE 19.6 Arteriovenous malformation. (a) Capsule endoscopy revealing a spider-like vascular lesion detected by the suspected blood indicator. (b) Active bleeding in the colon detected by the suspected blood indicator confirming the source of bleeding to be a colonic AVM.

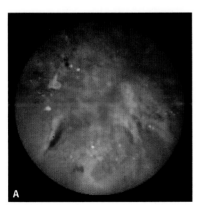
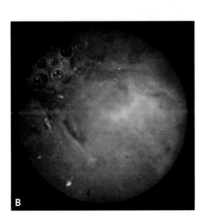

FIGURE 19.7 (a, b) Ulcerative colitis — capsule endoscopy showing erythema, erosions, and ulceration in the colon. The suspected blood indicator identified the presence of the abnormality in an unprepared colon.

therapy using 6-mercaptopurine or azathioprine, and biological therapy with infliximab. Surgery is limited to disease not responding to medical management or patients with toxic megacolon.[17]

Tumors

Tumors (large polyps and cancer) are a relatively less common but serious cause of GI bleeding. Bleeding occurs as the result of overlying erosion or ulceration and tends to be low-grade and recurrent. Right-sided lesions can present with maroon blood or melena and mimic upper or small bowel bleeding.

Diagnosis

Tumors are easily detected on colonoscopy, barium radiography, and computed tomography. However, all of these can miss both large colon polyps and colon cancer. The SBI can alert to the presence of tumors in the colon in a patient undergoing capsule endoscopy for obscure GI bleeding.[12] Right-sided lesions can also be detected on capsule endoscopy performed after colonic preparation in patients who may have had an incomplete colonoscopy (Figure 19.8).

Treatment

Treatment of colon cancer is surgical resection with adjuvant chemo-radiation for advanced disease. Endoscopic thermal therapy, argon plasma coagulation, endoscopic sclerosant injection, and angiographic embolization can be attempted to achieve acute hemostasis of malignant bleeding.[18]

Bleeding without a lesion

The SBI can detect areas of active bleeding in an unprepared colon. Although a distinct lesion may not be seen, this can point to a colonic source of bleeding. Likely lesions associated with colonic bleeding which can be missed on colonoscopy include AVMs, Dieulafoy lesion in the colon, and diverticula. This finding can prompt the physician to re-evaluate the colon for possible bleeding sources and also point to the segment of colon where the source may be located.[12]

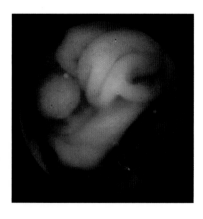

FIGURE 19.8 Colon polyp in the ascending colon seen on small bowel capsule endoscopy in a patient who had an incomplete colonoscopy.

Conclusion

Capsule endoscopy currently is indicated for the evaluation of esophageal and small bowel diseases. However, important gastric and colonic findings can be identified in patients undergoing esophageal or small bowel capsule endoscopy. The suspected blood indicator may alert the capsule readers to findings in the stomach and colon. Future development of specific capsule endoscopes for viewing the stomach and colon will improve our ability to diagnose disease of these organs using capsule endoscopy.

References

1. Iddan G, Meron G, Glukhovsky A, Swain P. Wireless capsule endoscopy. Nature 2000;405:417.

2. Marmo R, Rotondano G, Piscopo R, Bianco MA, Cipolletta L. Meta-analysis: capsule enteroscopy vs. conventional modalities in diagnosis of small bowel diseases. Aliment Pharmacol Ther 2005;22:595–604.

3. Carlo JT, DeMarco D, Smith BA, et al. The utility of capsule endoscopy and its role for diagnosing pathology in the gastrointestinal tract. Am J Surg 2005;190:886–90.

4. Peter S, Heuss LT, Beglinger C, Degen L. Capsule endoscopy of the upper gastrointestinal tract — the need for a second endoscopy. Digestion 2005;72:242–7.

5. Thuluvath P, Yoo HY. Portal hypertensive gastropathy. Am J Gastroenterol 2002;97:2973–8.

6. Rondonotti E, Villa F, Signorelli C, de Franchis R. Portal hypertensive enteropathy. Gastrointest Endosc Clin N Am 2006;16:277–86.

7. Eisen GM, Eliakim R, Zaman A, et al. The accuracy of PillCam ESO capsule endoscopy versus conventional upper endoscopy for the diagnosis of esophageal varices: a prospective three-center pilot study. Endoscopy 2006;38:31–5.

8. Sebastian S, O'Morain CA, Buckley MJ. Review article: current therapeutic options for gastric antral vascular ectasia. Aliment Pharmacol Ther 2003;18:157–65.

9. Pavey DA, Craig PI. Endoscopic therapy for upper-GI vascular ectasias. Gastrointest Endosc 2004;59:233–8.

10. Wells CD, Harrison ME, Gurudu SR, Sharma VK. Endoscopic band ligation is superior to endoscopic thermal therapy for the treatment of gastric antral vascular ectasia — a case control study (Abstract 1373). Am J Gastroenterol 2006;101:S526.

11. Schulmann K, Schmiegel W. Capsule endoscopy for small bowel surveillance in hereditary intestinal polyposis and non-polyposis syndromes. Gastrointest Endosc Clin N Am 2004;14:149–58.

12. Kitiyakara T, Selby W. Non-small-bowel lesions detected by capsule endoscopy in patients with obscure GI bleeding. Gastrointest Endosc 2005;62:234–8.

13. Parra-Blanco A. Colonic diverticular disease: pathophysiology and clinical picture. Digestion 2006;73(Suppl 1):47–57.

14. Fishman SJ, Fox VL. Visceral vascular anomalies. Gastrointest Endosc Clin N Am 2001;11:813–34.

15. Kwan V, Bourke MJ, Williams SJ, et al. Argon plasma coagulation in the management of symptomatic gastrointestinal vascular lesions: experience in 100 consecutive patients with long-term follow-up. Am J Gastroenterol 2006;101:58–63.

16. Chutkan RK, Sherl E, Waye JD. Colonoscopy in inflammatory bowel disease. Gastrointest Endosc Clin N Am 2002;12:463–83.

17. Egan LJ, Sandborn WJ. Advances in the treatment of Crohn's disease. Gastroenterology 2004;126:1574–81.

18. Green BT, Rockey DC. Lower gastrointestinal bleeding — management. Gastroenterol Clin N Am 2005;34:665–78.

CHAPTER **20**

Esophageal Capsule Endoscopy

Glenn M Eisen

KEY POINTS

1. An esophageal capsule endoscope is now available that can provide wireless imaging of the esophagus.

2. The esophageal capsule is the same size and shape as the small bowel capsule but has cameras on either end each obtaining 7 frames per second.

3. Esophageal capsule endoscopy may be useful in screening at-risk patient populations for Barrett's esophagus and esophageal varices.

Introduction

Small bowel capsule endoscopy has proven to be the gold standard for evaluating the small intestine, surpassing the extent of examination and accuracy of both endoscopic and radiological imaging modalities. The capsule is ingested and despite passing through the esophagus on its way to the more distal bowel, images of this part of the gastrointestinal (GI) tract are often incomplete. This is due to the small bowel capsule endoscope capturing only 2 images per second and the rapid esophageal transit, which is due in part to patient positioning at the time of ingestion. Although the esophagus is readily visualized during esophagogastroduodenoscopy (EGD), many patients may not undergo this procedure because of concerns about invasiveness, discomfort, and sedation issues. Recently, an esophageal capsule has been developed to potentially serve as an alternative imaging procedure to traditional upper endoscopy.

The Given Diagnostic System Pillcam ESO is comprised of three major components: an ingestible esophageal capsule; a data recorder, which includes a recorder belt and sensor array; and a RAPID workstation. Federal Drug Administration (FDA) clearance for this device was granted in November of 2004. The ingestible, disposable Pillcam ESO is an $11 \times 26\,mm$ capsule and is able to acquire images from both ends of the device during passage through the esophagus at a rate of 7 frames/second from each end of the capsule (Figure 20.1). Therefore, 14 frames/second are captured, as compared to 2 frames/second for Pillcam SB. The capsule transmits the acquired images via digital radiofrequency communication channel to the data recorder unit residing outside the study subject. The data recorder is an external receiving/recording unit that receives all data transmitted by the capsule. After completion of the 20-minute examination, the accumulated data can be transferred from the recording unit to the RAPID workstation for processing and interpretation.

Pillcam ESO has been developed to visualize the esophagus, although both the stomach and proximal duodenum may be visualized. However, the capsule battery life may end prior to the capsule passing through the pylorus, and significant parts of the stomach may also not be visualized. The potential complication of capsule retention requiring endoscopic or surgical extraction is the same as for Pillcam SB, but it is anticipated that this rate will be significantly lower than for patients with suspected small bowel disease. Nonetheless, an accurate history should be obtained to minimize this potential risk.

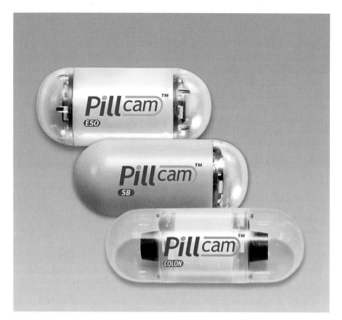

The PillCam™ COLON capsule is an investigational device, not yet cleared for marketing in the USA.

FIGURE 20.1 Given Imaging capsule endoscopes. Top: PillcamEso (esophageal imaging: note the optical domes on each end of the device). Middle: PillcamSB (small bowel imaging: note the single optical dome). Bottom: Pillcam colon (colonic imaging; this device is investigational).

Procedure

Patients are instructed to fast for at least 4 hours prior to undergoing the Pillcam procedure. Following setup of the system, the patient swallows the capsule using a standardized Pillcam ESO protocol. Each patient is allowed to ingest up to 100 mL of water to clear the esophagus of saliva. The patient may also ingest liquid simethicone as well, in order to reduce bubbles in the esophagus. After this, the patient ingests the capsule in the supine position with up to 10 mL of water. After swallowing the capsule, patients remain in the supine position for two minutes then are passively raised to 30° for two minutes, 60° for one minute, and sitting up for one minute. Patients are asked not to speak or make sudden movements during the 6-minute ingestion process. After this, patients are allowed to have sips of water to assure capsule passage into the stomach and resume normal activities for an additional 20 minutes until the capsule battery turns off.

A recent trial was performed to compare alternative methods for capsule ingestion with the intent of improving esophageal visualization. Nine variations were compared in healthy volunteers, and the best results were found when the subject lay in the right decubitus position, drank 100 mL of water, then, after pill ingestion, drank 15 mL of water through a straw twice a minute for 5 minutes. This simplified ingestion procedure (SIP) allowed greater visualization of the z line with less bubbles and saliva as compared to other variations, including the procedure utilized in current studies.[1] It should be noted that at the time of writing this chapter, all clinical trials and published data have used the ingestion protocol first mentioned in

this section. It is likely that by the time of publication of this chapter numerous trials will have begun to use the simplified ingestion protocol.

Screening for esophageal disease

The World Health Organization (WHO) has enumerated several principles that should be met in order for a screening intervention to be successful[2]: (1) the target disease should have a high associated morbidity or mortality; (2) effective intervention, capable of reducing morbidity and mortality, should be available; and (3) screening procedures should be acceptable, safe, and relatively inexpensive.

Currently, traditional EGD has been used as a screening tool of the esophagus for primarily two disorders: chronic gastroesophageal reflux, which places patients at increased risk of developing Barrett's esophagus and esophageal adenocarcinoma, and chronic liver disease, leading to portal hypertension and the development of esophageal varices. Esophageal capsule endoscopy (ECE) has recently been introduced as a potential alternative to EGD for screening, since it is acceptable to patients, safe, and less invasive than EGD. This chapter will discuss the accumulating data and indications for ECE since its FDA clearance in November 2004.

A significant economic burden is imposed by chronic gastroesophageal reflux (GERD). It has been estimated that almost 20% of the U.S. population experiences GERD symptoms weekly and up to 60% monthly.[3] It is also estimated that the direct and indirect costs of GERD are almost $10 billion annually in the U.S.[4] It is now well studied and accepted that chronic GERD increases the likelihood of developing esophageal adenocarcinoma (relative risk, 40–125× the general population). The incidence of this malignancy has risen significantly over the past 30 years.[5] Current Gastroenterology Society recommendations suggest endoscopic screening for Barrett's esophagus in patients with long-standing reflux symptoms.[6] A recent cost-effectiveness analysis confirmed that endoscopic screening of individuals with long-standing GERD might be reasonable compared to other screening practices in medicine.[7] Despite Society endorsement of endoscopic screening and the rising risk of esophageal adenocarcinoma, the majority of individuals at risk still remain unscreened.

Chronic liver disease is also a clinically and economically significant health-care problem in the United States, affecting 360 per 100 000 persons in the general adult population and costing over $2 billion per year.[8] The most advanced stage of chronic liver disease is cirrhosis, and up to half of patients with Child's class A or B cirrhosis have moderate or large underlying esophageal varices.[9,10] Once esophageal varices form, the risk of variceal bleeding within 2 years is 20–35%, and the mortality risk of the index hemorrhage may be as high as 50%.[11,12] Both pharmacologic (non-selective beta blockade) and endoscopic (band ligation) prophylactic therapies appear to decrease the risk of hemorrhage in patients with esophageal varices (relative risk reduction 40–48%, as compared to placebo, number needed to treat 8.4–10).[13] Given that there are effective therapies, both American and European societies have endorsed universal endoscopic screening of patients with cirrhosis.[3,7,14] Conventional upper endoscopy (EGD) may be inconvenient and unpleasant for patients. In addition, most cases require conscious sedation, which may lead to decreased work productivity as well as a small but not insignificant risk of complications.[15] The risk of complications may be even higher in individuals with cirrhosis. Despite the attendant risks of variceal bleeding and societal endorsement of endoscopic screening, there remains debate as to whether this is an appropriate or cost-effective practice.[16–18] Also, as with screening individuals with chronic GERD, the majority (over 50%) remain unevaluated.[19]

ECE has the potential to increase screening rates and improve outcomes in patients at risk for adverse sequelae from chronic GERD and liver disease.

Pillcam ESO

Screening for complications of chronic GERD

As noted above, there have been few published studies assessing Pillcam ESO. This novel, noninvasive diagnostic tool has been directly compared to traditional upper endoscopy (EGD) in the trials so far performed. The clinical endpoints have been concordance with endoscopy findings. Pillcam ESO potentially has a niche as a noninvasive tool for the diagnosis of esophagitis, suspected Barrett's esophagus, and esophageal varices. The appeal of Pillcam ESO as compared to endoscopy is that it can be office-based, is performed in less than 30 minutes, does not involve the costs, risks, and inconvenience of conscious sedation, and may increase patient acceptability for being screened. The pilot trial of Pillcam ESO involved 17 patients who underwent both EGD and capsule endoscopy.[20] Twelve of the 17 patients examined had esophageal findings using the endoscope as the gold standard. The positive predictive value of the capsule for any esophageal pathology was 92% and the negative predictive value was 100%. Esophageal capsule sensitivity was 100% and specificity 80%. A larger followup trial confirmed these results in 106 patients.[21] Sixty-six of 106 patients had positive esophageal findings and Pillcam ESO identified abnormalities in 61 (sensitivity 92%, specificity 95%). Positive and negative predictive values were between 94% and 99% for both suspected Barrett's esophagus and esophagitis (see Figures 20.2 and 20.3 for representative images of Barrett's esophagus and esophagitis). It should be noted that both the pilot trial and this larger study utilized a capsule that captured images at 4 frames per second.

The next trial published was a direct comparison between the 4 frame per second (fps) capsule and the now utilized 14 fps capsule.[22] All patients underwent EGD, while 25 patients ingested the 4 fps device and another 25 ingested the 14 fps device. The diagnostic miss rate (compared to EGD as the gold standard) was 18% (5/27) for the 4 frame per second capsule versus 0% (0/23) (p < 0.02).

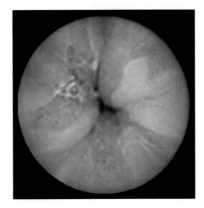

FIGURE 20.2 Barrett's esophagus as seen with the Pillcam ESO.

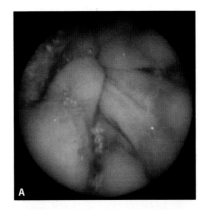

FIGURE 20.3 (a, b) Esophagitis as seen with the Pillcam ESO.

A

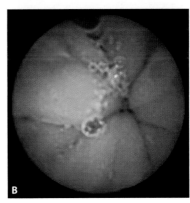

B

A recently presented trial has called into question the initial results just described. Lin et al evaluated 90 patients who, similar to the previous studies, underwent both EGD and Pillcam ESO for chronic GERD screening or Barrett's surveillance.[23] The authors found that 21 patients had biopsy proven Barrett's esophagus. The prior trials only utilized suspected Barrett's as a finding. Test characteristics showed that, for screened patients, the sensitivity and specificity of Pillcam ESO (14 fps) for Barrett's was 67% and 84%, respectively. The positive predictive value was 22% and the negative predictive value 98%. The sensitivity for Barrett's esophagus (assuming detection would occur if the patient was sent for EGD based on the capsule findings) was 81%.

A second study of an enriched Barrett population (41 of 78 had suspected Barrett's by EGD) that remains in abstract form as of this writing, found that overall sensitivity and specificity for suspected Barrett's by capsule was 73% and 86%.[24] The sensitivity of capsule was not surprisingly higher for long segment as compared to short segment Barrett's (67% vs. 86%).

The results of the trials raise provocative issues regarding the accuracy of Pillcam ESO in its current form, as well as general issues with diagnosing Barrett's esophagus. The new simplified ingestion protocol has demonstrated that improved visualization of the distal esophagus can be achieved by altering this process. Adequate visualization of the z line in its entirety is needed to best assess for possible Barrett's esophagus, especially short segment. This protocol needs to be validated in patients with chronic GERD, as well as those suspected to harbor varices. It should be noted that even endoscopic accuracy in short segment Barrett's is questionable, and it is likely that neither endoscopy nor capsule is likely to be infallible. Future trials could consider unblinding capsule results so that if the capsule reading suggests Barrett's then the endoscopist could take a closer look.

A second issue is the choice of study populations. In order to best assess Pillcam ESO's accuracy, a true screening population (no patient with known Barrett's) should be studied. Enriched populations may afford a better sense of the ability to detect Barrett's but could lead to an inaccurate assessment of the device's test characteristics. It is also likely that with future iterations of Pillcam ESO, which may have a faster frame rate, better optics, and a wider field of view, the device will prove to be a reasonable alternative to traditional endoscopy for population screening.

Screening for esophageal varices

Utilizing Pillcam ESO for esophageal varices screening is potentially attractive as a first-line screening tool since it does not require sedation and also, if varices are found, therapy can be instituted (non-selective beta blockade). It is also possible that patients with end-stage liver disease might be more amenable to this type of screening. Of course, this remains hypothetical since it has not been formally studied. Two recently published pilot trials have assessed the diagnostic capabilities of Pillcam ESO versus EGD.[25,26] The U.S. pilot trial assessed 32 patients with both Pillcam ESO and EGD. Twenty-three of 32 patients were found to have esophageal varices on both EGD and Pillcam. The overall diagnostic concordance was 96.9% for esophageal varices and 90.6% for portal hypertensive gastropathy (see Figure 20.4 for an example of esophageal varices on Pillcam ESO). The European trial assessed 21 patients in a similar fashion and found concordance of 84.2%.[23] In addition, Pillcam correctly indicated the need for primary prophylaxis (esophageal varices grade 2 or more and/or red signs) in 100% of cases. This is a promising start, but remains preliminary. A large-scale international trial designed to validate these early findings is ongoing. Interim results of this trial were presented at ICCE 2006.[27]

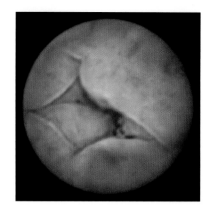

FIGURE 20.4 Esophageal varices as seen with the Pillcam ESO.

The data on the first 97 patients entering the study were presented. This study utilized patients who were presenting for a clinically indicated EGD (for variceal screening or surveillance). This differs from the pilot U.S. trial, which was enriched with surveillance patients in order to ensure that varices would frequently be seen. The findings were comparable to the pilot trial as the sensitivity and specificity for esophageal varices was 86.6% and 86.7%.

Conclusions

The potential benefits for screening patients with Pillcam ESO are several: (1) convenience; (2) patient acceptability; (3) safety; (4) tolerability; (5) administration by a non-physician provider; (6) potentially increased adherence to screening recommendations.

With regard to screening/surveillance for varices, the preliminary results from the two pilot trials are encouraging. The ongoing prospective large-scale trial may provide validation of diagnosis and grading. Ultimately, ECE may have a role in screening and surveillance of varices in patients with cirrhosis.

However, several issues remain before utilization of this capsule can be broadly recommended as an alternate screening tool. Endoscopists generally utilize insufflation to better appreciate the 'true' size of varices in the esophagus. Large appearing varices sometimes diminish greatly in size when insufflation is applied. Grading the size of varices is important since it is accepted that medium and large varices should be treated either medically or with band ligation, while small varices require continued surveillance.

A second potential issue is the presence or absence of gastric varices and the ability of Pillcam ESO to visualize this reliably. Although capsule endoscopy may not always visualize the proximal stomach, the new simplified ingestion protocol increases this likelihood. Also, only a small minority of patients will have isolated gastric varices, without esophageal varices being seen.

Regarding the use of Pillcam ESO for screening patients with chronic GERD, this practice cannot be endorsed at this time due to the recently presented results, which are at odds with the initial data. The middling accuracy of Pillcam ESO for Barrett's esophagus in the two studies only in abstract form may be due to visualization issues, which may make accurate interpretation difficult. However, the altered ingestion protocol, as well as technological advances, may well significantly improve the accuracy of Pillcam. This will need to be assessed in a large-scale study directly comparing EGD with the newer device.

References

1. Gralnek IM, Rabinowitz R, Afik D, Eliakim R. A simplified ingestion procedure for esophageal capsule endoscopy: initial evaluation in healthy volunteers. Endoscopy 2006;38:913–8.

2. World Health Organization: screening — general considerations. Available at: http://www.who.int/cancer/detection/variouscancer/en/index.html. Accessed June 2006.

3. Locke GR III, Talley NJ, Fett SL, Zinsmeister AR, Melton LJ. Prevalence and clinical spectrum of gastroesophageal reflux: a population-based study in Olmstead County, Minnesota. Gastroenterology 1997;112:1448–56.

4. Sandler RS, Everhart JE, Donowitz M, et al. The burden of selected digestive diseases in the United States. Gastroenterology 2002;122:1500–11.

5. Eisen GM, Lieberman DA, Fennerty MB, Sonnenberg A. Screening and surveillance in Barrett's esophagus: A call to action. Clin Gastroenterol Hepatol 2004;2:861–4.

6. Devault KR, Castell DO. Updated guidelines for the diagnosis and treatment of gastroesophageal reflux disease. Am J Gastroenterol 2005;100:190–200.

7. Inadomi JM, Sampliner R, Lagergren J, Lieberman D, Fendrick AM, Vakil N. Screening and surveillance for Barrett esophagus in high-risk groups: a cost-utility analysis. Ann Intern Med 2003;138:176–86.

8. Dufour MC. Chronic liver disease and cirrhosis. In: Everhart JE, ed. Digestive diseases in the United States: Epidemiology and impact. US Dept of Health and Human Services, Washington, DC, 1994. NIH publication 94-1447, pp. 615–645.

9. Cales P, Desmorat H, Vinel JP, et al. Incidence of large oesophageal varices in patients with cirrhosis: application to prophylaxis of first bleeding. Gut 1990;31:1298–302.

10. Zaman A, Becker T, Lapidus J, Benner K. Risk factors for the presence of varices in cirrhotic patients without a history of variceal hemorrhage. Arch Intern Med 2001;161:2564–70.

11. The North Italian Endoscopic Club for the Study and Treatment of Esophageal Varices. Prediction of the first variceal hemorrhage in patients with cirrhosis of the liver and esophageal varices. A prospective multicenter study. N Engl J Med 1988;319:983–9.

12. Gores GJ, Weisner RH, Dickson ER, Zinmeister AR, Jorgensen AR, Langworthy A. Prospective evaluation of esophageal varices in primary biliary cirrhosis: development, natural history and influence in survival. Gastroenterology 1989;96:1552–9.

13. De Franchis R. Updating consensus in portal hypertension: report of the Baveno III consensus workshop on definitions, methodology and therapeutic strategies in portal hypertension. J Hepatol 2000;33:846–52.

14. Grace ND. Practice guidelines: diagnosis and treatment of gastrointestinal bleeding secondary to portal hypertension. Am J Gastroenterol 1997;92:1081–91.

15. Eisen G, Baron TH, Dominitz J. American Society for Gastrointestinal Endoscopy. Complications of upper GI endoscopy. Gastrointest Endosc 2002;55:784–93.

16. Spiegel BMR, Targownik LE, Karsan HA, Dulai GS, Gralnek IM. Endoscopic screening for esophageal varices in cirrhosis: is it ever cost-effective? Hepatology 2003;37:366–77.

17. Arguedas MR, Heudebert GR, Eloubeidi MA, Abrams GA, Fallon MB. Cost-effectiveness of screening, surveillance, and primary prophylaxis strategies for esophageal varices. Am J Gastroenterol 2002;97:2441–52.

18. Saab S, DeRosa V, Nieto J, Durazo F, Han S, Roth B. Costs and clinical outcomes of primary prophylaxis of variceal bleeding in patients with hepatic cirrhosis: a decision analytic model. Am J Gastroenterol 2003;98:763–70.

19. Arguedas MR, McGuire BM, Fallon MB, Abrams GA. The use of screening and preventive therapies for gastroesophageal varices in patients referred for evaluation of orthotopic liver transplantation. Am J Gastroenterol 2001;96:833–7.

20. Eliakim R, Yassin K, Shlomi I, Suissa A, Eisen G. A novel diagnostic tool for detecting oesophageal pathology: the PillCam oesophageal video capsule. Aliment Pharmacol Ther 2004;20:1083–9.

21. Eliakim R, Sharma VK, Yassin K, et al. A prospective study of the diagnostic accuracy of PillCam ESO esophageal capsule endoscopy versus conventional upper endoscopy in patients with chronic gastroesophageal reflux diseases. J Clin Gastroenterol 2005;39:572–8.

22. Koslowsky B, Jacob H, Eliakim, R, Adler SN. Pillcam ESO in esophageal studies: improved diagnostic yield of 14 frames per second(fps) compared to 4(fps). Endoscopy 2006;38:27–30.

23. Lin O, Schembre D, Kozarek R. Blinded comparison of esophageal capsule endoscopy versus conventional endoscopy for diagnosis of Barrett's esophagus in patients with chronic gastroesophageal reflux. Gastrointest Endosc 2006;63:AB103.

24. Sharma P, Rastogi A, Esquivel R, et al. Accuracy of wireless capsule endoscopy for the detection of Barrett's esophagus. Gastroenterology 2006;130 suppl 2:A262.

25. Eisen GM, Eliakim R, Zaman A, et al. The accuracy of PillCam ESO capsule endoscopy versus conventional upper endoscopy for the diagnosis of esophageal varices: a prospective three-center pilot study. Endoscopy 2006;38:31–5.

26. Lapulus MG, Dumortier J, Fumex F, et al. Esophageal capsule endoscopy versus esophagogastroduodenoscopy for evaluating portal hypertension: a prospective comparative study of performance and tolerance. Endoscopy 2006;38:36–41.

27. Eisen GM, Eliakim R, Defranchis R, et al. Interim analysis of the evaluation of Pillcam ESO in the detection of esophageal varices. 2006 Mar ICCE.

Index